Current Technologies to Increase the Transdermal Delivery of Drugs

(Volume 2)

Physical Penetration Enhancers: Therapeutic Applications and Devices

Edited by

José Juan Escobar-Chávez

Universidad Nacional Autónoma de México
Facultad de Estudios Superiores Cuautitlán
Unidad de Investigación Multidisciplinaria
Laboratorio 12: Sistemas transdérmicos y materiales nanoestructurados
Av. Cuautitlán-Teoloyucan. San Sebastián Xhala
Cuautitlán Izcalli, Estado de México. C.P 54714 México

Bentham Science Publishers Ltd.
Executive Suite Y - 2
PO Box 7917, Saif Zone
Sharjah, U.A.E.
Email: subscriptions@benthamscience.org

BENTHAM SCIENCE

CONTENTS

FOREWORD

Pharmaceutical knowledge has grown exponentially over the last 40 years. We now have a much clearer understanding of how drugs are absorbed into, distributed within, and cleared from the body.

The potency of agents with which we deal continues to increase, and our ability to unravel mechanisms of action proceeds. New drugs –in particular peptides, proteins and other biological response modifiers- are being developed and new challenges await pharmaceutical scientists. Controlled drug delivery represents a field that must keep pace with changing nature of chemotherapy. Tighter control of drug input into the body in both quantitative and temporal senses is crucial, and design *of new delivery systems* must respond to this demand for increased sophistication. For this purpose, scientists have used new technologies to improve the penetration rate of drugs. These technologies include physical and electrical methods that include iontophoresis (small direct current), sonophoresis (mainly by low frequency ultrasound energy), electroporation (by application of short micro to milli-second electrical pulses), radiofrequency (laser-generated stress), microneedles and also the use of nanocarriers alone or in combination with the use of the above mentioned physical enhancers. These biophysical techniques have many others therapeutical applications that include physiotherapy, gene delivery, DNA based vaccination, drug administration, diagnosis, dentistry, *etc*.

The development of technology has permitted the generation of devices that involve the use of physical enhancers for many of the mentioned therapeutical applications.

The objective of this book is to provide a general and an updated overview of the theoretical and practical aspects of iontophoresis, electroporation, sonophoresis, microneedles, radiofrequency and transdermal nanocarrier systems on the delivery of transdermal drugs. Such a generalized approach would be helpful in medicine, pharmacy, drug discovery, drug delivery, drug design and toxicological research.

The contributors to this text have been directed to emphasize updates on above mentioned technologies involved in therapeutic applications and devices. Authors were selected for their knowledge and reputation in their subject area, and for their ability to address objectively the topics of this book. I believe that they have performed this task effectively, producing a text that will facilitate and optimize future developmental programs in pharmacy, medicine and pharmaceutical technology.

Dr. Amparo Nácher Alonso
Department of Pharmacy and Pharmaceutical Technology
University of Valencia,
Spain

SPECIAL ACKNOWLEDGEMENTS

- **PAPIIT IT 200115,** PAPIIT IT 200115: "Diseño, desarrollo y caracterización de microagujas poliméricas biodegradables y geles termorreversibles cargados de sustancias de interés terapéutico para el tratamiento de enfermedades como alternativas a la vía oral".
- **PAPIME 200414:** Diseño y Desarrollo de Prácticas Experimentales para la Elaboración del Manual de la Asignatura de Análisis de Medicamentos de la Carrera de Licenciatura en Farmacia de la FES Cuautitlán.
- **Cátedra PIAPIC:** Desarrollo de Formas Farmacéuticas No Convencionales para la Administración de Fármacos.

PREFACE

"*Physical penetration enhancers: Therapeutic applications and devices*", is the second volume of the series "*Current technologies to increase the transdermal delivery of drugs*" from Bentham Science Publishers. This book provides an overview of main current physical enhancers in the therapeutical and pharmacy field. The importance of therapeutical applications of physical enhancers, and devices existing in the market will be addressed in each chapter. Exclusive chapters on Iontophoresis, Sonophoresis, Electroporation, Microneedles, Radiofrequency and more recently the use of nanoparticles in combination with the above mentioned physical enhancers, highlighting their main therapeutic applications will be included in this book.

Currently, there are no unique books available on therapeutical applications of physical penetration enhancers and currently devices in the market. Brief chapters and books describing only one of the physical enhancers or only one of the therapeutical applications (*i.e.*, transdermal drug delivery) of these enhancers are available to readers in some drug delivery or toxicology books. For these reasons, more detailed information about therapeutical applications (drug delivery, gene therapy, physiotherapy, skin disorders, vaccination, *etc.*) is now needed. This book presents a general overview of the theoretical and therapeutic aspects of iontophoresis, electroporation, sonophoresis, microneedles, radiofrequency and nanocarriers systems in combination with physical enhancers. Such a generalized approach would be helpful in medicine, pharmacy, drug discovery, drug delivery and toxicological research.

A comprehensive book which provides the basis and updated therapeutical research information is necessary. For this fact, this e-book will be an interesting option that could be used by students and academics of medicine, biopharmacy, pharmaceutical technology, design and development of drugs, pharmacology, by physicians, dermatologists, scientists and pharmaceutical R & Ds. The book also will be useful for medicine, pharmacy, pharmacology and pharmaceutical technology departments of different Universities all over the world.

In summary, this e-book reviews the therapeutical uses of physical enhancers such as iontophoresis, sonophoresis, electroporation, microneedles, radiofrequency and nanocarriers in combination with physical enhancers. After an introduction, definition, mechanisms of action, the focus turns to the relevance of therapeutical applications studies and finally the different physical enhancer devices in the market.

Dr. José Juan Escobar-Chávez
Universidad Nacional Autónoma de México
Facultad de Estudios Superiores Cuautitlán
Unidad de Investigación Multidisciplinaria
Laboratorio 12: Sistemas transdérmicos y materiales nanoestructurados
Av. Cuautitlán-Teoloyucan. San Sebastián Xhala
Cuautitlán Izcalli, Estado de México. C.P 54714,
México

List of Contributors

Alicia López Castellanos	Instituto de Ciencias Biomédicas. Departamento de Farmacia, Facultad de Ciencias de la Salud. Universidad CEU Cardenal Herrera, 46113, Moncada, Spain
Alma Lidia Aguiñaga Mirelles	Unidad de Investigación Multidisciplinaria. Laboratorio 12: "Sistemas Transdérmicos y Nanomateriales", Facultad de Estudios Superiores Cuautitlán-Universidad Nacional Autónoma de México. Km 2.5 Carretera Cuautitlán–Teoloyucan, San Sebastián Xhala, Cuautitlán Izcalli, Estado de México, México
Clara Luisa Domínguez-Delgado	Unidad de Investigación Multidisciplinaria. Laboratorio 12: "Sistemas Transdérmicos y Nanomateriales", Facultad de Estudios Superiores Cuautitlán-Universidad Nacional Autónoma de México. Km 2.5 Carretera Cuautitlán–Teoloyucan, San Sebastián Xhala, Cuautitlán Izcalli, Estado de México, México
Cristina Balaguer-Fernández	Instituto de Ciencias Biomédicas, Departamento de Farmacia. Facultad de Ciencias de la Salud. Universidad CEU Cardenal Herrera, 46113 Moncada, Spain
Elizabeth García-García	Psicofarma S.A. de C.V., Calz. de Tlalpan 4369, Col, Toriello Guerra, Distrito Federal. C.P.14050, México
Isabel Marlen Rodríguez-Cruz	Hospital Regional de Alta Especialidad Zumpango. Unidad de Enseñanza e Investigación, Carretera Zumpango-Jilotzingo #400. Barrio de Santiago 2da Sección. Zumpango,, Estado de México. C.P. 55600, México
Jennyfer Cázares Delgadillo	R&I, L'Oreal, 188-200 rue Paul-Hochart, 94550 Chevilly-Larue, France
José Juan Escobar-Chávez	Unidad de Investigación Multidisciplinaria. Laboratorio 12: "Sistemas Transdérmicos y Nanomateriales", Facultad de Estudios Superiores Cuautitlán-Universidad Nacional Autónoma de México. Km 2.5 Carretera Cuautitlán–Teoloyucan, San Sebastián Xhala, Cuautitlán Izcalli, Estado de México, México
Kate Broderick	Inovio Pharmaceuticals, Inc., 660W. Germantown Pike, Suite 110, Plymouth Meeting, PA 19462, USA
Katherine Schultheis	Inovio Pharmaceuticals, Inc., 660W. Germantown Pike, Suite 110, Plymouth Meeting, PA 19462, USA
María Araceli Catalayud-Pascual	Instituto de Ciencias Biomédicas. Departamento de Farmacia, Facultad de Ciencias de la Salud. Universidad CEU Cardenal Herrera, 46113 Moncada, Spain

Miriam López-Cervantes Unidad de Investigación Multidisciplinaria. Laboratorio 12: "Sistemas Transdérmicos y Nanomateriales", Facultad de Estudios Superiores Cuautitlán-Universidad Nacional Autónoma de México. Km 2.5 Carretera Cuautitlán–Teoloyucan, San Sebastián Xhala, Cuautitlán Izcalli, Estado de México, México
Laboratorio de Farmacotecnia. Universidad Autónoma Metropolitana-Xochimilco, Calzada del Hueso 1100, Villa Quietud, Coyoacán, Distrito Federal,, México, C.P. 04960, México

Omar Rodrigo Guadarrama-Escobar Unidad de Investigación Multidisciplinaria. Laboratorio 12: "Sistemas Transdérmicos y Nanomateriales", Facultad de Estudios Superiores Cuautitlán-Universidad Nacional Autónoma de México. Km 2.5 Carretera Cuautitlán–Teoloyucan, San Sebastián Xhala, Cuautitlán Izcalli, Estado de México, México

Pablo Serrano Castañeda Unidad de Investigación Multidisciplinaria. Laboratorio 12: "Sistemas Transdérmicos y Nanomateriales", Facultad de Estudios Superiores Cuautitlán-Universidad Nacional Autónoma de México. Km 2.5 Carretera Cuautitlán–Teoloyucan, San Sebastián Xhala, Cuautitlán Izcalli, Estado de México, México

Patricia Ramírez Noguera Unidad de Investigación Multidisciplinaria, acultad de Estudios Superiores Cuautitlán, Universidad Nacional Autónoma de México,, Estado de México, México

Roberto Díaz-Torres Unidad de Investigación Multidisciplinaria, acultad de Estudios Superiores Cuautitlán, Universidad Nacional Autónoma de México,, Estado de México, México

Suohui Zhang Key Laboratory of Photochemical Conversion and Optoelectronic Materials, Technical Institute of Physics and Chemistry, Chinese Academy of Sciences, Beijing, 100190, China

Trevor R.F. Smith Inovio Pharmaceuticals, Inc., 660W, Germantown Pike, Suite 110, Plymouth Meeting, PA 19462, USA,

Virginia Merino Instituto Interuniversitario de Reconocimiento Molecular y Desarrollo Tecnológico, Centro Mixto Universidad Politécnica de Valencia-Universidad de Valencia. Departament de Farmàcia i Tecnologia Farmacèutica, Facultat de Farmacia, Universitat de València, 46100 Burjassot, Spain

Yunhua Gao Key Laboratory of Photochemical Conversion and Optoelectronic Materials, Technical Institute of Physics and Chemistry, Chinese Academy of Sciences, Beijing, 100190, China

Yuqin Qiu Key Laboratory of Photochemical Conversion and Optoelectronic Materials, Technical Institute of Physics and Chemistry, Chinese Academy of Sciences, Beijing, 100190, China

Current Technologies to Increase the Transdermal Delivery of Drugs

(Volume 2)

Physical Penetration Enhancers: Therapeutic Applications and Devices

To my Family and all my personal affections.

CHAPTER 1

Physical Penetration Enhancers: An Overview

Isabel Marlen Rodríguez-Cruz[1,2,*], Clara Luisa Domínguez-Delgado[3], José Juan Escobar-Chávez[3], Miriam López-Cervantes[3,4] and **Roberto Díaz-Torres[5]**

[1] *Hospital Regional de Alta Especialidad Zumpango. Unidad de Enseñanza e Investigación. Carretera Zumpango-Jilotzingo #400. Barrio de Santiago 2da Sección. Zumpango, Estado de México. C.P. 55600, México*

[2] *Laboratorio de Investigación en Citogenética Básica del CBT Dr. Alfonso León de Garay. Calle Fresnos S/N, San Mateo, Tequixquiac, Estado de México C.P.55657, México*

[3] *Unidad de Investigación Multidisciplinaria. Laboratorio 12: "Sistemas Transdérmicos y Nanomateriales". Facultad de Estudios Superiores Cuautitlán-Universidad Nacional Autónoma de México. Km 2.5 Carretera Cuautitlán–Teoloyucan, San Sebastián Xhala, Cuautitlán Izcalli, Estado de México, México CP. 54714, México*

[4] *Laboratorio de Farmacotecnia. Universidad Autónoma Metropolitana-Xochimilco. Calzada del Hueso 1100, Villa Quietud, Coyoacán, Distrito Federal, México, C.P. 04960, México*

[5] *Unidad de Investigación Multidisciplinaria. Laboratorio 9: "Toxicología y genética". Facultad de Estudios Superiores Cuautitlán-Universidad Nacional Autónoma de México, México*

Abstract: A number of physical methods for drug penetration enhancement and improve bioavailability of the stratum corneum (SC) such as micro-needles, heating, iontophoresis, electroporation, and ultrasound have also been evaluated in the last decade. On the other hand, nanotechnology has shown remarkable potential in target-specific delivery of drugs in the body. In this chapter, we discuss the role of overview about nanocarrier systems, physical enhancers and their possible combination in order to improve the passage of molecules through the organ systems. All these methods have their own advantages and disadvantages, nevertheless, novel developments are projected to be more adaptable to different needs.

[*] **Corresponding author Isabel Marlen Rodríguez-Cruz:** Hospital Regional de Alta Especialidad de Zumpango. Unidad de Enseñanza e Investigación, Zumpango, Estado de México. C.P.56600, México; & Laboratorio de Investigación en Citogenética Básica del CBT Dr. Alfonso León de Garay. Calle Fresnos S/N, San Mateo, Tequixquiac, Estado de México C.P.55657, México; Tel: +52 5513428688; E-mail: isabelmarlen@yahoo.com.mx

José Juan Escobar-Chávez (Ed.)

Keywords: Controlled release, Drug delivery, Nanocarrier systems, Nanomedicine, Nanoparticles, Nanopharmaceutics, Physical penetration enhancers, Synergism, Therapeutic applications.

1. INTRODUCTION

In order to improve the penetration ability of agents therapeutics into systemic circulation, numerous methodologies have been investigated, developed and patented such as physical enhancers: iontophoresis, electroporation, ultrasound, microneedles and radiofrequency [1 - 10]. Alternatively, nanocarrier systems are being used as drug transporter systems. In this review, the expression nanocarrier referred to nano-systems that are used for effective carriage of loaded drug to the target sites or cells such as nanoparticles (NP), nanoemulsions, nanosuspensions, liposomes, micelles, vesicles, dendrimers and transfersomes. In the case of NP, these are defined as nanospheres or nanocapsules which is different in the morphology and architecture. Nanospheres are prepared by a polymeric matrix and nanocapsules are made of an oil core delimited by a polymeric membrane [1].

Currently, in order to improve penetration of nanocarrier systems into organ systems, especially to increase the skin permeability of drugs, a number of methods have been developed including use of physical enhancers [10 - 15]. Particularly, the skin has become an important way of administration of therapeutics agents for dermal and transdermal drug delivery. Dermal and transdermal ways offer a viable non-invasive administration of drugs, and avoids the hepatic first-pass effect. Also, dermic drug delivery system localizes high concentrations of agent therapeutic at the site of action and consequently, decreasing the side effects [1].

Transdermal delivery involves increasing the penetration of a drug through the skin when a systemic effect is wanted. Though, the dermal and transdermal administration of drugs is influenced by on drug's physicochemical properties, for example, charge, solubility, diffusivity, molecular size, polarity and molecular weight [1]. This chapter reviews the combination of nanocarrier systems and physical enhancers in order to improve the delivery of therapeutic molecules in many ways. Additionally, potential therapeutically applications of these physical enhancers are reviewed in this chapter.

2. PHYSICAL ENHANCERS

2.1. General Aspects of Physical Enhancers

An enhancer is a technique that modify the penetration facility of drug chemically or physically. With the intention of increase the penetration ability of drugs into organ systems, numerous methodologies such as physical enhancers have been investigated, developed and patented (*e.g.* iontophoresis, electroporation, ultrasound, microneedles and radiofrequency) [4]. Tabel **1** shows the principal characteristics of these techniques.

Table 1. Physical enhancers.

Physical Enhancers	Definition	Characteristics	Refs
Sonophoresis	Sonophoresis is the application of ultrasonic energy that temporarily improves skin permeability.	Sonophoresis functions at frequencies of 20 kHz-16 MHz and intensities up to 14 W/cm^2 (spatial average pulse average intensity, ISAPA) to enhance skin permeability.	[7]
Iontophoresis	Iontophoresis is the use of slight electric current in order to improve the transport of drugs, which consists of an anode and a cathode deposited on a surface (*e.g.* skin).	Iontophoresis uses an electric current of ~ 0.5 A/cm). A drug can pass through the surface by electromigration, electroosmosis or passive diffusion.	[8]
Electroporation	The electroporation technique consists of the application of a high electrical field pulses with the purpose to create nano-sized pores in a cell membrane and thus, increase the passage of ions and macromolecules through the skin.	Electroporation can be reversible and irreversible.	[4, 5]
Microneedles	Microneedles are used to open holes into the skin to create a pathway for the following delivery of drugs.	Generally, microneedles have a length of 100-500 μm.	[4, 5]
Radiofrequency	Radiofrequency ablation (RF) is a simple, safe, and effective therapy for chronic radiation proctopathy.	The frequency is between 10 kHz and 900 MHz.	[9]

According to physical enhancers, one of the main routes of drug administration is the skin (topical and transdermal drug). In this sense, biological properties of the skin are described below.

Skin represents the largest organ of the body (10% of body mass) and which interacts directly with the environment. The main functions of the skin are protecting and maintaining homeostasis or sensing. Likewise, the skin is an organ that is in a continual state of regeneration and repair.

The thickness of skin is~ 2-3 mm. Skin consists of four layers: the stratum corneum (SC), the epidermis, the dermis, and the subcutaneous tissue. Additionally, there are associated appendages.

The SC is the upper layer of the skin (~15 μm thick) and this forms an obstacle to the permeation of external substances.

The SC consists of dead flattened, keratin rich cells and the corneocytes. The epidermis is composed by melanocytes (3%), Langerhans cells (2%), Merkel cells (0.5%) and keratinocytes (90-95% of cells). The epidermis plays a role in temperature, pressure, and pain regulation [2]. The dermis (0.1-0.5 cm thick depending of body site) is composed of collagenous (70%) and elastin fibers. Also, in this layer are included the appendages (sweat glands, pilosebaceous glands, blood vessels, lymphatic and nerves) [2].

Hypodermis is the innermost layer of the skin and is composed of lipocytes. Hypodermis acts as a heat insulator, a shock absorber and an energy storage region. Fibroblast and macrophages cells are included in this layer. The main function of this layer is to transport the vascular and neural systems for the skin.

Skin appendages consist of: hair follicles; sebaceous glands; eccrine and apocrine sweat glands; and nails. The hair follicles are present in all skin with the exception of the soles of the feet, the palms of the hand and the lips. Each follicle is associated with a sebaceous gland, these gland are not present on the palms, soles and nail beds. Sweat glands respond to temperature *via* parasympathetic nerves, except on palms, soles and axillae, where they respond to emotional stimuli *via* sympathetic nerves [2, 3, 5].

The nail is a keratinized epithelial structure. Nail consists of nail plate, nail matrix, nail folds and nail bed. The main appendage functions are protection (hair and nails) and lubrication (sebum) [2, 3, 5]. Due to the characteristics of the skin, it provides a useful way for drug delivery systems; however, is necessary to use different physical enhancer to achieve effective drug absorption.

2.2. Classification

2.2.1. Sonophoresis

Sonophoresis is the application of ultrasonic energy that temporarily improves skin permeability. Sonophoresis, which uses ultrasound (US) as a physical enhancer for systemic drug delivery, is efficiently to deliver several types of drugs regardless of their electrical characteristics. Ultrasound conditions are as follows: Diagnostic ultrasound (High frequency, 3-10 MHz); Therapeutic ultrasound (Medium frequency, 0.7-3 MHz); Regulator ultrasound (Low frequency, 18 to 100 KHz). The use of low-frequency is viable technique of local, regional, and systemic transdermal drug delivery, which lets the diminution of side effects associated with oral and intravenous delivery. When ultrasound passes through a medium, energy is partially absorbed. In the human body, US energy absorbed by tissue causes a local temperature increase that is dependent upon ultrasound frequency, intensity, area of the US beam, duration of exposure, and the rate of heat removal by blood flow or conduction. The resultant temperature increase of the skin may enhance permeability due to an increase in diffusivity of the skin [5, 7, 16 - 21].

When US passes through a medium, energy is partially absorbed. In the human body, ultrasound energy absorbed by tissue causes a local temperature increase that is dependent upon ultrasound frequency, intensity, area of the ultrasound beam, duration of exposure, and the rate of heat removal by blood flow or conduction. The resultant temperature increase of the skin may enhance permeability due to an increase in diffusivity of the skin [16, 21].

Numerous studies of sonophoresis have been shown to increase skin permeability to various drugs and therapeutic compounds, including hydrophilic and large molecular weight compounds, especially under low frequency sonophoresis. Although, the fundamental mechanism is still not clearly understood or characterized. Several proposed mechanisms of sonophoresis include thermal effects by absorption of ultrasound energy and cavitation effects caused by collapse and oscillation of cavitation bubbles in the ultrasound field. Between these two effects, cavitation is believed to be the predominant mechanism responsible for sonophoresis [4 - 7, 16 - 21].

2.2.2. Iontophoresis

Iontophoresis is a non-invasive technique that controls the rate and extent of drug delivery by modulation of the intensity and duration of current application [22]. Iontophoresis is the use of slight electric current (~ 0.5 A/cm^2) in order to improve the transport of drugs, *via* an electrical circuit constituted by two drug reservoirs (anode and cathode) deposited on skin surface. Iontophoresis, which utilizes small electric currents, can enhance transport across the skin by different mechanisms such as electromigration, electroosmosis or passive diffusion [1, 8].

Electromigration (electrorepulsion), in this mechanism, ions are repelled by the electrode of the same charge and attracted by the electrode of the opposite charge. In electroosmosis, neutral substances are transported with the solvent flow [1, 3, 22 - 25].

Iontophoresis looks to be appropriate for enhance the transdermal transport of drugs and even nanoparticles through the skin. Using of electric current at 0.5 mA/cm^2 for 24 hours not affect the morphology of the skin [3, 22, 23 - 25].

2.2.3. Electroporation

The electroporation technique consists of the application of a high electrical field pulses with the purpose to create nano-sized pores (20 to 200 nm) in a cell membrane and thus, increase the passage of ions and macromolecules through the skin [1, 4 - 5, 26 - 28].

In irreversible electroporation, the membrane permeabilization leads to cell death due to a magnitude which can cause a severe disruption of the cell homeostasis that can finally results in cell death, either necrotic or apoptotic. This is an innovative technique for the treatment for local solid tumors. Moreover, electroporation is used for sterilization in the alimentary industry and in medicine for tissue ablation. In reversible electroporation the electric pulse causes only a temporary increase in permeability and the cell survives. The reversible electroporation is used in biotechnology and medicine [27, 29 - 31].

2.2.4. Microneedles (MNs)

Microneedles are micron-sized needles, generally, microneedles have a length of 100-500 μm, made of a diversity of materials and shapes. Microneedles are used to open holes into the skin to create a pathway for the following delivery of drugs, and thus, microneedles can penetrate the higher layer of the skin without reaching the dermis and almost painless. Then, the drug diffuses through the rest of the epidermis into the dermis where it is absorbed into the blood circulation [4, 5, 32 - 35].

Numerous studies have proven that such devices improve transdermal delivery of large molecules and may be employed alone or with other methods (iontophoresis or nanocarrier systems) [4, 5, 32 - 35].

Flow resistance owing to dense dermal tissue compressed around microneedles tip during insertion, is a limitation for microneedles. Nevertheless, research has shown that partial needle retraction following insertion improved the fluid infusion due to relaxation of the compressed tissue and an increase in flow conductivity of skin beneath the microneedles tip. Additionally, skin deformation during needle insertion could possibly be minimized by application of microneedles *via* drilling or vibrating motion [1, 4, 5, 32 - 35].

2.2.5. Radiofrequency

Radiofrequency (RF) uses a range frequency of 10 kHz - 900 MHz [36]. Radiofrequency ablation (RFA) is a simple and safe technique, as well as an effective therapy for chronic radiation proctopathy. RF thermal ablation is used in electro-surgery and ablation of malignant tissues. RF is generally useful for the treatment of small hepatocellular carcinomas. This technique contains an electrode connected directly into the tumor, which the ions inside the tissue try to follow the change in the direction of the alternating current, their movements result in frictional heating of the tumor, generating coagulative necrosis and cell ablation [9, 37]. This technology has been adapted as an optional physical enhancer of drug transport across the skin. Its potential in the creation of aqueous microchannels in the outer layer of the skin was studied [36, 38].

2.3. Therapeutic Applications

Physical enhancers have several therapeutic applications in order to improve the passage of molecules of drugs. For example, the main use of electroporation is for the introduction of DNA into cells.

Electrochemotherapy involves the use of electroporation with chemothrerapeutic agents for the treatment of cancer. The method consists of the systemic administration of anticancer agent followed by release of electric field pulses at the site of the cancer.

One of the main limitations of cancer drugs is that many of these substances are very poorly permeable into the tumor cells; nevertheless, pulsing the tumor site could increase the drug release into the tumor cells [4, 5, 7, 8].

Also, electroporation is used for transdermal drug delivery [29]. Becker *et al.* showed that is more efficient when low voltage pulses alone are applied than when high voltage pulses previous to the application of low voltage pulses are applied [4, 5, 29].

On the other hand, iontophoresis has been widely used for clinical dermatological applications for drug delivery. Dexamethasone with lidocaine is applied using iontophoresis to treat local inflammatory musculoskeletal conditions such as bursitis, tendinitis, arthritis, carpal tunnel syndrome, tennis elbow, and temporomandibular joint dysfunction. Likewise, lidocaine is applied using iontophoresis for local anesthesia for different routes of administration [4, 5]. Also, iontophoresis is used in the treatment of hyperhidrosis in different areas of the body (palms, soles and axillae) as well as in the diagnosis of cystic fibrosis. Moreover, different drugs are being investigated by ocular iontophoresis (gentamicin, cefazolin, fluorescein, tobramycin, lidocaine, epinephrine, timolol maleate, idoxuridine, dexamethasone) for numerous applications [2, 3, 6, 8, 9, 22, 23, 29]. Additionally, buccal iontophoresis have been investigated for delivery of chemotherapeutic agents to treat head and neck cancer [22]. Iontophoresis can be used for targeted topical delivery of chemotherapeutics to the buccal mucosa and may enable less invasive local therapy of head and neck cancers.

In other case, Malinovskaja *et al.* proved that the use of pulsed current offers significant advantages over constant current in transdermic iontophoresis for peptides which have the characteristic of adsorb into skin and impede the electroosmosis mechanism. Though, the use of pulsed current did not increase of transdermal flux of the cationic hydrophobic peptide leuprorelin acetate through porcine epidermis compared to constant current due to electroosmotic solvent flow [23].

In the case of microneedles, the therapeutic infusion rates of drugs vary from micro-liters per hour to several milliliters per hour and depend on the drug formulation and concentration. Microneedles have been considered for several biomedical applications such as immunization, skin rejuvenation, delivery of DNA to cells, delivery of drugs to eyes, to skin and as treatment of cancer. Also, drugs transported by microneedles have demonstrated their anticipated effects including protein, insulin, and vaccines [4, 5, 32].

Radiofrequency ablation (RFA) becomes the first choice loco-regional treatment. RFA is usually applied for the treatment of small hepatocellular carcinomas ($\leq$3 cm). Moreover, some procedures have been developed to avoid RFA-related complications, resulting in marked enhancement in the protection of liver RFA. Additionally, RF has been demonstrated to be more accurate and effective in detecting and preventing retained surgical sponge [36 - 38].

Alternatively, US has been used widely to improve transdermal drug delivery. For transdermal drug delivery there are studies assessed using different shapes of the cymbal transducers and different active ingredients such as insulin. In this sense, rectangular cymbal transducers showed to be effective and feasible of the light weight transducers for human applications [39, 40]. Nowadays SonoPrep® is approved by FDA and it was applied onto human skin to enhance the penetration of 5-Aminolevulinate (used for actinic keratosis and other non-melanoma skin cancers) showing a higher skin penetration, whereas in untreated skin it did not penetrate the skin at all [41].

As it was before mentioned, US has been used on the skin for different applications. Voigt *et al.* [42] applied US (20-30 kHz) as adjunctive treatment to increase the healing of chronic wounds. US affect the debridement of adherent necrotic fibrin, loose slough, and fragmentation of bacteria and biofilms on wound surfaces [42 - 45]. Also, US is used to remove localized fat deposits to improve body contours. Moreno-Moraga *et al.* showed that the use of US on human skin (abdomen) decreased the fat thickness after three treatments (one month intervals) by 2.28 ± 0.80 cm. Ascher presented similar results using the same system on Caucasian women (circumference reduced by 3.58 cm) [46]. Nevertheless, Shek *et al.* used the same system on 53 patients (51 females and 2 males) and found no effect on abdominal circumference and also reported poor satisfaction among patients [47]. On the other hand, US has also been used in other cosmetic applications such as in facial plastic surgery. White *et al.* and Gliklich *et al.* presented that high frequency of US (7.5 and 4.4 MHz, respectively) was used to induce thermal injury zones (TIZ). Noninvasive rejuvenation treatments are based on the ability to produce TIZs that trigger tissue remodeling and/or tightening [48 - 50]. Application of US has been shown to improve transdermal transport of numerous therapeutic agents. This type of enhancement is termed sonophoresis, indicating the enhanced transport of molecules under the influence of US [51]. In the last decade, the use of US at low-frequencies has developed a powerful tool for facilitating transport of different macromolecules across the skin including proteins as insulin for treating diabetes, oligonucleotides for gene delivery, as well as immunogens for vaccination. Normally, low-frequency sonophoresis has brought together a broad range of disciplines including physics, chemistry, engineering, pharmacology, biology and medicine [17, 18].

3. NANOCARRIER SYSTEMS

3.1. General Aspects of Nanocarrier Systems

Nanocarriers systems are colloidal drug delivery system. Nanoparticles (NP) have a size smaller than one micrometer [12]. Nanocarrier drug delivery systems must be manufactured from inert materials, biocompatible, biodegradable and available in pharmaceutical grade purity. These materials could be organic and inorganic [18]. The choice of materials depends on the route of administration, type of drug, type of nanocarrier and therapeutic objective [13]. Likewise, nanocarrier systems have several advantages such as improve the solubility, permeability, bioavailability and stability of drugs. However, these systems have a disadvantage which is the low drug loading capacity in most cases. Nanocarriers are a powerful weapon against a lot of illnesses since they are so small to be detected by immune system and they can deliver the drug in the target organ [3, 4, 10, 13, 14].

3.2. Biodistribution of Nanocarrier Systems

According to several researches, nanoparticles have been distributed in different areas of the body such as the colon, lungs, bone marrow, liver, spleen, and the lymphatics after intravenous injection [14]. NPs cross cells *via* endocytotic processes including clathrin-mediated endocytosis, potocytosis, pinocytosis, and phagocytosis [14, 52 - 55]. Following endocytosis, the material is delivered to the endosome and subsequently in the lysosome, which materials are exposed to hydrolytic enzymes that are active on proteins, polysaccharides and nucleic acid components [14, 56]. Distribution of drug is followed by rapid clearance from the systemic circulation [14, 55]. Clearance and opsonization the process that prepares foreign material to be more efficiently engulfed by macrophages occur under certain conditions for NP depending on size and surface characteristics [55, 57].

After oral exposure, NP distribute to the kidneys, liver, spleen, lungs, brain and the gastrointestinal tract [10, 14, 57 - 60]. A small number of studies have observed the clearance of NP from the gastrointestinal (GI) tract. Some NP can pass through the GI tract and are rapidly eliminated in feces and in urine, indicating that they can be absorbed across the GI barrier and into the systemic circulation. Drug stability in the stomach can be achieved by an enteric coating of the delivery system such as capsules or tablets for the nanocarrier systems [4, 5, 10, 14, 59 - 61].

When NP are inhaled, these are found to be distributed to the lungs, liver, heart, kidney, spleen and brain [5, 7, 51, 62]. NP are cleared in the alveolar region *via* phagocytosis by macrophages facilitated by chemotactic attraction of alveolar macrophages to the deposition site. NP have a half-life of ~700 days in humans in the respiratory tract [3, 14, 55]. The respiratory tract is divided in three regions: nasopharyngeal, tracheobronchial, and alveolar regions. Depending on particle size, NP can be deposited in different regions, for example, 90% of NP of 1 nm in diameter deposit in the nasopharyngeal region, whereas only 10% of these NP deposit in the tracheobronchial region and almost none reach the alveolar region. In comparison, 15% of NP of 20 nm in diameter deposit in the nasopharyngeal region, 15% in the tracheobronchial region, and approximately 50% in the alveolar region [14, 55, 60]. Nanocarrier system offer several benefits as the potential to achieve uniform distribution of drug dose among the alveoli, a sustained drug release and a decrease of side effects [4, 10].

About skin, one possibility for increasing the penetration of drugs across the skin is the use of vesicular/nano system such as nanoparticles, transfersomes and niosomes [27, 63 - 66]. In recent times, the hair follicles have proven to be an alternative to the penetration of drugs loaded nanoparticles [4 - 6, 34, 67, 68].

3.3. Toxicity of Nanocarrier System

At this time, nanocarrier systems toxicity is low. Nevertheless, Curtis *et al.* theorized possible mechanisms of toxicity for nanoparticles: 1) Toxicology of bulk materials is relatively defined as in the case of heavy metals as this toxicity is quite facile to quantify; 2) Nanomaterials can create reactive oxygen species and free radicals; 3) Toxicity of nanoparticles may be related to their size because these can cross the biological barriers and consequently affecting absorption, distribution, and excretion of these nanoparticles; 4) Shape may also be a feature that determines toxicity; for example, carbon nanotubes may be toxic due to their shape. 5) It has not been clearly delineated how nanoparticles can generate immune responses; however, there is a growing concern about their role in possible allergic reactions [10, 11, 13, 14, 54, 55, 69].

4. IMPORTANCE OF USING NANOCARRIER SYSTEMS WITH PHYSICAL ENHANCERS AND THERAPEUTIC APPLICATIONS

The combined usage of drug carriers systems with physical enhancers have demonstrated to offer many additional benefits. The combination of two or more drug delivery methods has proven to be more efficient than a method alone. This combination resulted in a synergistic effect of physical penetration enhancers with nanocarrier systems [21, 24, 27, 30, 31, 35]. Research continues to improve the bioavailability and the release of drugs into the human body; and thus achieve a better therapeutic effect. Physical enhancers (iontophoresis, ultrasound, electroporation, microneedles, radiofrequency) have been employed to improve bioavailability. These physical enhancers have some advantages such as short application process, abilities to modulate dosage and combine with other drug delivery systems, besides being a noninvasive technique. Among drug delivery systems are the nanocarier systems (liposomes, dendrimers, transfersomes, micelles, quantum dots, nanoemulsions, micro or nanoparticles) [16]. Nevertheless, NP offer several advantages as increasing half-life of drug, decreasing the peak concentration and toxicity, reducing dosing frequency, enhancing biocompatibility, and permeating together with drug molecule [21, 24, 27, 30, 31, 35].

The combinations of these technologies (physical enhancers and nanocarrier systems) have shown to provide a novel non-invasive administration of different drugs; additionally, the combinations of these technologies have been studied in order to improve the penetration and sustained release of drugs.

The combined use of drug nanocarriers systems and iontophoresis could offer various additional advantages. For example, Tomoda *et al.* evaluated estradiol-loaded PLGA-NP as a drug nanocarrier system for treatment of perimenopausal symptoms and osteoporosis.

The amount of estradiol into PLGA-NP delivered by simple diffusion through skin was higher than estradiol was free molecules. Though, the permeability of estradiol-loaded PLGA-NP was significantly increased when iontophoresis was applied. PLGA-NP were found to penetrate through follicles mainly. This effect was observed *in vivo*. The combination of charged NP system with iontophoresis is convenient for effective transdermal drug delivery [25]. Nevertheless, in other case, the application of cationic polymeric nanospheres (NS) combined with iontophoresis to improve the deposition of triclosan into the skin was evaluated by

Rodríguez-Cruz *et al.* [1]. They studied *in vitro* the passive diffusion and iontophoretic permeation of triclosan in solution and cationic triclosan-loaded NS in terms of the deposition of the drug into the skin for treatment of acne. These results confirmed that the deposition of triclosan within the human skin was greater when triclosan loaded cationic NS were employed than when a solution was administered by passive diffusion. Nevertheless, when iontophoresis was applied to NS, the amount of triclosan into the human skin was not increased; still, iontophoresis was effective in enhancing the passage of triclosan in solution through the skin [1]. For therapy cancer, the combination of iontophoresis with doxorubicin loaded solid lipid nanoparticles (SLNs) was also investigated; the cytotoxicity of doxorubicin was increased (50%) against malignant melanoma of the skin cells [70, 71].

In recent times, the combination of nanoparticles with iontophoresis has been investigated *via* ocular obtaining advantages as the penetration and controlled release of the drug; these advantages can be achieved by changing the particle size, particle charge and chemical properties of the nanoparticles or by using different ligands attached to the particle [72 - 78]. Positive NP seem to be better candidates for iontophoretic application due to the presence of positive charges that contributes to electrostatic interaction with the negatively charged corneal and conjunctival mucosa [79 - 82]. In other study, chitosan-coated NP (positively charged) compared with non-coated nanoparticles (negatively charged) confirmed faster corneal interaction and higher corneal penetration when using positively charged particles [81, 82]. Another study reported higher concentrations in all ocular tissues after iontophoresis of positive particles compared to no current application, except for the cornea and peripheral conjunctiva. Four hours after mock iontophoresis of positively charged particles, significant fluorescence traces were found only at the cornea [83].

With respect to electroporation, Lin *et al.* [27] studied a favorable tool for obtaining SERS (surface-enhanced Raman scattering) spectra of the cytoplasm of single living cells based on electroporation assisted by NP delivery. This method was validated using silver colloids delivered into three tumor cell lines. Electroporation based silver NP delivery combined with whole-cell SERS detection not only speeds up the test dramatically (a few minutes *versus* twenties hours), but also greatly improved the data reproducibility. These new methods possess great potential in biomedical applications such as for high-throughput cancer cell screening [27, 84].

A traditional approach for transferring load across cellular membranes is electroporation. Electroporation has been used previously to load exosomes with RNA load [85, 86] which is logical given that exosomes transport RNA naturally [87, 88]. Moreover, the use of electroporation for exosome studies minimizes perturbation of sensitive exosome components such as ligands and receptors. Electroporation relies on transient pore formation in the absence of chemical modification. However, while electroporation is traditionally considered as a means to introduce DNA, RNA, enzymes, drugs, or biochemical reagents into cells [89], it can also be used to produce fusion between cells to form hybrid cells as in the case of generating hybridomas for antibody production [90] or liposomes to study the electrofusion process [91]. Natural electrofusion occurs in living cells at the intracellular organelle level to facilitate the formation of vesicles during the exocytose process [92, 93].

Another application for drug delivery is the usage of microneedles devices, in which several studies have demonstrated that these devices increase the delivery of large molecules and may be employed alone or with other methods such as electroporation and iontophoresis, as well as with different drug carriers, as nanoparticles [4, 5, 32 - 35]. Zhang *et al.* [34] investigated the penetration and the distribution of PLGA-NP in the human skin using microneedles. Confocal laser scanning microscopy (CLSM) images exposed that NP were carried into the micro conduits created by microneedles and permeated into the epidermis and the dermis. The permeation of NP into the skin was improved by microneedles, but no NP reached the receptor solution. These results suggested that microneedles could enhance the intradermal delivery of PLGA-NP [34].

Paleco *et al.* [35] investigated the combination of MNs with lipid microparticles loaded with quercetin to increase the flavonoid permeability through the skin. The results of this study showed that MNs treatment did not affect the infiltration of free quercetin through porcine skin, whereas the use of the flavonoid-loaded lipid microparticles in association with microneedle insertion produced a pronounced enhancement of its percutaneous penetration. So, the combination of microneedles with lipid microparticles represents an effective delivery strategy for topical administration of quercetin [35].

One the other hand, recently was introduced the use of microneedles for minimally invasive, targeted the suprachoroidal space by injection [94, 95]. In this case, a single, hollow microneedle measuring less than 1 mm in length (*i.e.*, designed to match the scleral thickness) is pressed perpendicularly across the sclera to the sclera-choroid interface. A fluid formulation is then injected, and the hydrodynamic force of the injection opens the suprachoroidal space so that the fluid flows circumferentially around the eye between the sclera and choroid (*i.e.*, within the suprachoroidal space). Previously, microneedles have been shown to deliver nanoparticles and microparticles into rabbit, pig, and human eyes *ex vivo* [94, 96]. An *in vivo* study in the rabbit further showed microneedles can deliver particles as large as 10 μm to the posterior segment through the suprachoroidal space [95]. While these particles did not contain drug, their delivery provides information about how to deliver particles loaded with drug for localized controlled release. Another study tested particles injected into the suprachoroidal space can be localized at the site of injection or broadly distributed throughout the suprachoroidal space by controlling polymeric formulation properties. Single hollow microneedles were inserted into the sclera of New Zealand White rabbits and injected of non-biodegradable fluorescently tagged nanoparticles and microparticles suspended in polymeric formulations into the suprachoroidal space of the eye. The addition of hyaluronic acid to have moderately non-Newtonian solutions increased particle spread to up to 100% of the suprachoroidal space. This study demonstrated targeted particle delivery within the suprachoroidal space using polymer formulations that spread particles over the whole choroidal surface or localized them adjacent to the ciliary body after injection [97].

Huang *et al.* [16] investigated the use of silk fibroin-NP (SF-NP) for sustained drug delivery for ocular drug delivery with ultrasound (US). They use as a model drug a protein (Fluorescein isothiocynate labeled bovine serum albumin, FITC-BSA). The US application significantly enhanced the penetration efficiency of FITC-BSA-SF-NP compared with passive diffusion. This investigation proposed a non-invasive trans-scleral administration of macromolecular protein drugs using

SF-NP as carriers systems combining with US [16].

US treatment followed by the passive application of NP as nanocarriers system can be a good strategy, not only for transdermal drug delivery, but also for topical and ocular drug delivery and for transcutaneous immunization [21]. In another example, US was applied to transdermal mass transport of cationic, neutral, and anionic quantum dots and gold NP [98]. In this study, US also enhanced the permeability of gold NP [98, 99]. Moreover, US has also been used to facilitate the penetration of peptide dendrimers containing arginine and histidine (as terminal amino acids) with varying positive charges (up to 16+) and up to 2.2 kDa molecular mass. Also, another study showed that using smaller liposomes as a vaccine adjuvant were more effective when the skin was pre-treated by the US [100 - 107].

Gene therapy is other application which US is used [108 - 116]. Tran *et al.* presented that insonating melanocytic lesions followed by topical treatment of liposomal-siRNA complex (targeting V600EB-Raf gene) significantly decreased (~30-40%) cutaneous tumor development in animals [117]. US also has other applications as immunization, wound healing, vitiligo, melanoma, atomic dermatitis, and psoriasis [118 - 120].

According to many studies, US may be also used as hyperthermia for cancer therapy and this technology may also improve penetration of NP into carcinogenic cells [108, 121]. For cancer therapy, US may induce effects not only through heating, but also through non thermal mechanisms including ultrasonic cavitation, gas body activation, mechanical stress or other undetermined non thermal procedures [121].

The capacity to non-invasively target a specific position without increasing systemic exposure leads to the employment of US techniques as a novel strategy using physical energy to improve drug delivery, through sonophoresis, pulsed ultrasound, high intensity focused ultrasound (HIFU), MR-guided focused US (MRgFUS). In fact, US reduces the packing density of cells, which is a major blockade to the penetration of drugs into malignancies, through the cavitation of NP, which produce significant mechanical impacts on cells and extracellular matrix [120, 122 - 124].

In another example, microbubbles were used as drug carriers system which therapeutic molecules were integrated in the bubble shell or loaded into the interior of these particles in order to drugs may be released in the vascular compartment through US induced particle disruption [125, 126]. The main advantage of this drug delivery system is that requires very little amount of drug; therefore side effects are reduced [121, 127]. In addition, US mediated gene delivery with microbubbles has emerged as an attractive carrier system for site-specific and noninvasive gene therapy. Numerous preclinical studies have reported successful gene delivery into solid tumors with significant therapeutic effects using this novel system [128].

Recent research has exposed that hyperthermia cancer treatment has removed to the use of high intensity focused ultrasound (HIFU). Nevertheless, NP were used with US to increase the penetration and concentration of diagnostic and therapeutic NPs into skin cancer in the form of hyperthermia [122].

Likewise, irritation is a feature that should be considered before using enhancers or nanocarrier systems. The permeability of drugs through skin is improved by enhancers, but chemical enhancers induce irritation, cause damage, and reduce the skin barrier function. Up to date, more than 360 chemicals have been demonstrated to enhance the skin permeability. Though, irritation and damage to the skin barrier is predominantly associated with the use of chemical enhancers, mainly anionic and cationic surfactants [129, 130]. Non-ionic surfactants are generally considered to be less irritating than ionic surfactants [129]. Consequently, as a result of their incompatibility in the formulation or local irritation issues, few to date have been routinely incorporated in the currently marketed transdermal products [130]. Consequently it is necessary to release drugs across the SC keeping the normal skin barrier function without the assistance of chemical enhancers [25]. In addition to their favourable permeation enhancement properties, microemulsions and nanoemulsions may also reduce skin irritancy of certain excipients. For example, an aqueous solution containing 20% propylene glycol has been shown to cause irritation, but the same concentration of propylene glycol used as a cosurfactant in microemulsion formulations did not

[132]. Nonetheless, the combination of nanoparticle system and iontophoresis promoted permeability of drugs (triclosan, indomethacin) through skin synergistically [1, 25]. Typically, low amplitude direct current (0.5 mA/ cm^2) is applied to skin which generally causes no pain or irritation beyond mild erythema [1, 25]. In the case of ultrasound, several researches have reported that after ultrasound application, irritation was not observed on the skin surface [31, 133].

5. OVERALL COSTS

To our knowledge, at this time, there are not information about the comparison the overall cost of these physical penetration enhancers. Nevertheless, it is important to mention that in the case of microneedles, these are available at a reasonable cost. Though, the cost of production may also depend on the material of fabrication. For example, polymer microneedle fabrication, seems to be less expensive than silicon MNs fabrication [134]. In the case of RF, this is less invasive and has lower rates of complications and lower costs than surgery [135]. In the same sense, topical iontophoretic therapy would not only target the tumors and offer a non-invasive alternative to intravenous administration, but it would also reduce the dose administered concomitantly decreasing cost and the risk of systemic exposure [22]. In this way, local iontophoretic delivery of anti-cancer drugs could be an efficacious and safe alternative to systemic intravenous chemotherapy for patients who will receive radio-therapy or in whom surgery is not indicated, where surgical procedures would be much too invasive or limit normal physiological functions [22]. Furthermore, US is a very interesting method due to its accessibility, cost, and the possibility to combine imaging and therapeutic capabilities. On the other hand, in the case of nanocarrier systems, for example, niosomes compared with phospholipid-based vesicles, niosomes have a low cost of production, a higher chemical stability, and a larger membrane flexibility [136, 137]. Also, lipospheres have benefits as better physical stability, low cost, easy preparation and scale-up, high dispersibility in an aqueous medium, high entrapment capacity of hydrophobic drugs, controlled particle size, and extended release of entrapped drug after administration. In another case, lipid NP has the advantages as low cost production, clinical and large-scale production facilities, and accepted status of excipients.

Furthermore, their physical stability is a significant advantage as compared to other lipid base delivery systems [131]. Most of liposomes have been reported to have stability problem and high cost. The stability problems of liposomes are in the form of loss of entrapped drug, change in the size upon storage as well as chemical degradation of the lipid components [138]. In the case of quantum dots, these have advantages of optical imaging such as high resolution, high sensitivity, multiplexing, and in particular low cost [139].

CONCLUSION

This chapter has given an overview about, physical enhancers and nanocarrier systems as well as their possibly combination in order to improve the passage of molecules through the organ systems. Interesting and potential therapeutical applications of these physical enhancers and nanocarriers are being researching. All these methods have their own advantages and disadvantages, but a reality is that new developments are projected in the future to make these methods even more adaptable to different needs. The combination of these technologies has shown to provide a novel non-invasive administration of different drugs; additionally, the combination of these technologies has been studied in order to improve the penetration and sustained release of drugs.

CONFLICT OF INTEREST

The authors confirm that they have no conflict of interest to declare for this publication.

ACKNOWLEDGEMENTS

José Juan Escobar-Chávez wishes to acknowledge PAPIIT 200115, Cátedra PIAPI 1619 and PAPIME PE 200414. Roberto Díaz-Torres desires to acknowledge PAPITT IN219715.

REFERENCES

[1] Rodríguez-Cruz IM, Merino V, Merino M, Díez O, Nácher A, Quintanar-Guerrero D. Polymeric nanospheres as strategy to increase the amount of triclosan retained in the skin: passive diffusion *vs.* iontophoresis. J Microencapsul 2013; 30(1): 72-80. [http://dx.doi.org/10.3109/02652048.2012.700956] [PMID: 22746545]

[2] Escobar-Chávez JJ, Rodríguez-Cruz IM, Domínguez-Delgado CL, *et al.* Nanocarrier Systems for Transdermal Drug Delivery. Demir Sezer. Recent Advances in Novel Drug Carrier Systems. InTech 2012; pp. 201-40.

[3] Fang JY, Lin HH, Chen HI, Tsai YH. Development and evaluation on transdermal delivery of enoxacin *via* chemical enhancers and physical iontophoresis. J Control Release 1998; 54(3): 293-304. [http://dx.doi.org/10.1016/S0168-3659(98)00010-8] [PMID: 9766249]

[4] Escobar-Chávez JJ, Rodríguez-Cruz IM, Domínguez-Delgado CL. Chemical and Physical Enhancers for Transdermal Drug Delivery. Gallelli L. Pharmacology. InTech 2012; pp. 397-434.

[5] Domínguez-Delgado CL, Rodríguez-Cruz IM. López-Cervantes M. The skin a Valuable Route for Administration of Drugs. Escobar-Chávez JJ Current technologies to increase the transdermal delivery of drugs. Bentham Sciences 2010.

[6] Aldwaikat M, Alarjah M. Investigating the sonophoresis effect on the permeation of diclofenac sodium using 3D skin equivalent. Ultrason Sonochem 2015; 22: 580-7. [http://dx.doi.org/10.1016/j.ultsonch.2014.02.017] [PMID: 24916997]

[7] Escobar-Chávez JJ, Bonilla-Martínez D, Villegas-González MA, Rodríguez-Cruz IM, Domínguez-Delgado CL. The use of sonophoresis in the administration of drugs throughout the skin. J Pharm Pharm Sci 2009; 12(1): 88-115. [http://dx.doi.org/10.18433/J3C30D] [PMID: 19470295]

[8] Escobar-Chávez JJ, Merino V, López-Cervantes M, Rodríguez-Cruz IM, Quintanar-Guerrero D, Ganem-Quintanar A. The use of iontophoresis in the administration of nicotine and new non-nicotine drugs through the skin for smoking cessation. Curr Drug Discov Technol 2009; 6(3): 171-85. [http://dx.doi.org/10.2174/157016309789054924] [PMID: 19496753]

[9] Rustagi T, Corbett FS, Mashimo H. Treatment of chronic radiation proctopathy with radiofrequency ablation (with video). Gastrointest Endosc 2015; 81(2): 428-36. [http://dx.doi.org/10.1016/j.gie.2014.04.038] [PMID: 24973172]

[10] Bernkop-Schnürch A. Nanocarrier systems for oral drug delivery: do we really need them? Eur J Pharm Sci 2013; 49(2): 272-7. [http://dx.doi.org/10.1016/j.ejps.2013.03.008] [PMID: 23537503]

[11] Garnett MC, Kallinteri P. Nanomedicines and nanotoxicology: some physiological principles. Occup Med (Lond) 2006; 56(5): 307-11. [http://dx.doi.org/10.1093/occmed/kql052] [PMID: 16868128]

[12] Moghimi SM, Hunter AC, Murray JC. Nanomedicine: current status and future prospects. FASEB J 2005; 19(3): 311-30. [http://dx.doi.org/10.1096/fj.04-2747rev] [PMID: 15746175]

[13] Curtis J, Greenberg M, Kester J, Phillips S, Krieger G. Nanotechnology and nanotoxicology: a primer for clinicians. Toxicol Rev 2006; 25(4): 245-60. [http://dx.doi.org/10.2165/00139709-200625040-00005] [PMID: 17288496]

[14] Vega-Villa KR, Takemoto JK, Yáñez JA, Remsberg CM, Forrest ML, Davies NM. Clinical toxicities of nanocarrier systems. Adv Drug Deliv Rev 2008; 60(8): 929-38. [http://dx.doi.org/10.1016/j.addr.2007.11.007] [PMID: 18313790]

[15] Domínguez-Delgado CL, Rodríguez-Cruz IM, Escobar-Chávez JJ, Calderón-Lojero IO, Quintanar-Guerrero D, Ganem A. Preparation and characterization of triclosan nanoparticles intended to be used for the treatment of acne. Eur J Pharm Biopharm 2011; 79(1): 102-7. [http://dx.doi.org/10.1016/j.ejpb.2011.01.017] [PMID: 21295142]

[16] Huang D, Wang L, Dong Y, Pan X, Li G, Wu C. A novel technology using transscleral ultrasound to deliver protein loaded nanoparticles. Eur J Pharm Biopharm 2014; 88(1): 104-15. [http://dx.doi.org/10.1016/j.ejpb.2014.04.011] [PMID: 24833007]

[17] Agrawal U, Sharma R, Gupta M, Vyas SP. Is nanotechnology a boon for oral drug delivery? Drug Discov Today 2014; 19(10): 1530-46. [http://dx.doi.org/10.1016/j.drudis.2014.04.011] [PMID: 24786464]

[18] Polat BE, Deen WM, Langer R, Blankschtein D. A physical mechanism to explain the delivery of chemical penetration enhancers into skin during transdermal sonophoresis - Insight into the observed synergism. J Control Release 2012; 158(2): 250-60. [http://dx.doi.org/10.1016/j.jconrel.2011.11.008] [PMID: 22100440]

[19] Park D, Park H, Seo J, Lee S. Sonophoresis in transdermal drug deliverys. Ultrasonics 2014; 54(1): 56-65. [http://dx.doi.org/10.1016/j.ultras.2013.07.007] [PMID: 23899825]

[20] Maynard AD, Michelson E. The Nanotechnology Consumer Products Inventory. Woodrow Wilson International Center for Scholars 2005; pp. 1-8.

[21] Lopez RF, Seto JE, Blankschtein D, Langer R. Enhancing the transdermal delivery of rigid nanoparticles using the simultaneous application of ultrasound and sodium lauryl sulfate. Biomaterials 2011; 32(3): 933-41. [http://dx.doi.org/10.1016/j.biomaterials.2010.09.060] [PMID: 20971504]

[22] Gratieri T, Kalia YN. Targeted local simultaneous iontophoresis of chemotherapeutics for topical therapy of head and neck cancers. Int J Pharm 2014; 460(1-2): 24-7. [http://dx.doi.org/10.1016/j.ijpharm.2013.10.053] [PMID: 24219856]

[23] Malinovskaja K, Laaksonen T, Hirvonen J. Controlled transdermal delivery of leuprorelin by pulsed iontophoresis and ion-exchange fiber. Eur J Pharm Biopharm 2014; 88(3): 594-601. [http://dx.doi.org/10.1016/j.ejpb.2014.08.010] [PMID: 25173088]

[24] Liu KC, Green CR, Alany RG, Rupenthal ID. Synergistic effect of chemical penetration enhancer and iontophoresis on transappendageal transport of oligodeoxynucleotides. Int J Pharm 2013; 441(1-2): 687-92. [http://dx.doi.org/10.1016/j.ijpharm.2012.10.027] [PMID: 23099122]

[25] Tomoda K, Watanabe A, Suzuki K, Inagi T, Terada H, Makino K. Enhanced transdermal permeability of estradiol using combination of PLGA nanoparticles system and iontophoresis. Colloids Surf B Biointerfaces 2012; 97: 84-9. [http://dx.doi.org/10.1016/j.colsurfb.2012.04.002] [PMID: 22609586]

[26] Agarwal A, Zudans I, Weber EA, Olofsson J, Orwar O, Weber SG. Effect of cell size and shape on single-cell electroporation. Anal Chem 2007; 79(10): 3589-96. [http://dx.doi.org/10.1021/ac062049e] [PMID: 17444611]

[27] Lin J, Chen R, Feng S, *et al.* Rapid delivery of silver nanoparticles into living cells by electroporation for surface-enhanced Raman spectroscopy. Biosens Bioelectron 2009; 25(2): 388-94. [http://dx.doi.org/10.1016/j.bios.2009.07.027] [PMID: 19699079]

[28] Kammona O, Kiparissides C. Recent advances in nanocarrier-based mucosal delivery of biomolecules. J Control Release 2012; 161(3): 781-94. [http://dx.doi.org/10.1016/j.jconrel.2012.05.040] [PMID: 22659331]

[29] Becker S, Zorec B, Miklavčič D, Pavšelj N. Transdermal transport pathway creation: Electroporation pulse order. Math Biosci 2014; 257: 60-8. [http://dx.doi.org/10.1016/j.mbs.2014.07.001] [PMID: 25017876]

[30] Jourabchi N, Beroukhim K, Tafti B, Kee S, Lee E. Irreversible electroporation (NanoKnife) in cancer treatment. Gastrointest Interv 2014; 3: 8-18. [http://dx.doi.org/10.1016/j.gii.2014.02.002]

[31] Banga AK, Bose S, Ghosh TK. Iontophoresis and electroporation: comparisons and contrasts. Int J Pharm 1999; 179(1): 1-19. [http://dx.doi.org/10.1016/S0378-5173(98)00360-3] [PMID: 10053197]

[32] Yan XX, Liu JQ, Jiang SD, Yang B, Yang CS. Fabrication and testing analysis of tapered silicon microneedles for drug delivery applications. Microelectron Eng 2013; 111: 33-8. [http://dx.doi.org/10.1016/j.mee.2013.04.039]

[33] Domínguez-Delgado CL, Rodríguez-Cruz IM, Fuentes-Prado E, *et al.* Drug carrier systems using chitosan for non parenteral routes. Lee, Pharmacology. Europe, InTech 2014. [http://dx.doi.org/10.5772/57235]

[34] Zhang W, Gao J, Zhu Q, *et al.* Penetration and distribution of PLGA nanoparticles in the human skin treated with microneedles. Int J Pharm 2010; 402(1-2): 205-12. [http://dx.doi.org/10.1016/j.ijpharm.2010.09.037] [PMID: 20932886]

[35] Paleco R, Vučen SR, Crean AM, Moore A, Scalia S. Enhancement of the *in vitro* penetration of quercetin through pig skin by combined microneedles and lipid microparticles. Int J Pharm 2014; 472(1-2): 206-13. [http://dx.doi.org/10.1016/j.ijpharm.2014.06.010] [PMID: 24928134]

[36] Cardinal J, Klune JR, Chory E, *et al.* Noninvasive radiofrequency ablation of cancer targeted by gold nanoparticles. Surgery 2008; 144(2): 125-32. [http://dx.doi.org/10.1016/j.surg.2008.03.036] [PMID: 18656617]

[37] Yamakado K, Takaki H, Nakatsuka A, *et al.* Radiofrequency ablation for hepatocellular carcinoma. Gastrointest Interv 2014; 3: 35-9. [http://dx.doi.org/10.1016/j.gii.2014.04.002]

[38] Sintov AC, Krymberk I, Daniel D, Hannan T, Sohn Z, Levin G. Radiofrequency-driven skin microchanneling as a new way for electrically assisted transdermal delivery of hydrophilic drugs. J Control Release 2003; 89(2): 311-20. [http://dx.doi.org/10.1016/S0168-3659(03)00123-8] [PMID: 12711453]

[39] Park EJ, Werner J, Smith NB. Ultrasound mediated transdermal insulin delivery in pigs using a lightweight transducer. Pharm Res 2007; 24(7): 1396-401.

[http://dx.doi.org/10.1007/s11095-007-9306-4] [PMID: 17443398]

[40] Luis J, Park EJ, Meyer RJ, Smith NB. Rectangular cymbal arrays for improved ultrasonic transdermal insulin delivery. J Acoust Soc Am 2007; 122(4): 2022-30.
[http://dx.doi.org/10.1121/1.2769980] [PMID: 17902839]

[41] Krishnan G, Grice JE, Roberts MS, Benson HA, Prow TW. Enhanced sonophoretic delivery of 5-aminolevulinic acid: preliminary human *ex vivo* permeation data. Skin Res Technol 2013; 19(1): e283-9.
[http://dx.doi.org/10.1111/j.1600-0846.2012.00640.x] [PMID: 22672142]

[42] Voigt J, Wendelken M, Driver V, Alvarez OM. Low-frequency ultrasound (20-40 kHz) as an adjunctive therapy for chronic wound healing: a systematic review of the literature and meta-analysis of eight randomized controlled trials. Int J Low Extrem Wounds 2011; 10(4): 190-9.
[http://dx.doi.org/10.1177/1534734611424648] [PMID: 22184750]

[43] Bond LJ, Cimino WW. Physics of ultrasonic surgery using tissue fragmentation: Part II. Ultrasound Med Biol 1996; 22(1): 101-17.
[http://dx.doi.org/10.1016/0301-5629(95)02022-5] [PMID: 8928307]

[44] Gurfinkel R, Lavon I, Cagnano E, *et al.* Combined ultrasonic and enzymatic debridement of necrotic eschars in an animal model. J Burn Care Res 2009; 30(3): 505-13.
[http://dx.doi.org/10.1097/BCR.0b013e3181a28d89] [PMID: 19349883]

[45] Moreno-Moraga J, Valero-Altés T, Riquelme AM, Isarria-Marcosy MI, de la Torre JR. Body contouring by non-invasive transdermal focused ultrasound. Lasers Surg Med 2007; 39(4): 315-23.
[http://dx.doi.org/10.1002/lsm.20478] [PMID: 17457840]

[46] Ascher B. Safety and efficacy of UltraShape Contour I treatments to improve the appearance of body contours: multiple treatments in shorter intervals. Aesthet Surg J 2010; 30(2): 217-24.
[http://dx.doi.org/10.1177/1090820X09360692] [PMID: 20442099]

[47] Shek S, Yu C, Yeung CK, Kono T, Chan HH. The use of focused ultrasound for non-invasive body contouring in Asians. Lasers Surg Med 2009; 41(10): 751-9.
[http://dx.doi.org/10.1002/lsm.20875] [PMID: 20014261]

[48] White EA, Horne A, Runciman J, *et al.* On the correlation between single-frequency impedance measurements and human skin permeability to water. Toxicol In Vitro 2011; 25(8): 2095-104.
[http://dx.doi.org/10.1016/j.tiv.2011.09.011] [PMID: 21963824]

[49] Gliklich RE, White WM, Slayton MH, Barthe PG, Makin IR. Clinical pilot study of intense ultrasound therapy to deep dermal facial skin and subcutaneous tissues. Arch Facial Plast Surg 2007; 9(2): 88-95.
[http://dx.doi.org/10.1001/archfaci.9.2.88] [PMID: 17372061]

[50] White WM, Makin IR, Barthe PG, Slayton MH, Gliklich RE. Selective creation of thermal injury zones in the superficial musculoaponeurotic system using intense ultrasound therapy: a new target for noninvasive facial rejuvenation. Arch Facial Plast Surg 2007; 9(1): 22-9.
[http://dx.doi.org/10.1001/archfaci.9.1.22] [PMID: 17224484]

[51] Mitragotri S, Kost J. Low-frequency sonophoresis: a review. Adv Drug Deliv Rev 2004; 56(5): 589-601.
[http://dx.doi.org/10.1016/j.addr.2003.10.024] [PMID: 15019748]

[52] Ganta S, Devalapally H, Shahiwala A, Amiji M. A review of stimuli-responsive nanocarriers for drug and gene delivery. J Control Release 2008; 126(3): 187-204. [http://dx.doi.org/10.1016/j.jconrel.2007.12.017] [PMID: 18261822]

[53] Escobar-Chávez JJ, Díaz-Torres R, Rodríguez-Cruz IM, Domínguez-Delgado CL, *et al.* Nanocarriers for transdermal drug delivery. Res Reports Transdermal Drug Deliv 2012; 1: 3-17. [http://dx.doi.org/10.2147/RRTD.S32621]

[54] Kagan VE, Bayir H, Shvedova AA. Nanomedicine and nanotoxicology: two sides of the same coin. Nanomedicine 2005; 1(4): 313-6. [PMID: 17292104]

[55] Fabian E, Landsiedel R, Ma-Hock L, Wiench K, Wohlleben W, van Ravenzwaay B. Tissue distribution and toxicity of intravenously administered titanium dioxide nanoparticles in rats. Arch Toxicol 2008; 82(3): 151-7. [http://dx.doi.org/10.1007/s00204-007-0253-y] [PMID: 18000654]

[56] Oberdörster G, Oberdörster E, Oberdörster J. Nanotoxicology: an emerging discipline evolving from studies of ultrafine particles. Environ Health Perspect 2005; 113(7): 823-39. [http://dx.doi.org/10.1289/ehp.7339] [PMID: 16002369]

[57] Kurath M, Maasen S. Toxicology as a nanoscience?--disciplinary identities reconsidered. Part Fibre Toxicol 2006; 3: 6. [http://dx.doi.org/10.1186/1743-8977-3-6] [PMID: 16646961]

[58] Ma T, Wang L, TingyuanYang , Wang D, Ma G, Wang S. PLGA-lipid liposphere as a promising platform for oral delivery of proteins. Colloids Surf B Biointerfaces 2014; 117: 512-9. [http://dx.doi.org/10.1016/j.colsurfb.2014.02.039] [PMID: 24698146]

[59] Italia JL, Bhatt DK, Bhardwaj V, Tikoo K, Kumar MN. PLGA nanoparticles for oral delivery of cyclosporine: nephrotoxicity and pharmacokinetic studies in comparison to Sandimmune Neoral. J Control Release 2007; 119(2): 197-206. [http://dx.doi.org/10.1016/j.jconrel.2007.02.004] [PMID: 17399839]

[60] Hagens WI, Oomen AG, de Jong WH, Cassee FR, Sips AJ. What do we (need to) know about the kinetic properties of nanoparticles in the body? Regul Toxicol Pharmacol 2007; 49(3): 217-29. [http://dx.doi.org/10.1016/j.yrtph.2007.07.006] [PMID: 17868963]

[61] Medina C, Santos-Martinez MJ, Radomski A, Corrigan OI, Radomski MW. Nanoparticles: pharmacological and toxicological significance. Br J Pharmacol 2007; 150(5): 552-8. [http://dx.doi.org/10.1038/sj.bjp.0707130] [PMID: 17245366]

[62] Kooiman K, Vos HJ, Versluis M, de Jong N. Acoustic behavior of microbubbles and implications for drug delivery. Adv Drug Deliv Rev 2014; 72: 28-48. [http://dx.doi.org/10.1016/j.addr.2014.03.003] [PMID: 24667643]

[63] Escobar-Chávez JJ, Domínguez-Delgado CL, Rodríguez-Cruz IM. Targeting nicotine addiction: the possibility of a therapeutic vaccine. Drug Des Devel Ther 2011; 5: 211-24. [http://dx.doi.org/10.2147/DDDT.S10033] [PMID: 21607018]

[64] Zhong X, Han M, Dong Z, White TJ, Knoll W. Composition-tunable Zn(x)Cd(1-x)Se nanocrystals with high luminescence and stability. J Am Chem Soc 2003; 125(28): 8589-94.

[http://dx.doi.org/10.1021/ja035096m] [PMID: 12848567]

[65] Xu BB, Zhang YL, Zhang R, Wang L, Xiao XZ, Xia H, *et al.* Programmable assembly of CdTe quantum dots into microstructures by femtosecond laser direct writing. J Mater Chem C Mater Opt Electron Devices 2013; 1: 4699-704.
[http://dx.doi.org/10.1039/c3tc30666f]

[66] Rojas-Oviedo I, Salazar-López RA, Reyes-Gasga J, Quirino-Barreda CT. Elaboration and structural analysis of aquasomes loaded with indomethacin. Eur J Pharm Sci 2007; 32(3): 223-30.
[http://dx.doi.org/10.1016/j.ejps.2007.07.008] [PMID: 17905573]

[67] Gupta PN, Mishra V, Rawat A, *et al.* Non-invasive vaccine delivery in transfersomes, niosomes and liposomes: a comparative study. Int J Pharm 2005; 293(1-2): 73-82.
[http://dx.doi.org/10.1016/j.ijpharm.2004.12.022] [PMID: 15778046]

[68] Chaudhary H, Kohli K, Kumar V. Nano-transfersomes as a novel carrier for transdermal delivery. Int J Pharm 2013; 454(1): 367-80.
[http://dx.doi.org/10.1016/j.ijpharm.2013.07.031] [PMID: 23871739]

[69] Oberdörster G, Oberdörster E, Oberdörster J. Nanotoxicology: an emerging discipline evolving from studies of ultrafine particles. Environ Health Perspect 2005; 113(7): 823-39.
[http://dx.doi.org/10.1289/ehp.7339] [PMID: 16002369]

[70] Taveira SF, De Santana DC, Araújo LM, Marquele-Oliveira F, Nomizo A, Lopez RF. Effect of iontophoresis on topical delivery of doxorubicin-loaded solid lipid nanoparticles. J Biomed Nanotechnol 2014; 10(7): 1382-90.
[http://dx.doi.org/10.1166/jbn.2014.1834] [PMID: 24804558]

[71] Simões MC, Sousa JJ, Pais AA. Skin cancer and new treatment perspectives: a review. Cancer Lett 2015; 357(1): 8-42.
[http://dx.doi.org/10.1016/j.canlet.2014.11.001] [PMID: 25444899]

[72] Eljarrat-Binstock E, Domb AJ. Iontophoresis: a non-invasive ocular drug delivery. J Control Release 2006; 110(3): 479-89.
[http://dx.doi.org/10.1016/j.jconrel.2005.09.049] [PMID: 16343678]

[73] Behar-Cohen FF, El Aouni A, Gautier S, *et al.* Transscleral Coulomb-controlled iontophoresis of methylprednisolone into the rabbit eye: influence of duration of treatment, current intensity and drug concentration on ocular tissue and fluid levels. Exp Eye Res 2002; 74(1): 51-9.
[http://dx.doi.org/10.1006/exer.2001.1098] [PMID: 11878818]

[74] Eljarrat-Binstock E, Domb AJ, Orucov F, Frucht-Pery J, Pe'er J. Methotrexate delivery to the eye using transscleral hydrogel iontophoresis. Curr Eye Res 2007; 32(7-8): 639-46.
[http://dx.doi.org/10.1080/02713680701528674] [PMID: 17852187]

[75] Eljarrat-Binstock E, Raiskup F, Stepensky D, Domb AJ, Frucht-Pery J. Delivery of gentamicin to the rabbit eye by drug-loaded hydrogel iontophoresis. Invest Ophthalmol Vis Sci 2004; 45(8): 2543-8.
[http://dx.doi.org/10.1167/iovs.03-1294] [PMID: 15277475]

[76] Halhal M, Renard G, Courtois Y, BenEzra D, Behar-Cohen F. Iontophoresis: from the lab to the bed side. Exp Eye Res 2004; 78(3): 751-7.
[http://dx.doi.org/10.1016/j.exer.2003.10.017] [PMID: 15106955]

[77] Parkinson TM, Ferguson E, Febbraro S, Bakhtyari A, King M, Mundasad M. Tolerance of ocular iontophoresis in healthy volunteers. J Ocul Pharmacol Ther 2003; 19(2): 145-51. [http://dx.doi.org/10.1089/108076803321637672] [PMID: 12804059]

[78] Vollmer DL, Szlek MA, Kolb K, Lloyd LB, Parkinson TM. *In vivo* transscleral iontophoresis of amikacin to rabbit eyes. J Ocul Pharmacol Ther 2002; 18(6): 549-58. [http://dx.doi.org/10.1089/108076802321021090] [PMID: 12537681]

[79] Calvo P, Thomas C, Alonso MJ, Vila Jato JL, Robinson JR. Study of the mechanism of interaction of poly(e-caprolactone) nanocapsules with the cornea by confocal laser scanning microscopy. Int J Pharm 1994; 55: 283-91. [http://dx.doi.org/10.1016/0378-5173(94)90179-1]

[80] Lehr CM, Bouwstra JR, Schacht EH, Junginger HE. *In vitro* evaluation of mucoadhesive properties of chitosan and some other natural polymers. Int J Pharm 1992; 78: 43-8. [http://dx.doi.org/10.1016/0378-5173(92)90353-4]

[81] Calvo P, Vila-Jato JL, Alonso MJ. Evaluation of cationic polymer-coated nanocapsules as ocular drug carriers. Int J Pharm 1997; 153: 41-50. [http://dx.doi.org/10.1016/S0378-5173(97)00083-5]

[82] De Campos AM, Sánchez A, Gref R, Calvo P, Alonso MJ. The effect of a PEG versus a chitosan coating on the interaction of drug colloidal carriers with the ocular mucosa. Eur J Pharm Sci 2003; 20(1): 73-81. [http://dx.doi.org/10.1016/S0928-0987(03)00178-7] [PMID: 13678795]

[83] Eljarrat-Binstock E, Orucov F, Aldouby Y, Frucht-Pery J, Domb AJ. Charged nanoparticles delivery to the eye using hydrogel iontophoresis. J Control Release 2008; 126(2): 156-61. [http://dx.doi.org/10.1016/j.jconrel.2007.11.016] [PMID: 18201790]

[84] Arena CB, Neal RE II, Davalos RV. Electroporation Therapy. Reference module in biomedical sciences, from comprehensive biomedical physics 2014; 10: 269-87. [http://dx.doi.org/10.1016/B978-0-444-53632-7.01016-9]

[85] Alvarez-Erviti L, Seow Y, Yin H, Betts C, Lakhal S, Wood MJ. Delivery of siRNA to the mouse brain by systemic injection of targeted exosomes. Nat Biotechnol 2011; 29(4): 341-5. [http://dx.doi.org/10.1038/nbt.1807] [PMID: 21423189]

[86] Wahlgren J, De L Karlson T, Brisslert M, *et al.* Plasma exosomes can deliver exogenous short interfering RNA to monocytes and lymphocytes. Nucleic Acids Res 2012; 40(17): e130. [http://dx.doi.org/10.1093/nar/gks463] [PMID: 22618874]

[87] Valadi H, Ekström K, Bossios A, Sjöstrand M, Lee JJ, Lötvall JO. Exosome-mediated transfer of mRNAs and microRNAs is a novel mechanism of genetic exchange between cells. Nat Cell Biol 2007; 9(6): 654-9. [http://dx.doi.org/10.1038/ncb1596] [PMID: 17486113]

[88] Keller S, Ridinger J, Rupp AK, Janssen JW, Altevogt P. Body fluid derived exosomes as a novel template for clinical diagnostics. J Transl Med 2011; 9: 86. [http://dx.doi.org/10.1186/1479-5876-9-86] [PMID: 21651777]

[89] Weaver JC. Electroporation: a general phenomenon for manipulating cells and tissues. J Cell Biochem

1993; 51(4): 426-35.
[http://dx.doi.org/10.1002/jcb.2400510407] [PMID: 8496245]

[90] Sugar IP, Förster W, Neumann E. Model of cell electrofusion. Membrane electroporation, pore coalescence and percolation. Biophys Chem 1987; 26(2-3): 321-35.
[http://dx.doi.org/10.1016/0301-4622(87)80033-9] [PMID: 3607233]

[91] Stoicheva NG, Hui SW. Electrofusion of cell-size liposomes. Biochim Biophys Acta 1994; 1195(1): 31-8.
[http://dx.doi.org/10.1016/0005-2736(94)90005-1] [PMID: 7522568]

[92] Ramos C, Teissié J. Electrofusion: a biophysical modification of cell membrane and a mechanism in exocytosis. Biochimie 2000; 82(5): 511-8.
[http://dx.doi.org/10.1016/S0300-9084(00)00200-5] [PMID: 10865136]

[93] Hood JL, Scott MJ, Wickline SA. Maximizing exosome colloidal stability following electroporation. Anal Biochem 2014; 448: 41-9.
[http://dx.doi.org/10.1016/j.ab.2013.12.001] [PMID: 24333249]

[94] Patel SR, Lin AS, Edelhauser HF, Prausnitz MR. Suprachoroidal drug delivery to the back of the eye using hollow microneedles. Pharm Res 2011; 28(1): 166-76.
[http://dx.doi.org/10.1007/s11095-010-0271-y] [PMID: 20857178]

[95] Patel SR, Berezovsky DE, McCarey BE, Zarnitsyn V, Edelhauser HF, Prausnitz MR. Targeted administration into the suprachoroidal space using a microneedle for drug delivery to the posterior segment of the eye. Invest Ophthalmol Vis Sci 2012; 53(8): 4433-41.
[http://dx.doi.org/10.1167/iovs.12-9872] [PMID: 22669719]

[96] Kim YC, Edelhauser HF, Prausnitz MR. Particle-stabilized emulsion droplets for gravity-mediated targeting in the posterior segment of the eye. Adv Healthc Mater 2014; 3(8): 1272-82.
[http://dx.doi.org/10.1002/adhm.201300696] [PMID: 24652782]

[97] Kim YC, Oh KH, Edelhauser HF, Prausnitz MR. Formulation to target delivery to the ciliary body and choroid *via* the suprachoroidal space of the eye using microneedles. Eur J Pharm Biopharm 2015; 95(Pt B): 398-406.
[http://dx.doi.org/10.1016/j.ejpb.2015.05.020] [PMID: 26036448]

[98] Seto JE, Polat BE, Lopez RF, Blankschtein D, Langer R. Effects of ultrasound and sodium lauryl sulfate on the transdermal delivery of hydrophilic permeants: Comparative *in vitro* studies with full-thickness and split-thickness pig and human skin. J Control Release 2010; 145(1): 26-32.
[http://dx.doi.org/10.1016/j.jconrel.2010.03.013] [PMID: 20346994]

[99] Terentyuk GS, Genina EA, Bashkatov AN, *et al.* Use of fractional laser microablation and ultrasound to facilitate the delivery of gold nanoparticles into skin *in vivo.* Quantum Electron 2012; 42: 471.
[http://dx.doi.org/10.1070/QE2012v042n06ABEH014882]

[100] Mutalik S, Nayak UY, Kalra R, Kumar A, Kulkarni RV, Parekh HS. Sonophoresis-mediated permeation and retention of peptide dendrimers across human epidermis. Skin Res Technol 2012; 18(1): 101-7.
[http://dx.doi.org/10.1111/j.1600-0846.2011.00539.x] [PMID: 21507071]

[101] Gockel CM, Bao S, Beagley KW. Transcutaneous immunization induces mucosal and systemic

immunity: a potent method for targeting immunity to the female reproductive tract. Mol Immunol 2000; 37(9): 537-44.
[http://dx.doi.org/10.1016/S0161-5890(00)00074-2] [PMID: 11163403]

[102] Romani N, Holzmann S, Tripp CH, Koch F, Stoitzner P. Langerhans cells - dendritic cells of the epidermis. APMIS 2003; 111(7-8): 725-40.
[http://dx.doi.org/10.1034/j.1600-0463.2003.11107805.x] [PMID: 12974775]

[103] Stoitzner P, Holzmann S, McLellan AD, *et al.* Visualization and characterization of migratory Langerhans cells in murine skin and lymph nodes by antibodies against Langerin/CD207. J Invest Dermatol 2003; 120(2): 266-74.
[http://dx.doi.org/10.1046/j.1523-1747.2003.12042.x] [PMID: 12542532]

[104] Glenn GM, Scharton-Kersten T, Vassell R, Mallett CP, Hale TL, Alving CR. Transcutaneous immunization with cholera toxin protects mice against lethal mucosal toxin challenge. J Immunol 1998; 161(7): 3211-4.
[PMID: 9759833]

[105] Glenn GM, Kenney RT. Mass Vaccination: Solutions in the Skin. Berlin, Heidelberg: Springer 2006; pp. 247-6.

[106] Tezel A, Paliwal S, Shen Z, Mitragotri S. Low-frequency ultrasound as a transcutaneous immunization adjuvant. Vaccine 2005; 23(29): 3800-7.
[http://dx.doi.org/10.1016/j.vaccine.2005.02.027] [PMID: 15893617]

[107] Dahlan A, Alpar HO, Murdan S. An investigation into the combination of low frequency ultrasound and liposomes on skin permeability. Int J Pharm 2009; 379(1): 139-42.
[http://dx.doi.org/10.1016/j.ijpharm.2009.06.011] [PMID: 19539736]

[108] Cao T, Wang XJ, Roop DR. Regulated cutaneous gene delivery: the skin as a bioreactor. Hum Gene Ther 2000; 11(16): 2297-300.
[http://dx.doi.org/10.1089/104303400750035843] [PMID: 11084689]

[109] Featherstone C, Uitto J. *Ex vivo* gene therapy cures a blistering skin disease. Trends Mol Med 2007; 13(6): 219-22.
[http://dx.doi.org/10.1016/j.molmed.2007.03.006] [PMID: 17416553]

[110] Frerichs DM, Ellingsworth LR, Frech SA, *et al.* Controlled, single-step, stratum corneum disruption as a pretreatment for immunization *via* a patch. Vaccine 2008; 26(22): 2782-7.
[http://dx.doi.org/10.1016/j.vaccine.2008.02.070] [PMID: 18455283]

[111] Uitto J, Pulkkinen L. The genodermatoses: candidate diseases for gene therapy. Hum Gene Ther 2000; 11(16): 2267-75.
[http://dx.doi.org/10.1089/104303400750035807] [PMID: 11084685]

[112] Hammond SA, Guebre-Xabier M, Yu J, Glenn GM. Transcutaneous immunization: an emerging route of immunization and potent immunostimulation strategy. Crit Rev Ther Drug Carrier Syst 2001; 18(5): 503-26.
[http://dx.doi.org/10.1615/CritRevTherDrugCarrierSyst.v18.i5.30] [PMID: 11763499]

[113] Özbaş-Turan S, Akbuğa J. Plasmid DNA-loaded chitosan/TPP nanoparticles for topical gene delivery. Drug Deliv 2011; 18(3): 215-22.

[http://dx.doi.org/10.3109/10717544.2010.544688] [PMID: 21226549]

[114] Tran MA, Gowda R, Sharma A, *et al.* Targeting V600EB-Raf and Akt3 using nanoliposomal-small interfering RNA inhibits cutaneous melanocytic lesion development. Cancer Res 2008; 68(18): 7638-49.
[http://dx.doi.org/10.1158/0008-5472.CAN-07-6614] [PMID: 18794153]

[115] Zheng D, Giljohann DA, Chen DL, *et al.* Topical delivery of siRNA-based spherical nucleic acid nanoparticle conjugates for gene regulation. Proc Natl Acad Sci USA 2012; 109(30): 11975-80.
[http://dx.doi.org/10.1073/pnas.1118425109] [PMID: 22773805]

[116] Ritprajak P, Hashiguchi M, Azuma M. Topical application of cream-emulsified CD86 siRNA ameliorates allergic skin disease by targeting cutaneous dendritic cells. Mol Ther 2008; 16(7): 1323-30.
[http://dx.doi.org/10.1038/mt.2008.91] [PMID: 18461054]

[117] Tran MA, Gowda R, Park E, *et al.* Noninvasive drug delivery using ultrasound: targeting melanoma using siRNA against mutant (V600E) B-Raf. AIP Conf Proc 2009; 1113: 423-9.
[http://dx.doi.org/10.1063/1.3131463]

[118] Geusens B, Strobbe T, Bracke S, *et al.* Lipid-mediated gene delivery to the skin. Eur J Pharm Sci 2011; 43(4): 199-211.
[http://dx.doi.org/10.1016/j.ejps.2011.04.003] [PMID: 21515366]

[119] Liu Y, Yan J, Prausnitz MR. Can ultrasound enable efficient intracellular uptake of molecules? A retrospective literature review and analysis. Ultrasound Med Biol 2012; 38(5): 876-88.
[http://dx.doi.org/10.1016/j.ultrasmedbio.2012.01.006] [PMID: 22425381]

[120] Kievit FM, Zhang M. Cancer nanotheranostics: improving imaging and therapy by targeted delivery across biological barriers. Adv Mater 2011; 23(36): H217-47.
[http://dx.doi.org/10.1002/adma.201102313] [PMID: 21842473]

[121] Miller DL, Smith NB, Bailey MR, Czarnota GJ, Hynynen K, Makin IR. Overview of therapeutic ultrasound applications and safety considerations. J Ultrasound Med 2012; 31(4): 623-34.
[PMID: 22441920]

[122] Grainger SJ, Serna JV, Sunny S, Zhou Y, Deng CX, El-Sayed ME. Pulsed ultrasound enhances nanoparticle penetration into breast cancer spheroids. Mol Pharm 2010; 7(6): 2006-19.
[http://dx.doi.org/10.1021/mp100280b] [PMID: 20957996]

[123] Guzmán HR, McNamara AJ, Nguyen DX, Prausnitz MR. Bioeffects caused by changes in acoustic cavitation bubble density and cell concentration: a unified explanation based on cell-to-bubble ratio and blast radius. Ultrasound Med Biol 2003; 29(8): 1211-22.
[http://dx.doi.org/10.1016/S0301-5629(03)00899-8] [PMID: 12946524]

[124] Deng CX, Sieling F, Pan H, Cui J. Ultrasound-induced cell membrane porosity. Ultrasound Med Biol 2004; 30(4): 519-26.
[http://dx.doi.org/10.1016/j.ultrasmedbio.2004.01.005] [PMID: 15121254]

[125] Unger EC, Porter T, Culp W, Labell R, Matsunaga T, Zutshi R. Therapeutic applications of lipid-coated microbubbles. Adv Drug Deliv Rev 2004; 56(9): 1291-314.
[http://dx.doi.org/10.1016/j.addr.2003.12.006] [PMID: 15109770]

[126] Ferrara K, Pollard R, Borden M. Ultrasound microbubble contrast agents: fundamentals and application to gene and drug delivery. Annu Rev Biomed Eng 2007; 9: 415-47. [http://dx.doi.org/10.1146/annurev.bioeng.8.061505.095852] [PMID: 17651012]

[127] Tartis MS, McCallan J, Lum AF, *et al.* Therapeutic effects of paclitaxel-containing ultrasound contrast agents. Ultrasound Med Biol 2006; 32(11): 1771-80. [http://dx.doi.org/10.1016/j.ultrasmedbio.2006.03.017] [PMID: 17112963]

[128] Panje CM, Wang DS, Willmann JK. Ultrasound and microbubble-mediated gene delivery in cancer: progress and perspectives. Invest Radiol 2013; 48(11): 755-69. [http://dx.doi.org/10.1097/RLI.0b013e3182982cc1] [PMID: 23697924]

[129] Lane ME. Skin penetration enhancers. Int J Pharm 2013; 447(1-2): 12-21. [http://dx.doi.org/10.1016/j.ijpharm.2013.02.040] [PMID: 23462366]

[130] Chen Y, Quan P, Liu X, Wang M, Fang L. Novel chemical permeation enhancers for transdermal drug delivery. Asian J Pharm Sci 2014; 9: 51-64. [http://dx.doi.org/10.1016/j.ajps.2014.01.001]

[131] Elgart A, Cherniakov I, Aldouby Y, Domb AJ, Hoffman A. Lipospheres and pro-nano lipospheres for delivery of poorly water soluble compounds. Chem Phys Lipids 2012; 165(4): 438-53. [http://dx.doi.org/10.1016/j.chemphyslip.2012.01.007] [PMID: 22342324]

[132] Abd E, Namjoshi S, Mohammed YH, Roberts MS, Grice JE. Synergistic skin penetration enhancer and nanoemulsion formulations promote the human epidermal permeation of caffeine and naproxen. J Pharm Sci 2016; 105(1): 212-20. [http://dx.doi.org/10.1002/jps.24699] [PMID: 26554868]

[133] Mitragotri S. Devices for overcoming biological barriers: the use of physical forces to disrupt the barriers. Adv Drug Deliv Rev 2013; 65(1): 100-3. [http://dx.doi.org/10.1016/j.addr.2012.07.016] [PMID: 22960787]

[134] Olatunji O, Das DB, Nassehi V. Modelling transdermal drug delivery using microneedles: effect of geometry on drug transport behaviour. J Pharm Sci 2012; 101(1): 164-75. [http://dx.doi.org/10.1002/jps.22736] [PMID: 22109688]

[135] Ja-Der L, Xiao-Ou P, Yi-Ju T, Guan-Tarn H, Lai F, Pei-Ming Y. Recurrence predictive models for patients with hepatocellular carcinoma after radiofrequencyablation using support vector machines with feature selection methods, computer methods and programs in biomedicine. Comput Methods Programs Biomed 2014; 117(3): 425-34. [http://dx.doi.org/10.1016/j.cmpb.2014.09.001] [PMID: 25278224]

[136] Rapoport N, Nam KH, Gupta R, *et al.* Ultrasound-mediated tumor imaging and nanotherapy using drug loaded, block copolymer stabilized perfluorocarbon nanoemulsions. J Control Release 2011; 153(1): 4-15. [http://dx.doi.org/10.1016/j.jconrel.2011.01.022] [PMID: 21277919]

[137] Yeom S, Shin BS, Han S. An electron spin resonance study of non-ionic surfactant vesicles (niosomes). Chem Phys Lipids 2014; 181: 83-9. [http://dx.doi.org/10.1016/j.chemphyslip.2014.03.004] [PMID: 24721595]

[138] El Maghraby GM, Ahmed AA, Osman MA. Penetration enhancers in proniosomes as a new strategy

for enhanced transdermal drug delivery. Saudi Pharm J 2015; 23(1): 67-74.
[http://dx.doi.org/10.1016/j.jsps.2014.05.001] [PMID: 25685045]

[139] Probst CE, Zrazhevskiy P, Bagalkot V, Gao X. Quantum dots as a platform for nanoparticle drug delivery vehicle design. Adv Drug Deliv Rev 2013; 65(5): 703-18.
[http://dx.doi.org/10.1016/j.addr.2012.09.036] [PMID: 23000745]

CHAPTER 2

Iontophoresis

María Aracely Calatayud-Pascual[1], **Cristina Balaguer-Fernández**[1], **Alicia López-Castellano**[1] and **Virginia Merino**[2,*]

[1] *Instituto de Ciencias Biomédicas. Departamento de Farmacia. Facultad de Ciencias de la Salud. Universidad CEU Cardenal Herrera, 46113 Moncada, Spain*

[2] *Instituto Interuniversitario de Reconocimiento Molecular y Desarrollo Tecnológico, Centro Mixto Universidad Politécnica de Valencia-Universidad de Valencia. Departament de Farmàcia i Tecnologia Farmacèutica i Parasitologia, Facultat de Farmacia, Universitat de València, 46100 Burjassot, Spain*

Abstract: Transdermal administration offers an interesting alternative to oral and parenteral drug administration; nevertheless, skin is an important barrier for drug absorption. Iontophoresis, a technique that consist of the application of low current density across a membrane can facilitate drug entrance through it. Iontophoresis can be used for local effects on skin, nail, eye or ear and it can also be used for systemic delivery when applied through skin. In this chapter, the mechanisms involved in drug transport during iontophoresis application and factors affecting its efficacy are reviewed. Examples of the use of iontophoresis in different fields are presented together with the most recent research.

Keywords: Ear permeation, Electric current treatment, Electromotive drug delivery, Eye permeation, Iontophoresis, Iontophoretic devices, Low current treatment, Nail permeation, Physical permeation enhancement, Transdermal absorption.

1. INTRODUCTION

Epithelia general properties limit passive delivery of most compounds across

* **Corresponding author Virginia Merino:** Departament de Farmàcia i Tecnologia Farmacèutica i Parasitologia, Facultat de Farmacia, Vicente Andrés Estellés sn, 46100 Burjassot, Spain; Tel: +34963543324; Fax: +34963544911; E-mail: merinov@uv.es

them. To overcome this barrier limitation several passive and active strategies have been attempted to ensure safe delivery and to improve efficacy of drugs as well as patient compliance.

Passive procedures, as optimization of formulation or drug carrying vehicles to increase permeability, in general do not greatly enhance the drug permeation of molecules with molecular weights higher than 500 Daltons. Active methods such as sonophoresis, iontophoresis, electroporation and other techniques such as laser microporation and microneedless produce superior enhancement of drug transport through the membranes. These methods, physically or mechanically, facilitate the delivery of various lipophilicities and molecular weights drugs, including proteins, peptides, and oligonucleotides [1, 2].

Among the methodologies mentioned, iontophoresis is one of the best-known and represents a promising physical penetration method to enhance delivery of drugs, especially trough skin.

The application of low density electrical current, and voltage, through a membrane, called iontophoresis, promotes permeation of a therapeutic drug placed on the surface of the membrane.

Iontophoretic drug delivery through the skin offers several important advantages over more traditional dosage forms. First pass metabolism is avoided with iontophoretic transdermal administration and this technique usually increases patient compliance. Along with these advantages, iontophoresis provides additional ones:

- Delivery of both ionized and unionized polar drugs, that can have either low or high molecular weight.
- Continuous or pulsatile delivery of a drug can be selected, depending on the mode of current used.
- Permits ease ending of drug administration.
- Current mode, duration of the process and area of application, parameters that determine the amount of drug delivered, can be modified according to the needs.
- Easy skin recovery after application, since no severe irritation is produced.

- It can be used for systemic or local (topical) delivery of drugs.
- Inter and intra subject variability is considerably reduced compared with passive diffusion, since the rate of drug delivery is more dependent on applied current than on membrane characteristics.

Iontophoresis has been established as a safe, versatile and efficient enhancement technique and several iontophoretic devices have been marketed. Clinically, iontophoresis has been employed to deliver through skin fentanyl and lidocaine for pain relief [3, 4], pilocarpine to induce sweating (as a diagnostic test) [5], and tap water to treat hyperhidrosis [6]. Iontophoresis even has been used as a monitoring technique in diabetic patients, since it can be used to extract glucose from the skin [7]. Also, recently has seen an interest into the potential use of iontophoresis to deliver drugs through other membranes such as the nail and through the sclera and cornea, the two main barriers to eye drug delivery [8].

In this chapter basic concepts of iontophoresis will be discussed, examples of application of this delivery technique for drug application will be explained and currently existing iontophoretic devices for different treatments will be exposed.

2. MECHANISM OF ACTION AND THEORETICAL BASIS OF IONTOPHORESIS

During iontophoresis low density, and low voltage, current (less than 0.5 mA.cm^{-2}, 1-10 V) is applied through an electrical circuit which electrodes are placed on a membrane surface. This allows the propelled ions to pass through the membrane.

In the course of current application skin resistance is reduced. It may be due to micro- or nano-phores formation as a consequence of proteins and lipids, present in the stratum corneum, reorientation under the application of the electric field; or it may be caused by the ions flux into stratum corneum (either from beneath the stratum corneum or from the formulation on it). Local changes can also take place in hair follicles and sweat glands. As a result the originated pores, negatives in charge considering the permselectivity of skin at physiological pH, may have different diameters and structures. Nevertheless, after current cessation skin resistance is recovered so it can be considered that skin alterations under iontophoresis are reversible [9].

Under electrical current application electromigration, electroosmosis or passive diffusion are the possible mechanisms used by a drug to pass through skin (**Fig. 1**).

Simple electric repulsion of similar charges force ionised drugs across the membrane (electromigration). Thereby, anionic molecules cross the membrane by applying them in the electrode negatively charged. Likewise, positively charged drugs must be placed on the anode [10]. It has been observed that under iontophoresis conducted at pH 7.4 small cations flux (*i.e.* Na^+) is higher than that of anions (Cl^-), suggesting a permselectivity of skin to cations in this conditions. It is therefore accepted that the pores created into skin are mainly negative in charge and skin therefore behaves as a negatively charged membrane at pHs above its isoelectric point (4-4.5) [11, 12]. Consequently, cations that have been repelled by the anode are delivered through the skin more successfully than anions.

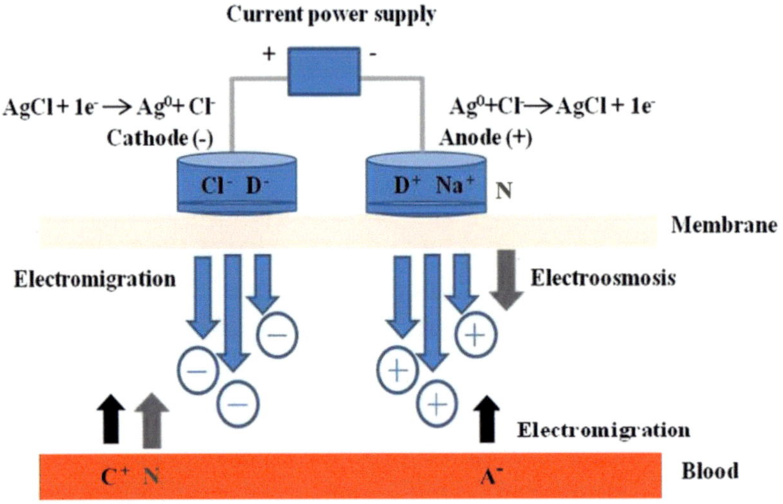

Fig. (1). Diagram of the direction of movement of substances during the application of iontophoresis technique. ($D^{-/+}$: drug negatively or positively charged, N: neutral substances; C^+ and A^- represent cations and anions in blood, respectively).

Once the barrier layer has been overcome by a drug, the later can easily reach the systemic circulation. Simultaneously, ions placed in or beneath the membrane, are attracted into the electrode chambers.

During iontophoresis application transport of drugs is also produced by passive diffusion and electroosmosis. The voltage difference produced across a charged porous membrane generates a flow of ions, and consequently of fluid, called electroosmosis. This flow includes movement of drugs not dependent on their concentration gradient and is a significant factor affecting iontophoresis of neutral substances, and in a minor manner of charged ones.

Accordingly, flux measured during iontophoresis corresponds to the sum of the fluxes due to electromigration, electroosmotic drug flux and change in the barrier permeability due to the electric field applied (passive) [13 - 15].

$$Jiontophoresis = Jelectromigration + Jelectrosmosis + Jpassive$$

Jelectromigration is the flux due to electric current application. Different mathematical models have been proposed to describe transdermal electrotransport and one of the more extended is the derived from the Nernst-Planck equation [16]:

$$J_{electromigration(d)} = \frac{Z_d \cdot U_d \cdot C_d}{\sum Z_i \cdot U_i \cdot C_i} \cdot \frac{I}{Z_d \cdot F} = t_d \frac{I}{Z_d F}$$

Where *C, U* and *Z* represent concentration, mobility and electric valence of the drug (*d*) and other ionic species present (*i*) and *F* is Faraday constant. In this expression t_d is the transport number of the drug considered, that is, the fraction of the total charge transported by the drug during iontophoresis.

Jelectrosmosis is the flux due to convective flow of the solvent:

$$Jelectrosmosis = Jw\ C$$

Where *Jw* is the water flux produced during iontophoresis and *C* is the concentration of the drug.

Jpassive, the flux due to passive delivery, is the minor contributing process, and is defined by:

$$Jpassive = K\ D\ dC/dh$$

Where K is the partition coefficient between donor solution and barrier layer, D the diffusivity across the barrier and dC/dh is the concentration gradient across the layer.

Small hydrophilic cations transport depends essentially on electromigration [17]. At very high concentration of the ionic drug it carries most of the current and consequently electroosmotic flow has no impact on drug flux.

On the contrary, electroosmosis effect becomes greater when large cations are considered. These compounds have low transport numbers compared with the small ions dissolved into the background solution; therefore current is transported by the competing ions and not by the drug. In this case electromigration is negligible compared with electroosmosis [17].

Various mathematical models have been proposed by different authors to describe iontophoretic transport kinetics, *in vitro* and *in vivo*. We highly recommend to the readers interested in this field the recent review of Gratieri and Kalia [16].

3. FACTORS INFLUENCING IONTOPHORETIC TRANSPORT

Different factors can influence the efficacy of iontophoresis. Molecular size, charge and concentration, are the main physicochemical properties of the drug influencing iontophoresis; background solution characteristics (type of the buffer, pH, presence of other compounds), electrical and technical factors (types of current, electrodes, treatment length, current density) and biological or physiological variations (site of application, pH and condition of the membrane, regional blood flow) are other factors of relevance on iontophoretic application (Table **1**).

The molecular size of the solute regulates the feasibility of iontophoretic delivery and hence the amount of drug transported. Generally, small ions are more mobile than large ones. Various studies indicate that smaller and more hydrophilic ions are transported at a faster rate than larger ions [18, 19]. The permeability coefficients of positively and negatively charged and also of uncharged solutes across membrane are a function of molecular size. In general, transport of drugs decreases when their molecular weight increases, if all other conditions are kept constant [20 - 23].

Table 1. Some relevant factors affecting iontophoretic transport.

Properties	Comments
Physicochemical properties of drug and formulation	
Molecular size Molecular weight	Higher transport is obtained with small molecules
Drug concentration	Its effect depends on the mechanism of transport (electrosmosis *vs* electromigration) and on the presence of competing ions
Polarity	Neutral molecules are transported by electrosmosis Ions are transported by electromigration
Charge of molecules	Positively charged drugs have higher transport
Ionic strength	Small competing ions reduce drug transport
Iontophoretic conditions	
Current strength Current density	Increasing current strength increases drug transport proportionally. A maximum of 0.5 mA·cm^{-2} is accepted to avoid skin damage
Type of current	The type of current can modulate the entrance of the drug into body. Constant or pulsatile current can be used.
Type of electrode	Some electrodes can alter pH of the media and modify drug transport during procedure
Biological or physiological variations	
Inter-intra subject variability	Lower than by passive diffusion
Regional blood flow	High blood flow favor drug absorption
Membrane pH	If the pH of the membrane is changed drug transport can be altered
Condition of barrier	Skin damage increase drug absorption
Area of the body	Modifying the size of the area of application the entrance flux can be modified

Iontophoretic mass transfer is driven principally by a potential gradient that generates a current flow from anode to the skin and then to the cathode. Nevertheless, if there are competing ions in the solution increasing drug concentration results in greater drug delivery (see equations above). As an example, in Fig. (**2**) can be seen that the transport number of sumatriptan drastically increases when the ionic strength of the media is reduced, and consequently the transdermal flux increases significantly. In these conditions of low ionic strength the fraction of charge transported by the drug during iontophoresis is higher (transport number, t_d is higher). Accordingly, the optimal situation for iontophoresis consists in avoiding competing co-ions. In this later condition, the drug reaches its maximal transport number and its flux is independent of concentration [17].

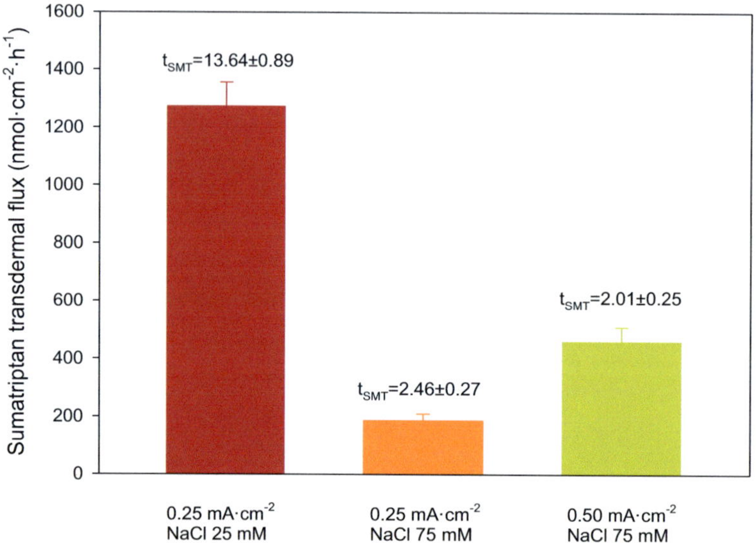

Fig. (2). Effect of ionic strength and the current density applied on sumatriptan transdermal flux (nmol/cm^2/h).

Under iontophoresis, charge of a molecule is an important physicochemical property that determines the mechanism by which it will be transported. Monovalent ions can be delivered more easily than divalent ones, even having similar molecular weight [24].

When a drug is in an ionized form its delivery under iontophoresis is maximal. This effect of pH was investigated with lignocaine, and it was observed that its transdermal flux under iontophoresis reached the maximal value when the drug was in an ionized form [25]. Since it is important to avoid competing ions in the media, additives used for controlling the pH (buffers) should be of a large molecular size (*i.e.* HEPES (N-[2-Hydroxiethyl] piperazine-N-[2-ethanesulfonic acid]) instead of phosphates).

The electrodes used can affect the iontophoresis process. Platinum or zinc/zinc chloride electrodes can produce pH changes during its use. On the contrary, Ag/AgCl electrodes do not cause pH changes, therefore are in general preferred over the former. The distribution of drug within the membrane depends on the size and position of the electrodes. They are usually selected according to individual needs [26].

The current strength applied (I in the equations above) plays an important role in drug penetration by iontophoresis administration. Some studies have demonstrated that there is a linear relationship between the flux of compound and the current applied (see equations above) [27]. However, the amount of current is limited by patient safety considerations, such as pain and possible electrical tissue damage due to burns or cell necrosis. In general, a maximum of 0.5 $mA \cdot cm^{-2}$ is accepted, although it depends on the treatment area and duration of current passage.

Current can be selected to control delivery of drugs to the body [28]. Either continuous or pulsatile (on-off periods) current can be used. This later allows skin to depolarize in the state "off" increasing its permeability.

4. REVERSE IONTOPHORESIS

Iontophoresis can be employed to assist the passage of the substances of a formulation across the skin or to extract from the body analytes representative of physiological or pathological circumstances. The first is known as direct iontophoresis and the later as reverse iontophoresis.

Reverse iontophoresis provides a convenient non-invasive method for extracting substances through skin, allowing this way sampling body fluids to monitor them efficiently. During current application negatively charged entities beneath the skin are attracted into the anode, while neutral and positively charged ones move into the cathode. Skin contains some of the entities to be analysed, therefore to correlate extracted levels of the analytes with levels in the blood it is necessary to withdraw skin reserves previously [7, 29 - 33]. Another limiting factor of reverse iontophoresis is the low levels extracted, which make it difficult to quantify the extracted molecules.

5. THERAPEUTICAL APPLICATIONS OF IONTOPHORESIS

Physical therapy, anaesthesiology, dermatology, dentistry and ophthalmology are some medical specialties that have adopted iontophoresis in their practice. Iontophoresis may be employed to administrate drugs for systemic or local therapy. In fact, cutaneous iontophoresis is the usual topical route and allows the administration of high concentrations in tissue while limiting the access of the drug to blood. The frequently polar and/or charged nature of biotechnology drugs makes them potentially well-suited candidates for electrically controlled drug delivery [34, 35]. In the following paragraphs some examples of use and ongoing research of iontophoresis are shown.

5.1. Iontophoresis for Topical Delivery

5.1.1. Corticosteroids

The primary drugs used with iontophoresis in physical therapy are corticosteroids. Dexamethasone sodium phosphate is frequently administrated by iontophoresis in the treatment of various musculoskeletal problems in physical therapy. The drug is used in clinical studies for the treatment of local pain and soft-tissue inflammation, employing different protocols, many of which have reported beneficial effects [36, 37] though improvement in the patient´s condition has not been always reported [38, 39]. Garrido *et al.* [40] reported that verapamil and dexamethasone iontophoresis is a safe and reliable treatment resolving painful erections in the acute phase of Peyronie's disease. A recent study concluded that dexamethasone iontophoresis may be a useful treatment of nail psoriasis [41]. Stefanou reported that lateral epicondylitis may be treated applying corticosteroid with iontophoresis technique [42].

Iontophoresis administration of other glucocorticoids has also been used in the treatment temporomandibular trismus and paresthesia [43] and for Peyronie's disease [44].

5.1.2. Anaesthetics

Iontophoresis of anaesthetics, for induction of local anaesthesia was one of the first therapeutical uses of this technique. In fact, iontophoresis is a chosen method for obtaining anaesthesia in surgical procedures in the external ear canal and tympanic membrane [45]. General sedation followed by infiltration anaesthesia can be painful due to the injection and is rather time-consuming. However the iontophoretic administration of local anaesthetics is satisfactory for the treatment of outpatients.

FDA approved the first combination of lidocaine and epinephrine for local anaesthesia in 1995 (Iontocaine®) and Emilidopel® and Lidosite® were approved in 2004. The anaesthetic action of lidocaine is extended, in a dose-dependent manner, by addition of epinephrine, since the later decreases skin blood flow [46, 47]. The current density of the lidocaine iontophoretic device Lidosite® is 0.35 $mA \cdot cm^{-2}$, and it is applied for 10 min with a patch electrode of a pH value of 4.5, at which both lidocaine and epinephrine are positively charged [48].

The pharmacokinetic of lidocaine applied with iontophoresis has been assessed in animals and humans. In an animal model to which lidocaine was applied it was observed that compared to passive drug administration iontophoresis at 0.15 $mA \cdot cm^{-2}$ resulted in a 40-fold increase in dermal lidocaine concentrations [49].

Furthermore iontophoresis has been very successful for induction of local anaesthesia in paediatric patients [50 - 52]. This population group suffers pain and anxiety associated to needle injections and topically applied anaesthetics take a long time to become effective (up to 1 hour) and often provide incomplete anaesthesia. Randomized studies have found lidocaine iontophoresis to be more effective than EMLA cream (eutectic mixture of local anaesthetics) or topical lidocaine for placement of paediatric intravenous catheters [52, 53]. Squire *et al.* [53] demonstrated that the time to accomplish topical anaesthesia was shorter with iontophoresis of 2% lidocaine with epinephrine 1:100000 (13 minutes) compared to a surface-applied EMLA cream (60 minutes) [53, 54]. Iontophoresis of lidocaine with epinephrine is a safe, rapid, and effective method of local anaesthesia delivery for paediatric procedures.

5.1.3. Hyperhidrosis

One of the oldest applications of iontophoresis is the treatment of hyperhidrosis

[55]. Hyperhidrosis, an abnormal and excessive rate of sweat secretion from the eccrine glands, is a disabling condition that affects both children and adults in various parts of the body, primarily the palms, soles and axillae. Different options have been considered in the treatment of hyperhidrosis: topical aluminium chloride, anti-cholinergics, botulinum toxin injections, local surgery, thoracic sympathectomy and iontophoresis. Either tap water, saline, botulinum toxin or anticholinergics have been applied with iontophoresis [56 - 58]. However, there is controversy about effectiveness; there is one study that defends that tap water is more effective than saline [59] while another study shows otherwise [60]. Iontophoresis of tap water is a safe, efficacious, and cost-effective primary treatment available of palmar and plantar hyperhidrosis [61], but the results are less rewarding concerning axillary hyperhidrosis [56, 58]. Iontophoresis has recently been shown to be more effective for the administration of botulinum toxin than for saline, because sweating is reduced more quickly without side-effects and for a longer period of time [62, 63].

5.1.4. Diagnosis

Diagnosis of ***cystic fibrosis*** is based on the induction of sweating. The application of pilocarpine by iontophoresis (2.5-3.0 mA of constant current for five minutes), in the arm or leg, is used to stimulate sweating, allowing sufficient amounts of sweat to be collected for the analysis of sodium and chloride concentration in sweat [5, 64, 65]. Furthermore, the use of pilocarpine iontophoresis may be extended for the diagnosis of other anomalies such as ***ectodermal dysplasia*** [66]. It is a genetic disorder affecting the skin, hair, nails, teeth and sweat glands. The clinical presentation is heterogeneous; however, hypohidrotic (reduced sweat) ectodermal dysplasia is the commonest. Sweat glands are sparse or rudimentary, leading to dysregulation of body temperature and episodes of uncontrolled hyperthermia.

5.1.5. Dentistry

One of the uses of iontophoresis in dentistry is for local application of ***anaesthetics*** prior to oral surgical procedures.

Moreover, sodium fluoride applied with iontophoresis has proved to be an effective treatment for ***dentin hypersensitivity*** [67 - 71]. Nevertheless, the mechanisms of action of sodium fluoride iontophoresis in this common clinical condition are not completely understood. One possible explication is that exposed dentin allows fluid movement through microtubules that stretch from the pulp. Occlusion of the patent dentinal tubules would appear to be one mechanism by which iontophoresis of sodium fluoride could be a successful therapy. Otherwise, Puapichartdumrong observed that iontophoresis could enhance the delivery of ionized drugs through intact and caries-affected dentine into the pulp [72].

The efficacy of topical treatment of ***Herpes labialis infection*** with traditional creams is in debate, due to limited improvement of the infection with commercial topical treatments of the antiretroviral drugs with respect to spontaneous recovery. The principal antiretroviral drug, acyclovir has a poor penetration through the skin and insufficient distribution to the targeted site of infection, the basal epidermis. The transdermal penetration enhancement of acyclovir has been widely studied involving chemical enhancers and electrical current. The use of iontophoresis to delivery acyclovir through the skin resulted in high drug levels in skin layers, which keep it up 2-3 days [73, 74]. As mentioned before, to delivery hydrophilic drug through the skin using iontophoresis is necessary to choose a proper formulation. This fact has been demonstrated in the iontophoretic delivery of acyclovir from different topical formulations. The results of the study carried by Shukla *et al.* showed that only when the drug is incorporated in the aqueous phase of the cream acyclovir was available for transport and pH 11 gels produced a statistically significant increase in the amount of acyclovir in the dermis compared with neutral creams [75].

5.1.6. Treatment of Nail Diseases

For effective topical therapy, ungual drug permeation must be enhanced, and, among other possible strategies, iontophoresis has been assayed. Hao *et al.* [76, 77] used as model compounds tetraethylammonium, manitol and urea to demonstrate that the main mechanism of transport of small ions during ungual iontophoresis is electromigration and that the contribution of electroosmotic flow to the overall iontophoretic flux is low. Their results also indicated that transungual electroosmosis was affected by the ionic strength and that a decrease in solution ionic strength enhanced the electrosmotic transport of the drug. Nail electrical resistance increased with decreasing thc ionic strength; nevertheless, a maximal value was obtained at ionic strength around 0.07 M. Their results are consistent with the existence of both proton-donating and -accepting functional groups in the nail plates and an isoelectric point of approximately 5. All these results are in accordance with transdermal iontophoresis.

Onychomycosis is a very common nail condition which implies that fungal pathogens colonize the nail creating an infection [78, 79]. The treatment for onychomycosis is difficult because the incapability to completely penetrate the nail plate [80]. Treatments could be more successful if it could be guaranteed that the drug administered penetrates the nail. In this sense, iontophoresis is used for terbinafine application, because it has the highest antifungal effect on dermatophytes *in vitro* [81]. The application of iontophoresis enhances the terbinafine accumulated in the nail plate compared with a passive administration of drug [82 - 85]. The plate acts as a reservoir of terbinafine and the drug is then released into the nail bed and matrix over a period of time of approximately 60-70 days [85, 86]. The amount of terbinafine can be increased with iontophoresis by removal of the dorsal layer of the nail plate, or in the presence of keratolysis [86]. Nair *et al.* proved that two applicators, a "nail-only" applicator which delivers terbinafine only into a part of the nail plate and a "nail/skin" applicator which delivers terbinafine into the nail plate and surrounding soft tissues, provided high amounts of drug through and into the nail [83]. Two clinical trials (a phase I and a phase II (NCT00768768, NCT01484145)) have been completed using the Electrokinetic Transungual System (ETS)-Terbinafine Gel registered by NB Therapeutics, but data remain unpublished [87, 88].

5.1.7. Antineoplastic Drugs

There is great interest in studying the application of iontophoresis to administer antineoplastic drugs for the treatment of certain skin cancers because iontophoresis could avoid the adverse effects related with the systemic administration of antineoplastics. Furthermore, iontophoretic administration of antineoplastic drugs could be a good alternative to surgery and radiation therapy and could avoid possible complications. Chang *et al.* [89] reported visual improvements in the lesions of nine patients diagnosed with basal cell carcinoma following the administration of cisplatin by iontophoresis. The dose of cisplatin and current applied to the patients varied depending on the size of the lesion. Cisplatin was applied together with a vasoconstrictor drug, epinephrine hydrochloride, in the anode compartment. In this study most of the patients in treatment showed a reduction in lesion area. Systemic side effects were not reported and only some of the patients reported a small burning perception in the skin. The small lesions responded better than the biggest and the authors recommended a daily iontophoretic therapy with cisplatin during 20 or 30 minutes for 5 days followed by a period of 2 weeks without treatment for patient recovery. Years later, another study described the successful treatment of a 67-year-old male with a histologically confirmed basal cell carcinoma on his upper anterolateral left leg. The treatment consisted of four cycles of five successive days of cisplatin iontophoresis, with a 2-week rest period between cycles. The cisplatin solution (5 mL at 1 $mg \cdot mL^{-1}$) was used in combination with epinephrine hydrochloride. The effectiveness of the treatment was confirmed by post-treatment biopsies, which revealed granulation tissue scarring without evidence of basal cell carcinoma. Measurements of cellular proliferation were monitored immunohistochemically with Ki-67 and cell cycle distribution analyzed by flow cytometry [90].

Moreover, regarding the treatment of cutaneous lesions associated with Kaposi sarcoma in patients with immunodeficiency virus type 1 and who have cutaneous lesions of Kaposi sarcoma it was observed that the application of vinblastine solution by iontophoresis is well tolerated, there is a symptomatic improvement and a reduction in lesions [91].

Methotrexate is widely used in the treatment of rheumatoid arthritis and psoriasis. Nevertheless, since oral administration of methotrexate has low bioavailability and toxicity transdermal administration could be a good alternative. However the physicochemical characteristics of the drug, solubility and charge, limits its delivery to skin. The effect of iontophoresis in the transdermal flux of the antineoplastic drug methotrexate has been investigated by several authors [92 - 94]. The development of an iontophoretic device of methotrexate could be a good alternative for the treatment of psoriasis and it is important to note that the cathodal iontophoresis of the drug produces a higher flux through the skin than when the drug is delivered passively. Different strategies, alone or in combination, chemical percutaneous enhancers, the use of physical techniques such as iontophoresis, electroporation and ultrasound and microneedles are being explored to enhance methotrexate permeability.

Gratieri and Kalia [95] have explored the use of buccal iontophoresis for the simultaneous delivery of chemotherapeutic to developing a new approach to treat head and neck cancers. The iontophoresis of 5-fluorouracil and leucovorin at 1 $mA \cdot cm^{-2}$ for 10 or 20 min from aqueous solution was evaluated *in vitro* using bovine mucosa. No drug permeation was observed in either case concluding that iontophoresis can be used for topical delivery of chemotherapeutics to the buccal mucosa as a less invasive local therapy of head and neck cancers.

5.1.8. Proteins

The administration of a protein, ribonuclease A (RNAse; 13.6 kDa) though the skin by iontophoresis is reported in different studies [96, 97]. These studies demonstrate that iontophoresis can be used to deliver significant amounts of protein across skin. RNAse inhibits the translation of numerous genes and therefore, the topical introduction of RNAse targeted against genes involved in various cutaneous disorders represents a possibility in the treatment of hereditary skin diseases, viral infections, cancer and dermatitis.

5.1.9. Ophthalmic Applications

Some descriptions of ocular iontophoresis were reported in the first part of the twentieth century. Some of them include the application of zinc salts for the treatment of corneal ulcers by Wirtz [98], magnesium for treatment of glaucoma, ammonium chloride for treatment of cataract, and iontophoresis of phosphoric acid for treatment of optic atrophy by Morisot [99] and ocular iontophoresis delivery for different antibiotics by Witzel *et al.* [100].

Iontophoresis has to be either transcorneal or transscleral, depending on the site of action of the drug intended to deliver. Transcorneal iontophoresis delivers a high concentration of drug to the anterior segment of the eye: cornea, ciliary body, aqueous humour and lens. Transscleral iontophoresis can deliver high and sustained amounts of drugs in the vitreous and retina. For this later purpose the iontophoretic device has to be placed on the conjunctiva. There is literature concerning the use of iontophoresis for delivery of anaesthetics to the eye and in the treatment of glaucoma, ocular infections, ocular inflammation, and ocular herpes infection [101].

5.1.10. Iontophoresis for Systemic Delivery

In 2006 was approved Ionsys® (Janssen, Beerse, Belgium) in Europe for the management of acute moderate to severe postoperative pain. Ionsys® is an iontophoretic patient-controlled transdermal delivery system of ***fentanyl***. The device contained 10.8 mg of fentanyl hydrochloride (a water-soluble salt with pKa 8.4), and it was designed to deliver a 40 mcg dose of fentanyl over a 10 minute period upon each activation of the dose button [102]. The efficacy of fentanyl applied with iontophoresis was compared with intravenous patient-controlled analgesia with morphine in a controlled trial and the authors of the study concluded that there were no differences in the efficacy of both treatments [3]. Ionsys® was designed for use only in hospitalized patients. Due to some problems related with overdose in some patients the product was withdrawn from the market in Europe and in USA.

Agonists of the 5-HT_1 family receptors used as anti-migraine agents (*i.e.* triptans) have high interest. Indeed, subcutaneous administration of ***sumatriptan*** leads to a rapid but transient effect, whereas oral or nasal administration suffers from poor bioavailability. Previous *in vitro* [103] and *in vivo* [104] studies demonstrated that iontophoresis enhances the transdermal passage of sumatriptan and that this technique could be appropriate to reach adequate plasma levels for treatment of migraine. Pharmacokinetic studies in healthy subjects to whom sumatriptan was administered using iontophoresis (4 mA for 1h followed by 2 mA for 3h) showed comparable areas under the curve concentration over time to the subcutaneous route [105]. The iontophoretic device containing sumatriptan (Zecuity®, formerly Zelrix®; NuPathe Inc., Conshohocken, PA, USA) has been approved by the US Food and Drug Administration (FDA) in January 2013 [106].

The iontophoresis delivery of another drugs 5-HT_1 agonists, such as zolmitriptan or almotriptan, have been reported but only preclinical data are available and suggest that these molecules are also appropriate candidates for iontophoresis [107, 108].

The transdermal iontophoretic administration of ***anti-Parkinsonian drugs*** have been evaluated in different studies. The results of transdermal iontophoretic delivery of apomorphine for the treatment of idiopathic Parkinson´s in human subjects are so far encouraging [109] particularly if the skin is previously treated with surfactants [110]. Furthermore, the iontophoretic administration of the anti-Parkinsonian ropinirole hydrochloride has been studied *in vivo* in rats and the results reveal the possibility of achieving therapeutic plasma levels of the drug [111].

Proteins administration has elevated interest in the ultimate few years. Iontophoresis of human insulin (molecular weight ~6000 Daltons and negatively charged) has been studied since 1980, but a low penetration rate precluded its consideration for therapeutic use [112]. The iontophoretic administration of insulin has an important number of difficulties, for example the degradation of the molecule caused by contact with the anode, which can be resolved by placing the drug in the cathodal compartment. Different *in vitro* studies have demonstrated the delivery of insulin by means of iontophoresis in animal models, particularly rats, mice and rabbits [113 - 116]. As an example, a study in which insulin has been encapsulated into positively charged nanovesicles driven by iontophoresis through skin with microneedle-induced microchannels obtained glucose levels in rats comparable to those obtained after subcutaneous injection of insulin [117]. Although these studies prove that blood glucose levels can be controlled by iontophoretic administration of insulin, frequently after compromising the stratum corneum, their results need to be extrapolated to humans, to prove that an iontophoretic device of insulin can be a reality.

Transdermal iontophoretic administration of other peptides, such as calcitonin, luteinizing hormone-releasing hormone or vasopressin has also been investigated, but no clinical applications have obtained of these experiments [112].

There is also some research concerning the administration of different molecules with the aid of iontophoresis. As an example, iontophoresis has been suggested as a way of administrating ***nicotine*** in smoking cessation [118]. However, there are no clinical studies currently assessing the efficacy and safety of nicotine applied with iontophoresis. *In vitro* studies point out the potential of iontophoresis for administering ***ranitidine*** [119] or ***phenobarbital*** [120] in paediatric. But, to our knowledge, there are no clinical data yet.

The transdermal administration of drugs has some advantages with respect to oral therapy in treatment of ***Alzheimer's disease*** patients, since they have swallowing problems and moreover they have problems to cooperate in their treatment. Memantine is used in therapy treating advanced stages of Alzheimer's disease. Del Rio-Sancho *et al.* demonstrated *in vitro* that iontophoresis exhibits a great ability to enhance the flux of memantine with respect to passive diffusion of drug [121].

These later are examples of molecules that are potential candidates for incorporating in a transdermal administration system based on iontophoresis for reaching therapeutical blood levels. In this sense, recently, some research is focused on the combination of iontophoresis with other technologies, mainly microneedles, to enhance the transdermal penetration. Apart from the study with insulin mentioned above, for other molecules as diclofenac sodium [122] and the anti-muscarinic agent glycopyrrolate [123] it has been demonstrated at different levels, *i.e., in vivo* with the first and *in vitro* for the later, that the combination allows a further increase in the transdermal absorption of the molecule than that obtained with each technique separately.

5.1.11. Reverse Iontophoresis

The first approved use of reverse iontophoresis was the extraction of glucose from beneath the skin. GlucoWatch G2® Biographer (Cygnus Inc., Redwood City, CA, USA) is a device that permitted a non-invasive extraction of glucose across skin, allowing the glycaemia to be evaluated every 10 min over several hours. In this system, glucose was extracted in the cathode due to the electrosmotic flow generated by the application of a low level current and it was then quantified in the same chamber where extracted [124, 125].

Although the detection of glucose is the only application that reached the market, a great deal of research has been carried out in this field, and the results obtained with some analytes are encouraging. In this sense, aminoacids, urea, lactate, lithium, valproate, phenytoin and amikacine focus most of the attention.

Amino acids are biological markers, the plasma levels of which may be used to detect inherited metabolic diseases. They are excellent candidates for non-invasive monitoring *via* reverse iontophoresis due to their small molecular weight and polar nature. Different authors have shown how the transport of amino acids across the skin can be significantly enhanced by iontophoresis [30, 31, 126] and pilot studies in humans have demonstrated the correlation between the amount of aminoacids extracted and their levels in stratum corneum [127]. Nevertheless, there are high levels of some of the aminoacids in skin; this depot effect requires a long period of time to be extracted and makes it difficult to correlate the levels extracted by means of iontophoresis with blood levels [127].

Other analytes that can be extracted by reverse iontophoresis and whose potential utility in the field of diagnosis have been explored are urea, used for the non-invasive diagnosis of individuals with chronic kidney disease [128]; lactate, a widely used marker of tissue distress in critically ill patients and of sports performance [129]; and drugs such as lithium [32, 130], phenytoin [131], valproate [132] and amikacin [133], which require routine drug monitoring to assess adequate plasma levels.

6. IONTOPHORETIC DEVICES

Iontophoretic devices usually consist of a power supply used to deliver the current, a controller and the electrodes. In Fig. (**3**) is represented a schema of the design of an iontophoretic device. There are different kinds of electrodes, depending on the purpose of the iontophoretic devices. The most common electrodes used for iontophoresis are adhesive electrodes, electrodes palmar/plantar, ear electrodes and handpiece electrodes.

If the product is marketed as a complete system that includes together the device and drug, then it is regulated as a drug-device combination product. On the other hand, the device can be marketed separately from the drug; in that case it is regulated as a medical device. In Table **2** are shown the drug-device combination products approved by the FDA.

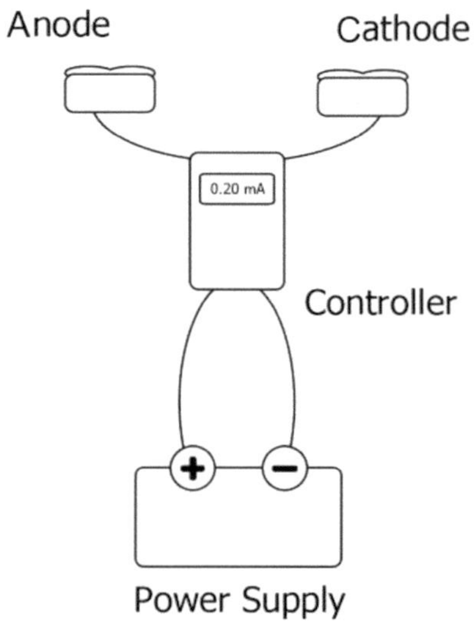

Fig. (3). Schema of the design of iontophoretic device.

FDA established three categories of devices concerning the controls needed to provide reasonable assurance of their safety and effectiveness. The three categories of devices are class I-III. In the class I are included the devices for which the general controls by themselves are sufficient to provide reasonable assurance of the safety and effectiveness.

Table 2. Drug-device combination products approved by the FDA.

Drug	Therapeutic Use	Commercial Name	Year of Approval
Lidocaine and epinephrine	Local dermal analgesia	Iontocaine	1995
		Empi Lidopel	2004
		LidoSite Topical System Kit	2004
Fentanyl	Short-term management of post-operative pain	IONSYS Fentanyl HCl	2006
Sumatriptan	Acute treatment of migraines	ZECUITY Transdermal System	2013

Class II includes the devices for which the general controls are insufficient to provide reasonable assurance of the safety and effectiveness but there is sufficient information to establish special controls to provide such assurance. In this group are included iontophoretic devices used in the diagnosis of cystic fibrosis or for use with a specific drug that has been approved for delivery by iontophoresis.

Other devices, for which there is no sufficient information to determine that general and special controls are sufficient to provide reasonable assurance of the safety and effectiveness, are included in class III, that is, devices not included in class I nor class II. This group includes devices indicated for use with a specific non-drug solution, for example the devices used for the treatment of hyperhidrosis.

Recently FDA has proposed that iontophoretic devices intended for any other purposes be reclassified from class III to class II designation due to the scientific evidences that demonstrate the safety and clinical effectiveness of these iontophoresis systems. In these devices, special controls proposed by the FDA can provide a reasonable assurance of effectiveness [134].

The two drug-device combination products containing lidocaine and fentanyl and the glucose monitoring system currently are unavailable. It has to be keeping in mind that it is not likely to launch a complex system (drug+delivery system) competitive in the market since technologically they are more difficult to obtain and their production is more expensive. Hopefully, incidents that finally determined their withdrawal from the market will not arrive to the recently approved sumatriptan system [135].

CONCLUSION

The scientific evidence and the results published since the use of iontophoresis demonstrates the safety and clinical effectiveness of the iontophoretic systems. The use of iontophoresis for topical delivery of drugs is well known in clinic. More recently, iontophoresis has been shown as an efficient technique for systemic delivery of drugs, and nowadays transdermal iontophoresis is a good alternative to parenteral administration of some drugs with the benefits for the patients, for example pain and discomfort associated with repeated injection.

Furthermore, various enhancement technologies, such microneedles, are being explored for use with iontophoresis to enhance skin permeability to macromolecules by disrupting the barrier property of the skin.

For all of these reasons it is palpable that iontophoresis holds a promise for the future of drug delivery.

CONFLICT OF INTEREST

The authors confirm that they have no conflict of interest to declare for this publication.

ACKNOWLEDGEMENTS

Declared none.

REFERENCES

[1] Brown MB, Traynor MJ, Martin GP, Akomeah FK. Transdermal drug delivery systems: skin perturbation devices. Methods Mol Biol 2008; 437: 119-39. [http://dx.doi.org/10.1007/978-1-59745-210-6_5] [PMID: 18369965]

[2] Rizwan M, Aqil M, Talegaonkar S, Azeem A, Sultana Y, Ali A. Enhanced transdermal drug delivery techniques: an extensive review of patents. Recent Pat Drug Deliv Formul 2009; 3(2): 105-24. [http://dx.doi.org/10.2174/187221109788452285] [PMID: 19519571]

[3] Viscusi ER, Reynolds L, Chung F, Atkinson LE, Khanna S. Patient-controlled transdermal fentanyl hydrochloride *vs* intravenous morphine pump for postoperative pain: a randomized controlled trial. JAMA 2004; 291(11): 1333-41. [http://dx.doi.org/10.1001/jama.291.11.1333] [PMID: 15026400]

[4] Kaya A, Kamanli A, Ardicoglu O, Ozgocmen S, Ozkurt-Zengin F, Bayik Y. Direct current therapy with/without lidocaine iontophoresis in myofascial pain syndrome. Bratisl Lek Listy (Tlacene Vyd) 2009; 110(3): 185-91. [PMID: 19507642]

[5] Gomez CC, Servidoni MdeF, Marson FA, *et al.* Pulsed direct and constant direct currents in the pilocarpine iontophoresis sweat chloride test. BMC Pulm Med 2014; 14(1): 198-208. [http://dx.doi.org/10.1186/1471-2466-14-198] [PMID: 25495771]

[6] Karakoç Y, Aydemir EH, Kalkan MT, Ünal G. Safe control of palmoplantar hyperhidrosis with direct electrical current. Int J Dermatol 2002; 41(9): 602-5. [http://dx.doi.org/10.1046/j.1365-4362.2002.01473.x] [PMID: 12358834]

[7] Potts RO, Tamada JA, Tierney MJ. Glucose monitoring by reverse iontophoresis. Diabetes Metab Res Rev 2002; 18 (Suppl. 1): S49-53. [http://dx.doi.org/10.1002/dmrr.210] [PMID: 11921430]

[8] Eljarrat-Binstock E, Raiskup F, Stepensky D, Domb AJ, Frucht-Pery J. Delivery of gentamicin to the rabbit eye by drug-loaded hydrogel iontophoresis. Invest Ophthalmol Vis Sci 2004; 45(8): 2543-8. [http://dx.doi.org/10.1167/iovs.03-1294] [PMID: 15277475]

[9] Curdy C, Kalia YN, Guy RH. Post-iontophoresis recovery of human skin impedance *in vivo*. Eur J Pharm Biopharm 2002; 53(1): 15-21. [http://dx.doi.org/10.1016/S0939-6411(01)00216-8] [PMID: 11777748]

[10] Sage BH. Iontophoresis. In: Swarbrick J, Boylan JC, Eds. Encyclopedia of pharmaceutical Technology. 1st ed. New York: Marcel Dekker Inc 1993; Vol. 8: pp. 217-47.

[11] Merino V, López A, Kalia YN, Guy RH. Electrorepulsion *versus* electroosmosis: effect of pH on the iontophoretic flux of 5-fluorouracil. Pharm Res 1999; 16(5): 758-61. [http://dx.doi.org/10.1023/A:1018841111922] [PMID: 10350021]

[12] Burnette RR, Ongpipattanakul B. Characterization of the permselective properties of excised human skin during iontophoresis. J Pharm Sci 1987; 76(10): 765-73. [http://dx.doi.org/10.1002/jps.2600761003] [PMID: 3123641]

[13] Srinivasan V, Higuchi WI. A model for iontophoresis incorporating the effect of convective solvent flow. Int J Pharm 1990; 60(2): 133-8. [http://dx.doi.org/10.1016/0378-5173(90)90298-I]

[14] Pikal MJ, Shah S. Transport mechanisms in iontophoresis II. Electroosmotic flow and transference number measurement for hairless mouse skin. Pharm Res 1990; 7: 313-21. [http://dx.doi.org/10.1023/A:1015898717936] [PMID: 2194197]

[15] Singh P, Maibach HI. Iontophoresis in drug delivery: basic principles and applications 1994.

[16] Gratieri T, Kalia YN. Mathematical models to describe iontophoretic transport *in vitro* and *in vivo* and the effect of current application on the skin barrier. Adv Drug Deliv Rev 2013; 65(2): 315-29. [http://dx.doi.org/10.1016/j.addr.2012.04.012] [PMID: 22626977]

[17] Marro D, Kalia YN, Delgado-Charro MB, Guy RH. Contributions of electromigration and electroosmosis to iontophoretic drug delivery. Pharm Res 2001; 18(12): 1701-8. [http://dx.doi.org/10.1023/A:1013318412527] [PMID: 11785689]

[18] Miller LL, Smith GA, Chang AC, Zhou QX. Electrochemically controlled release. J Control Release 1987; 6(1): 293-6. [http://dx.doi.org/10.1016/0168-3659(87)90082-4]

[19] Miller LL, Smith GA. Iontophoretic transport of acetate and carboxylate ions through hairless mouse skin. A cation exchange membrane model. Int J Pharm 1989; 49(1): 15-22. [http://dx.doi.org/10.1016/0378-5173(89)90147-6]

[20] Green PG, Hinz RS, Cullander C, Yamane G, Guy RH. Iontophoretic delivery of amino acids and amino acid derivatives across the skin *in vitro*. Pharm Res 1991; 8(9): 1113-20. [http://dx.doi.org/10.1023/A:1015894016235] [PMID: 1788156]

[21] Green PG, Hinz RS, Kim A, *et al.* Transdermal iontophoresis of amino acids and peptides *in vitro*. J Control Release 1992; 21(1-3): 187-90. [http://dx.doi.org/10.1016/0168-3659(92)90020-R]

[22] van der Geest R, Hueber F, Szoka FC Jr, Guy RH. Iontophoresis of bases, nucleosides, and nucleotides. Pharm Res 1996; 13(4): 553-8.
[http://dx.doi.org/10.1023/A:1016041904037] [PMID: 8710745]

[23] Burnette RR, Ongpipattanakul B. Characterization of the pore transport properties and tissue alteration of excised human skin during iontophoresis. J Pharm Sci 1988; 77(2): 132-7.
[http://dx.doi.org/10.1002/jps.2600770208] [PMID: 3361428]

[24] Shinde AJ, Shinde AL, Garala KC. Physical penetration enhancement by iontophoresis: a review. Int J Curr Pharmaceut Res 2010; 2(1): 1-9.

[25] Siddiqui O, Roberts MS, Polack AE. The effect of iontophoresis and vehicle pH on the *in-vitro* permeation of lignocaine through human stratum corneum. J Pharm Pharmacol 1985; 37(10): 732-5.
[http://dx.doi.org/10.1111/j.2042-7158.1985.tb04954.x] [PMID: 2867145]

[26] Khan A, Yasir M, Asif M, *et al.* Iontophoretic drug delivery: History and applications. J App Pharm Sci 2011; 1(3): 11-24.

[27] Femenía-Font A, Balaguer-Fernández C, Merino V, López-Castellano A. Iontophoretic transdermal delivery of sumatriptan: effect of current density and ionic strength. J Pharm Sci 2005; 94(10): 2183-6.
[http://dx.doi.org/10.1002/jps.20447] [PMID: 16136550]

[28] Suzuki Y, Iga K, Yanai S, *et al.* Iontophoretic pulsatile transdermal delivery of human parathyroid hormone (1-34). J Pharm Pharmacol 2001; 53(9): 1227-34.
[http://dx.doi.org/10.1211/0022357011776676] [PMID: 11578105]

[29] Wascotte V, Caspers P, de Sterke J, Jadoul M, Guy RH, Préat V. Assessment of the "skin reservoir" of urea by confocal Raman microspectroscopy and reverse iontophoresis *in vivo.* Pharm Res 2007; 24(10): 1897-901.
[http://dx.doi.org/10.1007/s11095-007-9314-4] [PMID: 17497081]

[30] Bouissou CC, Sylvestre JP, Guy RH, Delgado-Charro MB. Reverse iontophoresis of amino acids: identification and separation of stratum corneum and subdermal sources *in vitro.* Pharm Res 2009; 26(12): 2630-8.
[http://dx.doi.org/10.1007/s11095-009-9978-z] [PMID: 19806434]

[31] Sieg A, Jeanneret F, Fathi M, *et al.* Extraction of amino acids by reverse iontophoresis *in vivo.* Eur J Pharm Biopharm 2009; 72(1): 226-31.
[http://dx.doi.org/10.1016/j.ejpb.2008.12.012] [PMID: 19347973]

[32] Leboulanger B, Aubry JM, Bondolfi G, Guy RH, Delgado-Charro MB. Lithium monitoring by reverse iontophoresis *in vivo.* Clin Chem 2004; 50(11): 2091-100.
[http://dx.doi.org/10.1373/clinchem.2004.034249] [PMID: 15192031]

[33] Nair AB, Kumria R, Al-Dhubiab BE, Attimarad M, Harsha S. Noninvasive sampling of gabapentin by reverse iontophoresis. Pharm Res 2015; 32(4): 1417-24.
[http://dx.doi.org/10.1007/s11095-014-1546-5] [PMID: 25319106]

[34] Delgado-Charro MB, Guy RH. Iontophoresis of peptides. In: Berner B, Dinh SM, Eds. Electronically Controlled Drug Delivery. Boca Raton: CRC Press 1998; pp. 129-57.

[35] Green PG. Iontophoretic delivery of peptide drugs. J Control Release 1996; 41(1-2): 33-48.
[http://dx.doi.org/10.1016/0168-3659(96)01354-5]

[36] Nirschl RP, Rodin DM, Ochiai DH, Maartmann-Moe C. Iontophoretic administration of dexamethasone sodium phosphate for acute epicondylitis. A randomized, double-blinded, placebo-controlled study. Am J Sports Med 2003; 31(2): 189-95.
[PMID: 12642251]

[37] Li LC, Scudds RA, Heck CS, Harth M. The efficacy of dexamethasone iontophoresis for the treatment of rheumatoid arthritic knees: a pilot study. Arthritis Care Res 1996; 9(2): 126-32.
[http://dx.doi.org/10.1002/1529-0131(199604)9:2<126::AID-ANR1790090209>3.0.CO;2-K] [PMID: 8970271]

[38] Reid KI, Dionne RA, Sicard-Rosenbaum L, Lord D, Dubner RA. Evaluation of iontophoretically applied dexamethasone for painful pathologic temporomandibular joints. Oral Surg Oral Med Oral Pathol 1994; 77(6): 605-9.
[http://dx.doi.org/10.1016/0030-4220(94)90319-0] [PMID: 8065724]

[39] Runeson L, Haker E. Iontophoresis with cortisone in the treatment of lateral epicondylalgia (tennis elbow)-a double-blind study. Scand J Med Sci Sports 2002; 12(3): 136-42.
[http://dx.doi.org/10.1034/j.1600-0838.2002.02142.x] [PMID: 12135445]

[40] Garrido Abad P, Coloma A, Herranz LM, *et al.* Transdermal iontophoresis with verapamil and dexamethasone in the acute phase of peyronie's disease. Our experience. Arch Esp Urol 2012; 65(8): 745-51.
[PMID: 23117682]

[41] Le QV, Howard A. Dexamethasone iontophoresis for the treatment of nail psoriasis. Australas J Dermatol 2013; 54(2): 115-9.
[http://dx.doi.org/10.1111/ajd.12029] [PMID: 23425157]

[42] Stefanou A, Marshall N, Holdan W, Siddiqui A. A randomized study comparing corticosteroid injection to corticosteroid iontophoresis for lateral epicondylitis. J Hand Surg Am 2012; 37(1): 104-9.
[http://dx.doi.org/10.1016/j.jhsa.2011.10.005] [PMID: 22196293]

[43] Kahn J. Iontophoresis and ultrasound for postsurgical temporomandibular trismus and paresthesia. Phys Ther 1980; 60(3): 307-8.
[PMID: 7355161]

[44] Rothfeld SH, Murray W. The treatment of Peyronie's disease by iontophoresis of C21 esterified glucocortocoids. J Urol 1967; 97(5): 874-5.
[PMID: 6025934]

[45] Tolsdorff P. Iontophoresis-local anesthesia at the ear canal and tympanic membrane. Laryngol Rhinol Otol 1980; 59(2): 88-97.
[http://dx.doi.org/10.1055/s-2007-1008824]

[46] Riviere JE, Monteiro-Riviere NA, Inman AO. Determination of lidocaine concentrations in skin after transdermal iontophoresis: effects of vasoactive drugs. Pharm Res 1992; 9(2): 211-4.
[http://dx.doi.org/10.1023/A:1018985323001] [PMID: 1553344]

[47] Wakita R, Oono Y, Oogami S, Hayashi S, Umino M. The relation between epinephrine concentration and the anesthetic effect of lidocaine iontophoresis. Pain Pract 2009; 9(2): 115-21.
[http://dx.doi.org/10.1111/j.1533-2500.2008.00252.x] [PMID: 19019048]

[48] Lidosite®. Full Prescribing Information. Vyteris Inc 2004.

[49] Holovics HJ, Anderson CR, Levine BS, Hui HW, Lunte CE. Investigation of drug delivery by iontophoresis in a surgical wound utilizing microdialysis. Pharm Res 2008; 25(8): 1762-70. [http://dx.doi.org/10.1007/s11095-007-9490-2] [PMID: 18080730]

[50] DeCou JM, Abrams RS, Hammond JH, Lowder LR, Gauderer MW. Iontophoresis: a needle-free, electrical system of local anesthesia delivery for pediatric surgical office procedures. J Pediatr Surg 1999; 34(6): 946-9. [http://dx.doi.org/10.1016/S0022-3468(99)90765-0] [PMID: 10392910]

[51] Greenbaum SS, Bernstein EF. Comparison of iontophoresis of lidocaine with a eutectic mixture of lidocaine and prilocaine (EMLA) for topically administered local anesthesia. J Dermatol Surg Oncol 1994; 20(9): 579-83. [http://dx.doi.org/10.1111/j.1524-4725.1994.tb00150.x] [PMID: 8089357]

[52] Zempsky WT, Anand KJ, Sullivan KM, Fraser D, Cucina K. Lidocaine iontophoresis for topical anesthesia before intravenous line placement in children. J Pediatr 1998; 132(6): 1061-3. [http://dx.doi.org/10.1016/S0022-3476(98)70413-5] [PMID: 9627608]

[53] Squire SJ, Kirchhoff KT, Hissong K. Comparing two methods of topical anesthesia used before intravenous cannulation in pediatric patients. J Pediatr Health Care 2000; 14(2): 68-72. [http://dx.doi.org/10.1016/S0891-5245(00)79847-6] [PMID: 10736141]

[54] Galinkin JL, Rose JB, Harris K, Watcha MF. Lidocaine iontophoresis *versus* eutectic mixture of local anesthetics (EMLA) for IV placement in children. Anesth Analg 2002; 94(6): 1484-8. [PMID: 12032012]

[55] Sloan JB, Soltani K. Iontophoresis in dermatology. A review. J Am Acad Dermatol 1986; 15(4 Pt 1): 671-84. [http://dx.doi.org/10.1016/S0190-9622(86)70223-5] [PMID: 3534013]

[56] Kassan DG, Lynch AM, Stiller MJ. Physical enhancement of dermatologic drug delivery: iontophoresis and phonophoresis. J Am Acad Dermatol 1996; 34(4): 657-66. [http://dx.doi.org/10.1016/S0190-9622(96)80069-7] [PMID: 8601657]

[57] Stolman LP. Treatment of hyperhidrosis. Dermatol Clin 1998; 16(4): 863-9. [http://dx.doi.org/10.1016/S0733-8635(05)70062-0] [PMID: 9891696]

[58] Murphy R, Harrington CI. Treating hyperhidrosis. Iontophoresis should be tried before other treatments. BMJ 2000; 321(7262): 702-3. [letter]. [PMID: 11202931]

[59] Sato K, Timm DE, Sato F, *et al.* Generation and transit pathway of H^+ is critical for inhibition of palmar sweating by iontophoresis in water. J Appl Physiol 1993; 75(5): 2258-64. [PMID: 8307885]

[60] Yaghobi Z, Goljarian S, Oskouei AE. Comparison of tap water and normal saline iontophoresis in idiopathic hyperhidrosis: a case report. J Phys Ther Sci 2014; 26(8): 1313-5. [http://dx.doi.org/10.1589/jpts.26.1313] [PMID: 25202204]

[61] Pariser DM, Ballard A. Iontophoresis for palmar and plantar hyperhidrosis. Dermatol Clin 2014; 32(4): 491-4.

[http://dx.doi.org/10.1016/j.det.2014.06.009] [PMID: 25152342]

[62] Davarian S, Kalantari KK, Rezasoltani A, Rahimi A. Effect and persistency of botulinum toxin iontophoresis in the treatment of palmar hyperhidrosis. Australas J Dermatol 2008; 49(2): 75-9. [http://dx.doi.org/10.1111/j.1440-0960.2008.00441.x] [PMID: 18412805]

[63] Lakraj AA, Moghimi N, Jabbari B. Hyperhidrosis: anatomy, pathophysiology and treatment with emphasis on the role of botulinum toxins. Toxins (Basel) 2013; 5(4): 821-40. [http://dx.doi.org/10.3390/toxins5040821] [PMID: 23612753]

[64] Carter EP, Barrett AD, Heeley AF, Kuzemko JA. Improved sweat test method for the diagnosis of cystic fibrosis. Arch Dis Child 1984; 59(10): 919-22. [http://dx.doi.org/10.1136/adc.59.10.919] [PMID: 6497428]

[65] Hall SK, Stableforth DE, Green A. Sweat sodium and chloride concentrations-essential criteria for the diagnosis of cystic fibrosis in adults. Ann Clin Biochem 1990; 27(Pt 4): 318-20. [http://dx.doi.org/10.1177/000456329002700406] [PMID: 2403231]

[66] Basu S, Mitra M, Ghosh A. Evaluation of sweat production by pilocarpine iontophoresis: a noninvasive screening tool for hypohidrosis in ectodermal dysplasia. Indian J Clin Biochem 2013; 28(4): 433-5. [http://dx.doi.org/10.1007/s12291-013-0334-z] [PMID: 24426251]

[67] Gangarosa LP. Iontophoresis in Dental Practice. Chicago: Quintessence Publishing Co. Ltd. 1983; pp. 17-20.

[68] Aparna S, Setty S, Thakur S. Comparative efficacy of two treatment modalities for dentinal hypersensitivity: a clinical trial. Indian J Dent Res 2010; 21(4): 544-8. [http://dx.doi.org/10.4103/0970-9290.74213] [PMID: 21187622]

[69] Gangarosa LP, Park NH. Practical considerations in iontophoresis of fluoride for desensitizing dentin. J Prosthet Dent 1978; 39(2): 173-8. [http://dx.doi.org/10.1016/S0022-3913(78)80017-1] [PMID: 271732]

[70] Krauser JT. Hypersensitive teeth. Part II: Treatment. J Prosthet Dent 1986; 56(3): 307-11. [http://dx.doi.org/10.1016/0022-3913(86)90009-0] [PMID: 3528461]

[71] Singal P, Gupta R, Pandit N. 2% sodium fluoride-iontophoresis compared to a commercially available desensitizing agent. J Periodontol 2005; 76(3): 351-7. [http://dx.doi.org/10.1902/jop.2005.76.3.351] [PMID: 15857067]

[72] Puapichartdumrong P, Ikeda H, Suda H. Facilitation of iontophoretic drug delivery through intact and caries-affected dentine. Int Endod J 2003; 36(10): 674-81. [http://dx.doi.org/10.1046/j.1365-2591.2003.00712.x] [PMID: 14511224]

[73] Morrel EM, Spruance SL, Goldberg DI. Topical iontophoretic administration of acyclovir for the episodic treatment of herpes labialis: a randomized, double-blind, placebo-controlled, clinic-initiated trial. Clin Infect Dis 2006; 43(4): 460-7. [http://dx.doi.org/10.1086/505872] [PMID: 16838235]

[74] Siddoju S, Sachdeva V, Friden PM, Yu YY, Banga AK. Acyclovir skin depot characterization following *in vivo* iontophoretic delivery. Skin Res Technol 2011; 17(2): 234-44. [http://dx.doi.org/10.1111/j.1600-0846.2010.00490.x] [PMID: 21272079]

[75] Shukla C, Friden P, Juluru R, Stagni G. *In vivo* quantification of acyclovir exposure in the dermis following iontophoresis of semisolid formulations. J Pharm Sci 2009; 98(3): 917-25. [http://dx.doi.org/10.1002/jps.21474] [PMID: 18623192]

[76] Hao J, Li SK. Mechanistic study of electroosmotic transport across hydrated nail plates: effects of pH and ionic strength. J Pharm Sci 2008; 97(12): 5186-97. [http://dx.doi.org/10.1002/jps.21368] [PMID: 18386836]

[77] Hao J, Li SK. Transungual iontophoretic transport of polar neutral and positively charged model permeants: effects of electrophoresis and electroosmosis. J Pharm Sci 2008; 97(2): 893-905. [http://dx.doi.org/10.1002/jps.21025] [PMID: 17683062]

[78] Gupta AK, Drummond-Main C, Cooper EA, Brintnell W, Piraccini BM, Tosti A. Systematic review of nondermatophyte mold onychomycosis: diagnosis, clinical types, epidemiology, and treatment. J Am Acad Dermatol 2012; 66(3): 494-502. [http://dx.doi.org/10.1016/j.jaad.2011.02.038] [PMID: 21820203]

[79] Vander Straten MR, Hossain MA, Ghannoum MA. Cutaneous infections dermatophytosis, onychomycosis, and tinea versicolor. Infect Dis Clin North Am 2003; 17(1): 87-112. [http://dx.doi.org/10.1016/S0891-5520(02)00065-X] [PMID: 12751262]

[80] Murdan S. Enhancing the nail permeability of topically applied drugs. Expert Opin Drug Deliv 2008; 5(11): 1267-82. [http://dx.doi.org/10.1517/17425240802497218] [PMID: 18976136]

[81] Barsness M, Davis SP, Etheredge R, *et al.* Studies in drug transport *vs* current in iontophoretic onychomycosis treatment. Conf Proc IEEE Eng Med Biol Soc 2009; 289-94.

[82] Nair AB, Kim HD, Chakraborty B, *et al.* Ungual and trans-ungual iontophoretic delivery of terbinafine for the treatment of onychomycosis. J Pharm Sci 2009; 98(11): 4130-40. [http://dx.doi.org/10.1002/jps.21711] [PMID: 19340887]

[83] Nair AB, Kim HD, Davis SP, *et al.* An *ex vivo* toe model used to assess applicators for the iontophoretic ungual delivery of terbinafine. Pharm Res 2009; 26(9): 2194-201. [http://dx.doi.org/10.1007/s11095-009-9934-y] [PMID: 19582550]

[84] Amichai B, Mosckovitz R, Trau H, *et al.* Iontophoretic terbinafine HCL 1.0% delivery across porcine and human nails. Mycopathologia 2010; 169(5): 343-9. [http://dx.doi.org/10.1007/s11046-009-9265-x] [PMID: 20012894]

[85] Nair AB, Vaka SR, Murthy SN. Transungual delivery of terbinafine by iontophoresis in onychomycotic nails. Drug Dev Ind Pharm 2011; 37(10): 1253-8. [http://dx.doi.org/10.3109/03639045.2011.568946] [PMID: 21457120]

[86] Nair AB, Sammeta SM, Kim HD, Chakraborty B, Friden PM, Murthy SN. Alteration of the diffusional barrier property of the nail leads to greater terbinafine drug loading and permeation. Int J Pharm 2009; 375(1-2): 22-7. [http://dx.doi.org/10.1016/j.ijpharm.2009.03.012] [PMID: 19481686]

[87] A study of skin/nail sensation and the pharmacokinetics of the uptake of terbinafine in the great toe nail and systemically following treatment with the electrokinetic transungual system (ETS)-terbinafine gel in healthy normal voluneteers. Available from: http://clinicaltrials.gov/ct2/show/NCT00768768

2009.

[88] An unblinded clinical trial to evaluate the deposition of terbinafine in the nail bed after iontophoretic application of ETS terbinafine gel in subjects with distal subungual onychomycosis in the great toenail. Available from: http://clinicaltrials.gov/show/NCT01484145 2012.

[89] Chang BK, Guthrie TH Jr, Hayakawa K, Gangarosa LP Sr. A pilot study of iontophoretic cisplatin chemotherapy of basal and squamous cell carcinomas of the skin. Arch Dermatol 1993; 129(4): 425-7. [http://dx.doi.org/10.1001/archderm.1993.01680250033004] [PMID: 8466212]

[90] Bacro TR, Holladay EB, Stith MJ, Maize JC, Smith CM. Iontophoresis treatment of basal cell carcinoma with cisplatin: a case report. Cancer Detect Prev 2000; 24(6): 610-9. [PMID: 11198275]

[91] Smith KJ, Konzelman JL, Lombardo FA, *et al.* Iontophoresis of vinblastine into normal skin and for treatment of Kaposi's sarcoma in human immunodeficiency virus-positive patients. Arch Dermatol 1992; 128(10): 1365-70. [http://dx.doi.org/10.1001/archderm.1992.01680200075010] [PMID: 1417025]

[92] Alvarez-Figueroa MJ, Delgado-Charro MB, Blanco-Méndez J. Passive and iontophoretic transdermal penetration of methotrexate. Int J Pharm 2001; 212(1): 101-7. [http://dx.doi.org/10.1016/S0378-5173(00)00599-8] [PMID: 11165825]

[93] Prasad R, Koul V, Anand S, Khar RK. Effect of DC/mDC iontophoresis and terpenes on transdermal permeation of methotrexate: *in vitro* study. Int J Pharm 2007; 333(1-2): 70-8. [http://dx.doi.org/10.1016/j.ijpharm.2006.09.058] [PMID: 17116378]

[94] Prasad R, Anand S, Khar RK, Dinda AK, Koul V. Studies on *in vitro* and *in vivo* transdermal flux enhancement of methotrexate by a combinational approach in comparison to oral delivery. Drug Dev Ind Pharm 2009; 35(11): 1281-92. [http://dx.doi.org/10.3109/03639040902882322] [PMID: 19832628]

[95] Gratieri T, Kalia YN. Targeted local simultaneous iontophoresis of chemotherapeutics for topical therapy of head and neck cancers. Int J Pharm 2014; 460(1-2): 24-7. [http://dx.doi.org/10.1016/j.ijpharm.2013.10.053] [PMID: 24219856]

[96] Kigasawa K, Kajimoto K, Hama S, Saito A, Kanamura K, Kogure K. Noninvasive delivery of siRNA into the epidermis by iontophoresis using an atopic dermatitis-like model rat. Int J Pharm 2010; 383(1-2): 157-60. [http://dx.doi.org/10.1016/j.ijpharm.2009.08.036] [PMID: 19732811]

[97] Dubey S, Kalia YN. Non-invasive iontophoretic delivery of enzymatically active ribonuclease A (13.6 kDa) across intact porcine and human skins. J Control Release 2010; 145(3): 203-9. [http://dx.doi.org/10.1016/j.jconrel.2010.04.020] [PMID: 20423719]

[98] Wirtz R. Die Ionentherapie in der Augenheilkunde. Lin Monatsbl Augenheilkd 1908; 46: 543-73.

[99] Morisot L. L'iontherapie ou ionisation appliquee au traitement des affections ocu-laires. Clin Ophthalmol 1927; 31: 5-16.

[100] Fielding IZ, Ormsby HL, Witzel SH. Ocular penetration of antibiotics by iontophoresis. Am J Ophthalmol 1956; 42(4 Part 2): 89-95. [PMID: 13372658]

[101] Kang-Mieler JJ, Osswald CR, Mieler WF. Advances in ocular drug delivery: emphasis on the posterior segment. Expert Opin Drug Deliv 2014; 11(10): 1647-60. [http://dx.doi.org/10.1517/17425247.2014.935338] [PMID: 24975820]

[102] Ionsys. Available from: http://www.rxlist.com/ionsys-drug.htm 2015.

[103] Femenía-Font A, Balaguer-Fernández C, Merino V, López-Castellano A. Iontophoretic transdermal delivery of sumatriptan: effect of current density and ionic strength. J Pharm Sci 2005; 94(10): 2183-6. [http://dx.doi.org/10.1002/jps.20447] [PMID: 16136550]

[104] Siegel SJ, O'Neill C, Dubé LM, *et al.* A unique iontophoretic patch for optimal transdermal delivery of sumatriptan. Pharm Res 2007; 24(10): 1919-26. [http://dx.doi.org/10.1007/s11095-007-9317-1] [PMID: 17577644]

[105] Pierce M, Marbury T, O'Neill C, Siegel S, Du W, Sebree T. Zelrix: a novel transdermal formulation of sumatriptan. Headache 2009; 49(6): 817-25. [http://dx.doi.org/10.1111/j.1526-4610.2009.01437.x] [PMID: 19438727]

[106] [NuPathe's Zecuity approved by the FDA for the acute treatment of migraine]. Available from: http://www.marketwired.com/press-release/nupathes-zecuity-approved-by-the-fda-for-the-acute-treatment-of-migraine-nasdaq-path-1747184.htm 2015.

[107] Calatayud-Pascual MA, Balaguer-Fernández C, Serna-Jiménez CE, *et al.* Effect of iontophoresis on *in vitro* transdermal absorption of almotriptan. Int J Pharm 2011; 416(1): 189-94. [http://dx.doi.org/10.1016/j.ijpharm.2011.06.039] [PMID: 21736929]

[108] Patel SR, Zhong H, Sharma A, Kalia YN. Controlled non-invasive transdermal iontophoretic delivery of zolmitriptan hydrochloride *in vitro* and *in vivo.* Eur J Pharm Biopharm 2009; 72(2): 304-9. [http://dx.doi.org/10.1016/j.ejpb.2008.08.006] [PMID: 18771728]

[109] Boddé HE, Danhof M, Van der Geest R, Danhof M. An integrated pharmacokinetic-pharmacodynamic approach to optimization of R-apomorphine delivery in Parkinson's disease. Adv Drug Deliv Rev 1998; 33(3): 253-63. [http://dx.doi.org/10.1016/S0169-409X(98)00033-7] [PMID: 10837665]

[110] Li GL, de Vries JJ, van Steeg TJ, *et al.* Transdermal iontophoretic delivery of apomorphine in patients improved by surfactant formulation pretreatment. J Control Release 2005; 101(1-3): 199-208. [http://dx.doi.org/10.1016/j.jconrel.2004.09.011] [PMID: 15588905]

[111] Luzardo-Alvarez A, Delgado-Charro MB, Blanco-Méndez J. *In vivo* iontophoretic administration of ropinirole hydrochloride. J Pharm Sci 2003; 92(12): 2441-8. [http://dx.doi.org/10.1002/jps.10502] [PMID: 14603489]

[112] Gratieri T, Kalaria D, Kalia YN. Non-invasive iontophoretic delivery of peptides and proteins across the skin. Expert Opin Drug Deliv 2011; 8(5): 645-63. [http://dx.doi.org/10.1517/17425247.2011.566265] [PMID: 21428867]

[113] Pillai O, Borkute SD, Sivaprasad N, Panchagnula R. Transdermal iontophoresis of insulin. II. Physicochemical considerations. Int J Pharm 2003; 254(2): 271-80. [http://dx.doi.org/10.1016/S0378-5173(03)00034-6] [PMID: 12623203]

[114] Kari B. Control of blood glucose levels in alloxan-diabetic rabbits by iontophoresis of insulin. Diabetes 1986; 35(2): 217-21.

[http://dx.doi.org/10.2337/diab.35.2.217] [PMID: 3510926]

[115] Liu J, Sun Y, Siddiqui O, Chien Y, Shi W, Li J. Blood glucose control in diabetic rats by transdermal iontophoretic delivery of insulin. Int J Pharm 1988; 44: 197-204. [http://dx.doi.org/10.1016/0378-5173(88)90116-0]

[116] Rastogi SK, Singh J. Effect of chemical penetration enhancer and iontophoresis on the *in vitro* percutaneous absorption enhancement of insulin through porcine epidermis. Pharm Dev Technol 2005; 10(1): 97-104. [http://dx.doi.org/10.1081/PDT-200049679] [PMID: 15776817]

[117] Chen H, Zhu H, Zheng J, *et al.* Iontophoresis-driven penetration of nanovesicles through microneedle-induced skin microchannels for enhancing transdermal delivery of insulin. J Control Release 2009; 139(1): 63-72. [http://dx.doi.org/10.1016/j.jconrel.2009.05.031] [PMID: 19481577]

[118] Escobar-Chávez JJ, Merino V, López-Cervantes M, Rodríguez-Cruz IM, Quintanar-Guerrero D, Ganem-Quintanar A. The use of iontophoresis in the administration of nicotine and new non-nicotine drugs through the skin for smoking cessation. Curr Drug Discov Technol 2009; 6(3): 171-85. [http://dx.doi.org/10.2174/157016309789054924] [PMID: 19496753]

[119] Djabri A, Guy RH, Delgado-Charro MB. Transdermal iontophoresis of ranitidine: an opportunity in paediatric drug therapy. Int J Pharm 2012; 435(1): 27-32. [http://dx.doi.org/10.1016/j.ijpharm.2012.03.006] [PMID: 22429890]

[120] Djabri A, Guy RH, Delgado-Charro MB. Passive and iontophoretic transdermal delivery of phenobarbital: Implications in paediatric therapy. Int J Pharm 2012; 435(1): 76-82. [http://dx.doi.org/10.1016/j.ijpharm.2012.02.026] [PMID: 22387370]

[121] del Rio-Sancho S, Serna-Jiménez CE, Calatayud-Pascual MA, *et al.* Transdermal absorption of memantin--effect of chemical enhancers, iontophoresis, and role of enhancer lipophilicity. Eur J Pharm Biopharm 2012; 82(1): 164-70. [http://dx.doi.org/10.1016/j.ejpb.2012.06.005] [PMID: 22732268]

[122] Patel H, Joshi A, Joshi A, Stagni G. Effect of microporation on passive and iontophoretic delivery of diclofenac sodium. Drug Dev Ind Pharm 2015; 41(12): 1962-7. [http://dx.doi.org/10.3109/03639045.2015.1019353] [PMID: 25758411]

[123] Gujjar M, Banga AK. Iontophoretic and microneedle mediated transdermal delivery of glycopyrrolate. Pharmaceutics 2014; 6(4): 663-71. [http://dx.doi.org/10.3390/pharmaceutics6040663] [PMID: 25533309]

[124] Tierney MJ, Tamada JA, Potts RO, Jovanovic L, Garg S. Clinical evaluation of the GlucoWatch biographer: a continual, non-invasive glucose monitor for patients with diabetes. Biosens Bioelectron 2001; 16(9-12): 621-9. [http://dx.doi.org/10.1016/S0956-5663(01)00189-0] [PMID: 11679237]

[125] Pitzer KR, Desai S, Dunn T, *et al.* Detection of hypoglycemia with the GlucoWatch biographer. Diabetes Care 2001; 24(5): 881-5. [http://dx.doi.org/10.2337/diacare.24.5.881] [PMID: 11347748]

[126] Merino V, López A, Hochstrasser D, Guy RH. Noninvasive sampling of phenylalanine by reverse

iontophoresis. J Control Release 1999; 61(1-2): 65-9.
[http://dx.doi.org/10.1016/S0168-3659(99)00102-9] [PMID: 10469903]

[127] Sylvestre JP, Bouissou CC, Guy RH, Delgado-Charro MB. Extraction and quantification of amino acids in human stratum corneum *in vivo.* Br J Dermatol 2010; 163(3): 458-65.
[http://dx.doi.org/10.1111/j.1365-2133.2010.09805.x] [PMID: 20394632]

[128] Wascotte V, Rozet E, Salvaterra A, *et al.* Non-invasive diagnosis and monitoring of chronic kidney disease by reverse iontophoresis of urea *in vivo.* Eur J Pharm Biopharm 2008; 69(3): 1077-82.
[http://dx.doi.org/10.1016/j.ejpb.2008.02.012] [PMID: 18406585]

[129] Nixon S, Sieg A, Delgado-Charro MB, Guy RH. Reverse iontophoresis of L-lactate: *in vitro* and *in vivo* studies. J Pharm Sci 2007; 96(12): 3457-65.
[http://dx.doi.org/10.1002/jps.20989] [PMID: 17506512]

[130] Leboulanger B, Fathi M, Guy RH, Delgado-Charro MB. Reverse iontophoresis as a noninvasive tool for lithium monitoring and pharmacokinetic profiling. Pharm Res 2004; 21(7): 1214-22.
[http://dx.doi.org/10.1023/B:PHAM.0000033008.64915.c8] [PMID: 15290862]

[131] Leboulanger B, Guy RH, Delgado-Charro MB. Non-invasive monitoring of phenytoin by reverse iontophoresis. Eur J Pharm Sci 2004; 22(5): 427-33.
[http://dx.doi.org/10.1016/j.ejps.2004.04.010] [PMID: 15265512]

[132] Delgado-Charro MB, Guy RH. Transdermal reverse iontophoresis of valproate: a noninvasive method for therapeutic drug monitoring. Pharm Res 2003; 20(9): 1508-13.
[http://dx.doi.org/10.1023/A:1025730815971] [PMID: 14567648]

[133] Nicoli S, Santi P. Transdermal delivery of aminoglycosides: amikacin transport and iontophoretic non-invasive monitoring. J Control Release 2006; 111(1-2): 89-94.
[http://dx.doi.org/10.1016/j.jconrel.2005.11.008] [PMID: 16413081]

[134] Federal Register. Available from: www.gpo.gov/fdsys/pkg/FR-2014-09-22/html/2014-22453.htm 2015; 79(183): 56532-8.

[135] Wiedersberg S, Guy RH. Transdermal drug delivery: 30+ years of war and still fighting. J Control Release 2014; 190: 150-6.
[http://dx.doi.org/10.1016/j.jconrel.2014.05.022] [PMID: 24852092]

CHAPTER 3

Delivery of DNA-Based Vaccines with *In Vivo* Electroporation

Trevor R.F. Smith*, **Katherine Schultheis** and **Kate E. Broderick**

Inovio Pharmaceuticals, Inc., 660W. Germantown Pike, Suite 110, Plymouth Meeting, PA 19462, USA

Abstract: Recent technological advances have re-established the value of DNA-based vaccines in tackling unmet medical needs. Such advances include the optimization of DNA plasmid constructs, the addition of novel molecular adjuvants into the formulations, and the development of *in vivo* delivery strategies such as electroporation (EP). The combination of DNA-based vaccines with the delivery platform of EP has enhanced the antigen expression by up to 1000-fold higher than DNA injection alone, resulting in greatly enhanced immunogenicity of DNA-based vaccines. Pre-clinical EP-enhanced DNA-based vaccination has elicited robust functional host immune responses to a myriad of disease targets resulting in protection from viral challenge or tumor growth, depending on the disease model. Significantly, the problems encountered in translating these responses to the clinic have been overcome, and equally impressive immune responses are being observed in human beings when DNA-based vaccination is married with EP, as was observed in a recent clinical trial. In this review we will cover the principles of EP in respect to enhancing DNA-based vaccination protocols targeting pDNA delivery to the muscle or skin, and discuss the top line results that have revealed for the first time clinical efficacy of DNA-based vaccine candidates.

Keywords: DNA-based vaccines, Electroporation.

1. INTRODUCTION

Thirty years ago Neumann *et al.* reported on the successful delivery of genes into

* **Corresponding author Trevor R.F. Smith:** Inovio Pharmaceuticals, Inc., 660W. Germantown Pike, Suite 110, Plymouth Meeting, PA 19462, USA; E-mail: TSmith@inovio.com

José Juan Escobar-Chávez (Ed.)

cells in culture through the use of an electrical pulsing method [1]. This technique of gene delivery became known as electrotransfer or electroporation, and was quickly adapted to *in vivo* protocols to aide in the delivery of macromolecules, such as chemotherapeutics and plasmid DNA (pDNA), across the mammalian membrane of cells residing in a tissue rather than a culture dish. EP has been used in the clinic to efficiently deliver large molecule chemotherapeutics such as bleomycin in electrochemotherapy (ECT) [2], or high voltage irreversible EP (IRE) has proved efficacious at causing cancer cell death [3]. ECT and IRE have been reviewed in depth elsewhere [2, 3]. More recently, EP has been utilized to transfer nucleic acid constructs in gene therapy trials [4]. In this review we will focus on the use of EP to enhance the delivery of pDNA to elicit robust immune responses in DNA-based vaccination protocols.

1.1. DNA-based Vaccination: The Concept

Conceptually and experimentally, DNA-based vaccination is a very attractive platform. The vaccine construct is not an inactivated or attenuated version of a pathogen, or a pathogen-associated protein. The construct is designed to be a blue print of the antigen(s) of choice, which following nuclear delivery can be read by the host's own machinery, initiating its manufacture, processing and presentation. The major advantage of DNA-based vaccines over inactivated virus or viral protein-based vaccines is their ability to drive the generation of both T cell and B cell responses. This in conjunction with ease and speed of design and manufacture [5], and the stability of pDNA at room temperature, are some of the favorable traits associated with this technology [6]. Additionally, modern day genomics allows for customization of the vaccine, so scientists can marry molecular biology techniques with their understanding of the immune system to develop vaccines that encode novel antigens and/or combinations of antigens. DNA-based vaccination has the potential to harness the power of the immune system to tackle multiple unmet medical needs, such as HIV, RSV, Influenza, and various cancers.

1.2. DNA-based Vaccination: The Early Years

The first DNA-based vaccination studies were reported in the early 1990's, when multiple groups demonstrated the induction of immune responses following naked injection of pDNA into mouse muscle [7 - 9]. It was demonstrated that *in vivo* transfection of mouse muscle cells with pDNA encoding target infectious agent-associated antigens could drive robust T cell and antibody responses against the pathogens, and importantly protect against future challenge. For example, Ulmer *et al.* reported that *in vivo* transfection with pDNA encoding influenza A nucleoprotein raised a protective immune response against subsequent challenge with a heterologous strain of influenza A virus in mice [9]. Such studies demonstrated that vaccination of small animals with naked pDNA could protect against infectious agents or halt tumorigenic growth [9, 10].

However, historical attempts in the 1990's to translate these pDNA vaccine successes into large animal models or humans ended in disappointment [11, 12]. The robust immune responses observed in mice could not be replicated in non-human primates (NHPs) or humans. One of the major reasons cited for this was the inefficiency of the delivery of the pDNA into the host's cells. This appeared to be less of an issue for small animal studies that often compensated for this by using very high (dose by body weight) doses and by forced cellular transfection through hydrodynamic pressure.

1.3. DNA-based Vaccination: The Delivery

Even though the excitement associated with DNA-based vaccination waned during the first few years of this century, investigators that remained in the field focused their attention on further defining pDNA's interaction with the innate immune system, how and what adjuvants could be used in combination, and maybe most importantly, understanding how the use of certain modalities could enhance the delivery and cellular uptake of large (several kbp's) pDNA molecules. Platforms developed to enhance *in vivo* pDNA delivery included ballistic devices, polymers, bacteria, sonoporation and electroporation [6, 13 - 19].

As mentioned above, EP has been successfully employed to assist in the delivery of nucleic acids into cells, both *in vitro* and *in vivo*. EP achieves this by inducing transient perturbation in the cell membrane and an electrical gradient that permits entry of large molecules, such as pDNA vaccines, into the cell. Studies have described an increase in tissue gene expression by 100-1000 fold when reporter pDNA delivery was combined with EP, in contrast to naked pDNA injection alone [6]. *In vivo* animal studies analyzing T and B cell responses induced in immunization protocols performed in parallel with or without EP consistently revealed 10-100 fold higher responses when EP was employed [6]. Importantly, these EP + DNA-based vaccine responses have reached protective levels in challenge models in large animals [20 - 23]. For example, after EP-enhanced delivery of DNA vaccines into rhesus macaques, Laddy and colleagues demonstrated cross-reactive cellular and humoral responses that were protective against influenza virus infection [24]. Livingston *et al.* showed that addition of electroporation to an anthrax DNA vaccine protocol was associated with a 100-fold increased immunogenicity in NHPs as compared to conventional intramuscular injection, and long-lived protection against lethal Bacilius anthracis challenge [23]. Such impressive enhancement of host immunity upon the addition of EP to immunization regimens has led to multiple clinical trials being initiated using EP with DNA-based vaccination in both prophylactic and therapeutic settings [25 - 30].

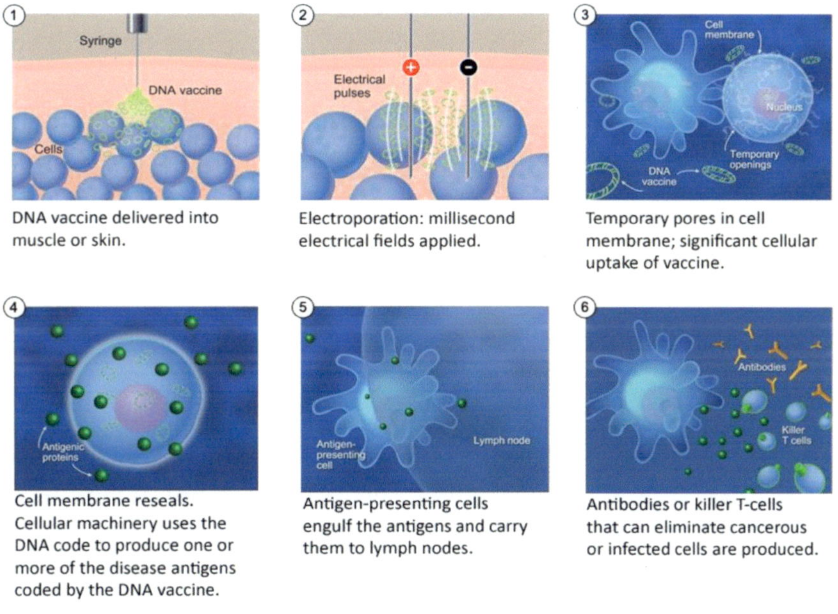

Fig. (1). Schematic depicting the *in vivo* electroporation process and delivery of DNA-based vaccines.

In this chapter we will review the studies that have been performed to understand the mechanisms involved in EP-enhanced delivery of pDNA, and how the technique is now being optimized (including development of EP devices and choice of sites of delivery) with the aim to improve the overall vaccination procedure in terms of tolerability and immunity generated. Even though there are many seminal *in vitro* studies concerning the intracellular delivery of large molecules by EP, we will focus on the use of EP to deliver pDNA-based vaccines *in vivo* (Fig. **1**).

2. MECHANISM OF pDNA TRANSFER BY ELECTROPORATION

The theory behind the marriage of electroporation to DNA-based vaccination is based on pDNA being a highly charged molecule, so its movement (*i.e.* across cell membranes) can be manipulated by electrophoretic forces [31]. However, before we consider the passage of pDNA across the cell membrane, it is important to consider the effect exposure to an electric field has on the cell. The aim of reversible electroporation is to manipulate the cell membrane using electric pulses to cause pores of suitable circumference and duration to form, subsequently allowing for the passage of pDNA into the cell. This can be achieved by the electric field generated by EP that will cause opposite charges at either side of the plasma membrane to accumulate, creating a transmembrane potential difference. Once the transmembrane potential difference reaches a certain threshold structural changes will occur at the cell surface. It is commonly theorized that this causes large hydrophobic pores to form, which then become hydrophilic as the phospholipid heads rotate between bilayers, resulting in the formation of large hydrophilic conductive conduits [32].

For DNA vaccination and other gene therapies it is essential that this process be reversible, as the cell must remain intact and capable of manufacturing protein. If the electrical field strength is too high the result is cell death – known as irreversible EP (used in the clinic to directly destroy tumors) [33]. If the electric field strength is too low the electrical stimulation will not cause sufficient pore formation. Due to the transient nature of the pore formation, pDNA is delivered to the tissue immediately before the EP procedure is activated. Studies have shown that delivery of pDNA to the tissue after EP results in no significant increase in transfection over pDNA delivery in the absence of EP [34, 35]. The duration of the pore opening may only be milliseconds, and is dependent on the electrical parameters used [36]. There is a current body of evidence that suggests short high intensity electrical pulses (*e.g.* 800 V/cm, 100 μs) increase the duration of the pore [34, 37]. On the other hand, long low voltage pulses (*e.g.* 80 V/cm, 100 ms), which may not be capable of inducing membrane pore formation, are favorable for the electrophoretic movement of pDNA across the opening in the cell membrane. EP pulse patterns that incorporate a short high-intensity series of pulses, followed by long low voltage pulses have been employed in protocols [38, 39]. However, such electrical parameters have yet to be universally applied to *in vivo* EP-enhanced DNA-based vaccination protocols and square wave parameters using constant current have been shown to be very effective in enhancing transfection and augmenting immunogenicity [6]. It is of absolute importance that appropriate electrical parameters are defined for each situation. For example, for optimal delivery of pDNA into muscle tissue the electrical parameters used will be different to those associated with delivery to another site (*e.g.* the skin) due to differences in tissue conductivity and cell size. Factors that affect the efficiency of pore formation in the cell membrane include electrical associated parameters such as voltages, frequencies, duration and numbers of pulses, and physical parameters of the device such as electrode size (length and perimeter) and spacing.

3. ELECTROPORATION DEVICES FOR THE *IN VIVO* DELIVERY OF DNA-BASED VACCINES

Devices for the *in vivo* delivery of nucleic acids have been designed with the aim of generating an appropriate electrical field to permit the efficient transfection of cells residing within the tissue of choice. Fortunately the tissues targeted for EP-enhanced DNA-based vaccination, the skin and muscle, are more accessible than those associated with other forms of gene therapy which may require gene delivery into deeper targets such as the heart or liver.

Historically skeletal muscle has been the tissue of choice for DNA vaccine delivery. Their size and long half-life endows myocytes with the ability to stably express the delivered gene for long durations of time and to translate high levels of protein. pDNA may be expressed for months in murine myocytes after initial electroporation [40]. In addition, the highly vascularized muscle environment allows for excellent systemic delivery of protein antigens. Clinically, the deltoid muscle is most often targeted for EP-enhanced DNA-based vaccine delivery. Many EP devices have been designed and developed with the aim of generating an appropriate electrical field for gene delivery in the human muscle. Such devices include Inovio's CELLECTRA®-5P device (Inovio.com), IGEA's CLINIPORATOR (Igeamedical.com) and the Ichor TriGrid™ (Ichorms.com). These devices are based on electrode array patterns that are fired in a predetermined order to create an optimal electric field in the muscle tissue surrounding the area where the pDNA has been injected. The EP-enhanced pDNA delivery process is outlined in Fig. (**1**). Intramuscular EP devices are currently being used in multiple clinical trials, delivering pDNA vaccines to treat pre-cancerous cervical lesions (NCT01304524), leukemia (NCT01334060), melanoma (NCT01138410), and infectious diseases: HIV (NCT01266616) and HCV (NCT01335711). Other clinical trials are outlined in Tables **1** and **2**.

In addition to the muscle, other EP delivery tissue targets are currently being investigated including skin [41], tumor [42], heart [43], cornea [44] and brain [45]. The skin is a very attractive immunization target, and is both easy to access and monitor. Most importantly it is a highly immunocompetent tissue that contains populations of dendritic cells that are vital in priming host immune responses [46]. Due to the ease of accessibility, non-invasive or minimally invasive EP devices have been designed to transfect the upper layers of the skin [41, 47 - 50]. Indeed fully contactless skin electrotransfer devices have also been investigated *e.g.* piezoelectric (static spark) [51] or helium-based plasma (corona charge) devices [52]. Early non-invasive or surface devices developed to achieve transfection of skin cells were metal plates or webs that lay on the skin. More recent and reliable device designs have been based on multiple electrode arrays [47, 49, 53]. In general, these platforms are placed in direct contact with the skin without rupturing the skin and operate at relatively high electric field strength to permit transfection of the upper layers of the skin. Invasive dermal EP devices have also been designed to consist of an array of needles that penetrate the skin. Such devices include the Easy Vax dermal electroporation system [54] and the

CELLECTRA®-3P [55]. Both devices have entered the clinical setting to assist in the delivery of prostate tumor antigen [41] and an influenza antigen DNA-based vaccine (ClinTrials.gov identifiers NCT01403155 and NCT01405885), respectively. The vaccination treatment procedure involved in delivering pDNA to the skin generally includes injection of a dose of pDNA by the Mantoux technique - similar to administration of the BCG vaccine. This technique results in the creation of a bleb in the skin. Surface EP (SEP) devices can be placed on top of this bleb and activated to generate an electric field that will span only as deep as the epidermis [47, 56]. On the other hand, the electrodes of penetrating devices are placed around the bleb and pushed into the skin, and upon activation generate an electric field that covers multiple layers of the skin including subdermal regions. Thus, skin devices have differing transfection patterns, with the non-invasive SEP devices targeting the epidermis and the penetrating device targeting deeper layers [47, 57, 58]. The advantage of a skin-penetrating device is that multiple layers of skin, and also underlying adipocytes and myocytes are transfected, resulting in a longer duration of gene expression than when SEP is used. However the non-invasive SEP device has obvious advantages in tolerability and safety due to use of lower voltages and electrodes not penetrating the skin. As this device allows for EP-enhanced transfection of only the epidermis, gene expression is short-lived (up to seven days in guinea pig skin) as the cells traverse up the epidermal layer and are sloughed off [56]. The transient gene expression enhances the safety profile of treatment protocols utilizing this delivery technique. As mentioned above, the Easy Vax and CELLECTRA®-3P I.D. devices have now entered clinical trials to enhance the delivery of a prostate antigen DNA vaccine [41] and an influenza DNA vaccine (NCT01405885), respectively. Pre-clinical studies are ongoing to determine optimal electrical parameters and appropriate antigen targets that will associate with the SEP device.

Table 1. Current clinical trials using EP-enhanced delivery of DNA-based vaccines to target tumor antigens.

Study Title	Phase	Target	Delivery route	Device	Estimated enrollment/status	ClinicalTrials. gov identifier	Sponsor
Dose-finding, Safety Study of Plasmid DNA Therapeutic Vaccine to Treat Cervical Intraepithelial Neoplasia	II	Cervical Intraepithelial Neoplasia	IM	TriGrid™ Delivery System (TDS)	72 (recruiting)	NCT02139267	Genexine, Inc.

(Table 1) contd.....

Study Title	Phase	Target	Delivery route	Device	Estimated enrollment/status	ClinicalTrials. gov identifier	Sponsor
Interleukin-12 Gene and *in vivo* Electroporation-Mediated Plasmid DNA Vaccine Therapy in Treating Patients With Merkel Cell Cancer	II	Neuroendocrine carcinoma of the skin/ Merkel cell cancer	Intra-tumor	Oncosec Medical System™ (OMS)	15 (ongoing, not recruiting)	NCT01440816	Oncosec Medical Incorporated, National Cancer Institute (NCI)
Safety Study of DNA Vaccine Delivered by Intradermal Electroporation to Treat Colorectal Cancer	I/II	Colorectal Cancer	ID	Derma Vax™	20 (ongoing, not recruiting)	NCT01064375	Karolinska Institutet, Swedish Institute for Infectious Disease Control, Cyto Pulse Sciences Inc.,
Safety of GX-188E DNA Therapeutic Vaccine Administered by Electroporation to Cervical Intraepithelial Neoplasia Grade 3	I	Cervical Intraepithelial Neoplasia 3	IM	TriGrid™ Delivery System (TDS)	9 (completed)	NCT01634503	Genexine Inc.
Safety and Efficacy of GX-188E DNA Therapeutic Vaccine Administered by Electroporation After Observation	I	Cervical Intraepithelial Neoplasia 3	IM	TriGrid™ Delivery System (TDS)	9 (ongoing, not recruiting)	NCT02100085	Genexine Inc.
Safety and Immune Response to a Mammaglobin-A DNA Vaccine In Breast Cancer Patients Undergoing Neoadjuvant Endocrine Therapy	I	Breast Cancer, Breast Carcinoma, Malignant Neoplasm of Breast	IM	?	12 (recruiting)	NCT02204098	Washington University School of Medicine
A Phase I/II Trial of SCIB1, a DNA Immunotherapy, in the Treatment of Patients With Malignant Melanoma	I/II	Malignant Melanoma	IM	TriGrid™ Delivery System (TDS)	54 (recruiting)	NCT01138410	Scanell Ltd
Dose Finding Study of a DNA Vaccine Delivered With Intradermal Electroporation in Patients With Prostate Cancer	I/II	Prostate Cancer	ID	Derma Vax™	15 (completed)	NCT00859729	Uppsala University
Pilot 2-Part Prospective Study of HPV Specific Immunotherapy in Patients With HPV Associated Head and Neck Squamous Cell Carcinoma (HNSCCa)	I/II	Head and Neck Squamos Cell Cancer	IM	CELLECTRA® -5P	20 (recruiting)	NCT02163057	Inovio Pharmaceuticals

(Table 1) contd.....

Study Title	Phase	Target	Delivery route	Device	Estimated enrollment/status	ClinicalTrials. gov identifier	Sponsor
Phase II Placebo Controlled Study of VGX-3100, (HPV16 E6/E7, HPV18 E6/E7 DNA Vaccine) Delivered IM Followed by Electroporation With Cellectra-5P for the Treatment of Biopsy-proven CIN 2/3 or CIN 3 With Documented HPV 16 or 18	II	Cervical Intraepithelial Neoplasia	IM	CELLECTRA® -5P	148 (ongoing, not recruiting)	NCT01304524	Inovio Pharmaceuticals
Safety and Immunogenicity of a Melanoma **DNA** Vaccine Delivered by **Electroporation**	I	Melanoma (Skin), Intraocular Melanoma	IM	TriGrid™ Delivery System (TDS)	24 (completed)	NCT00471133	Ichor Medical Systems Incorporated
Pilot Study of HPV Specific Immunotherapy in Subjects With HPV6 Associated Aerodigestive Malignancies	I	Aerodigestive Malignancies (*e.g.* Squamous Cell Carcinoma)	IM	CELLECTRA® -5P	6 (recruiting)	NCT02241369	Inovio Pharmaceuticals
Phase I of Human Papillomavirus (HPV) **DNA** Plasmid (VGX-3100) + **Electroporation** for CIN 2 or 3	I	Cervical Intraepithelial Neoplasia 2/3	IM	CELLECTRA® -5P	(completed)	NCT00685412	Inovio Pharmaceuticals
Phase II Intratumoral IL12 Plasmid **Electroporation** in Cutaneous Lymphoma (CTCL)	II	Cutaneous Lymphoma	IT	Oncosec Medical System™ (OMS)	34 (ongoing, not recruiting)	NCT01579318	OncoSec Medical Incorporated
Safety and Efficacy of GX-188E **DNA** Therapeutic Vaccine Administered by **Electroporation** After Observation	Follow up	Cervical Intraepithelial Neoplasia 3	IM	TriGrid™ Delivery System (TDS)	72 (recruiting)	NCT02411019	Genexine, Inc
Inovio TRT-001: Telomerase **DNA** Immunotherapy in Breast, Lung, and Pancreatic Cancers	I	Breast Cancer Lung Cancer Pancreatic Cancer	IM	CELLECTRA® -5P	54 (recruiting)	NCT02327468	Abramson Cancer Center of the University of Pennsylvania
A Study of INO-3112 **DNA** Vaccine With **Electroporation** in Patients With Cervical Cancer	I/II	Cervical Cancer	IM	CELLECTRA® -5P	30 (recruiting)	NCT02172911	Inovio Pharmaceuticals
INVAC-1 Anti-Cancer hTERT **DNA** Immunotherapy	I	Solid Tumors	ID		27 (recruiting)	NCT02301754	Invectys

(Table 1) contd.....

Study Title	Phase	Target	Delivery route	Device	Estimated enrollment/status	ClinicalTrials. gov identifier	Sponsor
A Study to Test the Tolerability of an Investigational **Electroporation** Device in Healthy Adults (V930-001)	I		IM	MedPulser DDS	(completed)	NCT00721461	Merck Sharp & Dohme Corp.
Trial of pIL-12 **Electroporation** Malignant Melanoma (IL-12MEL)	II	Melanoma	IT	Oncosec Medical System™ (OMS)	51 (recruiting)	NCT01502293	OncoSec Medical Incorporated
Trial of pIL-12 **Electroporation** in Squamous Cell Carcinoma of the Head and Neck (IL12HNSCC)	II	Head and Neck Squamous Cell Carcinoma	IT	Oncosec Medical System™ (OMS)	31 (recruiting)	NCT02345330	OncoSec Medical Incorporated
Safety and Immunogenicity of a Personalized Polyepitope **DNA** Vaccine Strategy in Breast Cancer Patients With Persistent Triple-Negative Disease Following Neoadjuvant Chemotherapy	I	Triple Negative Breast Cancer Triple-Negative Breast Cancer Triple Negative Breast Neoplasms	IM	TriGrid™ Delivery System (TDS)	15 (recruiting)	NCT02348320	Washington University School of Medicine
A Phase II Clinical Trial of Chemo-radiotherapy in Combination With INO-3112 in Patients With Locally Advanced Cervical Cancer	II	Uterine Cervical Neoplasms	IM	CELLECTRA® -5P	126 (not yet open for recruitment)	NCT02501278	European Organisation for Research and Treatment of Cancer - EORTC
Trial to Evaluate Safety and Immunogenicity of INO-5150 Alone or With INO-9012 in Men With Prostate Cancer	I	Prostate Cancer	IM	CELLECTRA® -5P	60 (recruiting)	NCT02514213	Inovio Pharmaceuticals

Table 2. Current clinical trials using EP-enhanced delivery of DNA-based vaccines to target infectious disease.

Study Title	Phase	Target	Delivery route	Device	Estimated enrollment/status	ClinicalTrials. gov identifier	Sponsor
Therapeutic Vaccine for HIV	I	Acute or early HIV-1 infection	IM	TriGrid™ Delivery System (TDS)	50 (recruiting)	NCT01859325	National Institute of Allergy and Infectious Diseases (NIAID), Profectus Biosciences Inc., Institutes of Health Clinical Center

(Table 2) contd.....

Study of PENNVAX™-B (Gag, Pol, Env) + Electroporation in HIV-1 Infected Adult Participants	I	HIV-1 infection	IM	CELLECTRA® -5P	12 (completed)	NCT01082692	Inovio Pharmaceuticals
Evaluating the Safety of and Immune Response to HIV-MAG DNA Vaccine With or Without Plasmid IL-12 Adjuvant Delivered Intramuscularly *Via* Electroporation Followed by VSV-gag HIV Vaccine Boost in Healthy, HIV-Uninfected Adults	I	HIV	IM	TriGrid™ Delivery System (TDS)	100 (active, not recruiting)	NCT01578889	National Institute of Allergy and Infectious Diseases (NIAID)
Tolerability, Immunogenicity and Efficacy of HB-110 Administered by Electroporation in Chronic Hepatitis B Patients	I	Chronic Hepatitis B infection	IM	TriGrid™ Delivery System (TDS)	9 (completed)	NCT01641536	Genexine, Inc.
Safety and Immunogenicity Study of HIV-MAG Vaccine +/- IL-12 and Ad35-GRIN/ENV in HIV-uninfected Volunteers	I	HIV	IM	TriGrid™ Delivery System (TDS)	75 (completed)	NCT01496989	International AIDS Vaccine Initiative, Profectus Biosciences, Inc., Ichor Medical Systems Incorporated
Multi-center, Open-label, Dose Escalation, Phase I Trial to Evaluate the Safety, Tolerability and Immunogenicity of VGX-6150 for Second-line Therapy of Chronic Hepatitis C Infection	I	Chronic Hepatitis C infection	IM	CELLECTRA® -5P	18 (ongoing, not recruiting)	NCT02027116	GeneOne Life Science, Inc., Inovio Pharmaceuticals (collaborator)

(Table 2) contd.....

A Phase I Study of the Safety and Immunogenicity of PENNVAX-G DNA (ENV & GAG) Administered by Intramuscular Biojector 2000 or CELLECTRA Intramuscular Electroporation Device Followed by MVA-CMDR (HIV-1 CM235 ENV/CM240 GAG/POL) Boost in Healthy, HIV Uninfected Adults	I	HIV infections	IM	CELLECTRA®-5P	92 (completed)	NCT01260727	National Institute of Allergy and Infectious Diseases (NIAID)
Phase I, Open Label Study to Evaluate Safety, Tolerability and Immunogenicity of Multiple Combinations of H1 and H5 Influenza Hemagglutinin Plasmids Administered ID Followed by *in vivo* Electroporation With CELLECTRA®-3P in Healthy Adults	I	Influenza	ID	CELLECTRA®-3P	116 (completed)	NCT01405885	Inovio Pharmaceuticals
A Phase II Trial to Assess the Safety and Immunogenicity of **DNA** Priming Administered by the ID Zetajet® With or Without ID Derma Vax™ **Electroporation** Followed by IM MVA Boosting in Healthy Volunteers in Tanzania and Mozambique (TaMoVac II)	II	HIV	ID	Derma Vax™	198 (completed)	NCT01697007	Muhimbili University of Health and Allied Sciences
Study of a **DNA**-based Venezuelan Equine Encephalitis Virus **DNA** Vaccine Administered by **Electroporation** in Healthy Volunteers	I	Venezuelan Equine Encephalitis Virus Infection	ID/IM	TriGrid™ Delivery System (TDS)	42 (completed)	NCT01984983	Ichor Medical Systems Incorporated

(Table 2) contd.....

Study of VGX-3400X, H5N1 Avian Influenza Virus **DNA** Plasmid + **Electroporation** in Healthy Adults	I	Influenza	IM	CELLECTRA® -5P	32 (completed)	NCT01142362	Inovio Pharmaceuticals
Study Of VGX-3400, H5N1 Avian Flu Virus Plasmid **DNA** With **Electroporation** Device In Healthy Adult Males	I	Influenza	IM	CELLECTRA® -5P	30 (completed)	NCT01184976	GeneOne Life Science, Inc.
Evaluating the Safety and Immunogenicity of PENNVAX®-GP **DNA** Vaccine and IL-12 Plasmid, Delivered *Via* Intradermal or Intramuscular **Electroporation** in Healthy, HIV-Uninfected Adults	I	HIV	ID/IM	CELLECTRA® -5P/-3P	94 (recruiting)	NCT02431767	National Institute of Allergy and Infectious Diseases
Fourth Dose of Human Papillomavirus (HPV) **DNA** Plasmid (VGX-3100) + EP in Adult Females Previously Vaccinated With Three Doses of VGX-3100	I	HPV	IM	CELLECTRA® -5P/-3P	14 (completed)	NCT01188850	Inovio Pharmaceuticals
EP1300 Polyepitope **DNA** Vaccine Against Plasmodium Falciparum Malaria	I	Malaria	IM		39 (completed)	NCT01169077	National Institute of Allergy and Infectious Diseases
Study of a Potential Preventive Vaccine Against HIV in Healthy Volunteers (ADVAX-EP)	I	HIV	IM	TriGrid™ Delivery System (TDS)	40 (completed)	NCT00545987	Rockefeller University
DNA-based Influenza Vaccine in the Elderly	I	Influenza	ID	CELLECTRA® -3P	50 (completed)	NCT01587131	University of Manitoba
Efficacy and Safety of Dual-plasmid Hepatitis B Virus **DNA** Vaccine in Chronic Hepatitis B Patients	II	Chronic Hepatitis B	IM		240 (unknown)	NCT01487876	Fuqiang Yang

(Table 2) contd.....

Study to Evaluate the Safety, Tolerability, and Immunogenicity of Hantaan and Puumala Virus **DNA** Vaccines (HTNV/PUUV)	I	Hemorrhagic Fever With Renal Syndrome	IM	TriGrid™ Delivery System (TDS)	31 (completed)	NCT01502345	U.S. Army Medical Research and Materiel Command
Safety of and Immune Response to the PENNVAX-B **DNA** Vaccine With and Without IL-12 in HIV-uninfected Adults	I	HIV			48 (completed)	NCT00991354	National Institute of Allergy and Infectious Diseases
Safety and Immunogenicity Study of AIDS Vaccine (Combined Use of **DNA** Vaccine and Recombinant Vaccinia Virus Tiantan)	II	AIDS			150 (completed)	NCT01705223	National Center for AIDS/STD Control and Prevention, China CDC
The Safety and Immunogenicity of the **DNA**-GTU Vaccine Administered to HIV-infected Patients on ART *vs* Placebo (CUTHIVTHER001)	I/II	HIV	IM	TriGrid™ Delivery System (TDS)	30 (recruiting)	NCT02457689	Imperial College London
Immunogenicity of Three HIV GTU® MultiHIV **DNA** Immunisations Administered *Via* Intramuscular, Intradermal and Transcutaneous Routes (CUT*HIVAC001)	I	HIV	IM	TriGrid™ Delivery System (TDS)	30 (recruiting)	NCT02075983	Imperial College London
A Follow-On Study With an H5 Influenza Vaccine for Subjects Who Participated in Study FLU-001	I	Influenza	ID	CELLECTRA® -3P	22 (completed)	NCT01403155	Inovio Pharmaceuticals

(Table 2) contd.....

Phase 2a Immunogenicity Study of Hantaan/Puumala Virus **DNA** Vaccine for Prevention of Hemorrhagic Fever	II	Hemorrhagic Fever With Renal Syndrome	IM	TriGrid™ Delivery System (TDS)	(recruiting)	NCT02116205	U.S. Army Medical Research and Materiel Command
Phase I/IIa Dose Ranging CHRONVAC-C® Study in Chronic HCV Patients	I/II	Chronic Hepatitis C Virus Infection	IM	CELLECTRA® -5P	12 (unknown)	NCT00563173	Tripep AB
Phase I Study of INO-1800 With or Without INO-9112 + EP in Chronic Hepatitis B Subjects	I	Hepatitis B	IM	CELLECTRA® -5P	126(recruiting)	NCT02431312	Inovio Pharmaceuticals
CHRONVAC-C Study Followed by Standard of Care in Chronic Hepatitis C Virus (HCV) Subjects	II	Chronic Hepatitis C	IM	CELLECTRA® -5P	32(unknown)	NCT01335711	ChronTech Pharma AB
Safety & Immunogenicity of HIV Vaccines in Healthy Kenyan Adults (HIV-CORE 004)	I/II	AIDS	IM	TriGrid™ Delivery System (TDS)	72 (ongoing, not recruiting)	NCT02099994	University of Oxford
Safety of and Immune Response to an Investigational HIV-1 Vaccine With or Without Interleukin-12 (IL-12) in HIV-1 Infected Adults	I	HIV Infections	IM		62 (completed)	NCT01266616	National Institute of Allergy and Infectious Diseases (NIAID)
Open-Label Study of INO-4212 With or Without INO-9012, Administered IM or ID Followed by Electroporation in Healthy Volunteers	I	Ebola	IM/ID	CELLECTRA® -5P/3P	75 (recruiting)	NCT02464670	Inovio Pharmaceuticals

4. THE SAFETY AND TOLERABILITY OF DNA-BASED VACCINATION COMBINED WITH ELECTROPORATION

Hundreds (379) of clinical trials were performed resulting in thousands of patients receiving DNA-based vaccinations, and the safety profile of this treatment has been exemplary. Toxicology studies performed both in animals and human clinical studies have not associated serious adverse events to DNA-based vaccination, performed either with or without EP. The biological distribution is limited to the treated tissue, plasmids are efficiently cleared from the body, and the fears of any integration into the host have proved unfounded.

The tolerability of the procedure (pDNA injection, followed by EP) has also been investigated. We recently compared the pain scores reported for both IM and ID procedures [55]. Using visual analog scale (VAS) where 0 = no pain, and 10 = the worst pain, patients were asked to record the pain they experienced after IM or ID pDNA injection followed by EP. After 1 ml saline injection into deltoid muscle followed by CELLECTRA®-5P EP, patients reported an immediate pain response that averaged a maximum of 6 on the pain score that fell to 1 by fifteen minutes post treatment. Following 0.15 ml saline injection into the forearm skin followed by CELLECTRA®-3P EP, patients reported an immediate pain response averaging 2.5 that fell to 0 at fifteen minutes post treatment. The results indicate the pain experienced after the use of either device was acute and rapidly dissipated. Furthermore, patient compliance to the vaccination regimens of a total of three vaccinations has been excellent. Thus, even though there is a transient pain associated with the procedure, it does not deter the patient from further treatments. The pain score results we recorded were in line with those reported by El-Kamary and colleagues, which demonstrated the Easy Vax dermal electroporation system to be both safe and well tolerated [41]. While significantly lower pain scores were reported for the ID procedure with the CELLECTRA®-3P compared to IM with the CELLECTRA®-5P [55], we have yet to determine the VAS pain scores for the non-invasive SEP device. The non-invasive nature and low electrical charge associated with the device strongly suggests it will be more tolerable.

5. ELECTROPORATION AUGMENTS THE IMMUNE RESPONSE

In simple terms, EP enhances immune responses associated with DNA vaccination by aiding the entry of plasmids into the cells. However, this is unlikely to be the limit to the assistance EP plays in driving host immune responses, as production and/or presentation of antigen alone by host cells do not always lead to productive host immune responses. Studies have described antigen presentation in the steady state will often lead to immune tolerance [59]. We believe two separate but complimentary aspects of EP-enhanced DNA-based vaccination protocols operate to drive productive over tolerogenic host immune responses. Firstly by increasing the efficiency of the entry of pDNA into the cell, the intracellular pDNA interactions with DNA sensors are increased. The entry of foreign DNA into the cell may lead to the activation of molecules such as STING (stimulator of interferon genes) and initiate an inflammatory response [60]. Secondly, the EP procedure will set up an appropriate milieu for the generation of productive host immune responses. EP causes low level damage to the tissue, and while on one hand this adds to the pain of the procedure, on the other it again creates an appropriate environment for driving immunity [61]. It has been shown that EP alone causes in influx of innate and adaptive immune cells such as macrophages and CD8+ T cells, that can potentially aide in the augmentation of an immune response [62] (unpublished data).

In comparison to the immune responses generated by pDNA delivery alone in pre-clinical disease models, the addition of EP to the delivery protocol has consistently enhanced responses against influenza antigens - generating protective levels of antibodies [20, 24], malaria antigens [63], anthrax [23], cancer antigens including HPV-associated oncoproteins E6 and E7 [64, 65], and prostate cancer antigens [54]. Both T cell and B cell immune compartments are enhanced. However, EP is not the only technology available to enhance DNA-based vaccine delivery and resulting immune responses. For EP to become widely accepted as a clinical pDNA delivery aide it must demonstrate advantages over other modalities, not just in terms of immunity, but safety, ease of use, and cost effectiveness. Pre-clinical studies have compared the immune responses generated by pDNA + EP with other antigen delivery strategies. In relevant non-human primate (NHP) models, Hirao *et al.* [66], evaluated the optimized naked SIV pDNA vaccine delivered with EP against the Merck Adenoviral serotype 5 (Ad5)-based SIV vaccine. T cell proliferative responses and IFN-γ production - benchmark assay for the analysis of CD8+ and T helper-1 cell responses after vaccination, were analyzed. Results revealed upon *ex vivo* SIV antigen stimulation that the magnitude of both T cell IFN-γ production and proliferation were greater in the SIV pDNA + EP delivery group. Additionally, this study highlighted an important consideration when using Ad5 viral vector delivery that these are subsequent immunizations after the prime failure to boost the immune response. On the other hand, responses in the SIV pDNA + EP delivery group were increased after each vaccination.

6. ELECTROPORATION-ENHANCED DNA-BASED VACCINE DELIVERY IN THE CLINIC

The plasticity of DNA vaccination allows for the technology to be applied against many disease targets, in both preventative and therapeutic clinical protocols. In this section we will outline the clinical trials that highlight the potential of EP-enhanced DNA-based vaccination protocols to tackle unmet disease targets in both the infectious disease and oncology arenas.

6.1. Cancer Immunotherapy

After years of disappointing clinical outcomes, immunotherapeutic strategies targeting tumors are finally realizing their promise. Checkpoint inhibitors, such as anti-PD1 and anti-CTLA-4 antibodies can block immunosuppressive signals, and have demonstrated efficacy in the treatment of a variety of cancers including melanoma, non-small-cell lung and renal cancer [67 - 69]. Adoptive transfers of chimeric antigen receptor (CAR) T cells have proved efficacious in the treatment of hematological malignancies [70, 71]. Thus, there is now strong clinical evidence demonstrating the immune cells can be targeted to treat cancer.

The goal of a DNA-based cancer vaccine is to elicit a functional immune response targeting specific tumor antigens (TA's) that will result in breaking established immune tolerance and the specific destruction of the tumor mass and subsequent protection from re-growth. To date, no vaccine has been able to fully achieve this in the clinical setting. However, there have been some promising recent advances in this field. In 2010 the first immunotherapeutic cancer vaccine was approved by the FDA [72]. Sipuleucel-T (Provenge™) treatment protocol, developed by Dendreon Corporation, achieved an increase in life expectancy of 4.1 months compared to placebo control in castration-resistent prostate cancer patients [73]. Thus, there is now proof of concept evidence that clinically efficacious anti-tumor responses can be generated by vaccination.

The signature CD8+T cell immune responses generated by EP-enhanced DNA-based vaccination are considered to have paramount therapeutic value, especially in the cancer setting. There is a plethora of pre-clinical data showing that DNA-based vaccination can drive the generation of robust T cell responses and can destroy and protect experimental animals from cancerous growth [74]. However, as mentioned above and in the cancer immunotherapeutic area in particular, the translation of pre-clinical successes with DNA-based vaccines into the clinical setting has generally led to disappointment. In this section we will focus on the recent promising interventions that have married DNA-based vaccine with EP-enhanced delivery platfroms to drive immune responses to TA. A recent search of thc ClinicalTrials.gov databasc rcvcalcd approximatcly half of thc ongoing trials testing pDNA vaccines used EP as a delivery tool. The immunotherapeutic targets of these trials included melanoma (NCT01138410), prostate cancer (NCT0085 9729), colorectal cancer (NCT01064375), breast cancer (NCT02204098), Merkel cell cancer (NCT01440816), head and neck squamous cell carcinoma (NCT0 2163057), cervical cancer (NCT02172911) and cervical intra-epithelial neoplasia (NCT02139267/NCT02100085). See Table **1** for further details.

In 2013 Erikkson and colleagues reported the findings of a phase I study testing a DNA-based vaccine in a cohort of fifteen patients with biochemical relapse of prostate cancer without macroscopic disease [75]. The DNA-based vaccine coded for rhesus prostate specific antigen (PSA) and was delived ID with skin EP. Safety assessment revealed no systemic toxicity or significant discomfort involved in the protocol that included a total of five vaccinations with EP. Vaccinations were performed at four week intervals. Increase in T cell reactivity to overlapping peptides representing the full length PSA protein were observed in some, but not all patients. Another phase I/II trial conducted at the University of Southampton, U.K., investigated a DNA fusion vaccine (fragment C of tetanus toxin conjugated to an HLA-A2-binding epitope from prostate-specific membrane antigen) delivered IM with or without EP [76]. The vaccination protocol was reported to be safe and well tolerated. Vaccine-induced T cell responses significantly above baseline levels were detected in the majority of the patients, trending higher for the patients that received EP. PSA doubling time increased significantly, but there was no clear differential effect of EP on this parameter.

Yuan *et al.* recently reported the results of a phase I study testing the *in vivo* electroporation of a xenogeneic melanosomal antigen DNA-based vaccine in malignant melanoma patients [77]. The treatment protocol was reported to be safe and CD8+ T cell responses against the vaccine antigen were detected in 6 of 15 patients in the cohort that received the highest dose of vaccine. Table **1** outlines current cancer immunotherapy DNA-based vaccine trials being performed using EP as a delivery enabling platform.

Inovio Pharmaceuticals recently completed a dose-escalating phase I clinical trial to determine the safety, tolerability and immunogenicity of a therapeutic DNA vaccine (VGX-3100) encoding the HPV 16/18-associated oncoproteins E6 and E7 delivered with CELLECTRA®-5P electroporation into the deltoid muscle [25]. The safety profile of the treatment was unremarkable, no SAEs or vaccine-related Grade 3 or 4 AEs were reported. ELISA and ELISpot analysis revealed robust humoral and T cell immune responses in 100% (ELISA) and 78% (IFN-γ ELISpot) of the patients. Importantly sophisticated flow cytometric analysis revealed the generation of effector CTL populations specifically targeting E6 and E7 oncoproteins and memory T cells. The breadth and level of the generated immune responses across the cohort were unprecedented. Subsequently, a phase II trial was performed to determine the clinical efficacy of VGX-3100 in clearing of HPV16 and 18 virus and pre-cancerous cervical lesions in stage CIN2/3 subjects. This study was recently un-blinded. Of the total 167 patients recruited, 125 received 3 doses of VGX-3100 and 42 placebo. Histological regression to CIN 1 or normal pathology was observed in 49.5% of the VGX-3100 and 30.6% of the placebo recipients (p=0.034). Furthermore regression and viral clearance was recorded in 40.2% of the VGX-3100 and 14.3% of the placebo recipients (p=0.003).Thus, the primary (histological regression) and secondary (concomitant histopathological regression and clearance of HPV-16 or HPV-18, or both) clinical efficacy endpoints were met [78]. In a separate small phase I/II study, Kim and colleagues also reported robust CD8+ T cell responses against E6/E7 antigens in CIN3 patients vaccinated with a HPV DNA-based vaccine delivered IM with EP [79]. Notably, eight of the nine patients in this study displayed regression of their lesions and HPV viral clearance. Importantly, these studies represent milestones for the field of DNA-based vaccines combined with EP in that they are the first demonstrations of clinical efficacy.

We are currently at a very exciting time in the field of immunotherapy. Monoclonal antibody treatments have demonstrated efficacy in both attenuating disease mediating immune responses to treat autoimmune diseases, *e.g.* Crohn's disease and rheumatoid arthritis [80, 81][REMOVED HYPERLINK FIELD], and conversely, allowing the immune system to respond to cancer antigens, for example anti-CTLA4 and anti-PD-1 antibody therapies [68, 69]. The combination of anti-cancer monoclonal antibody therapies with DNA-based vaccination is just beginning to be investigated and the prospect of unprecedented levels of clinical efficacy has now become a real possibility.

6.2. Infectious Disease Prophylaxis and Immunotherapy

EP has been combined with DNA-based vaccination to target many infectious disease agents. There is a plethora of data available demonstrating the induction of robust immune responses and/or disease protection in multiple pre-clinical models. These targets include HIV [82 - 85], HCV [86], HBV [87], influenza [24], malaria [88] and Ebola [89, 90]. The first demonstration that EP could be used in healthy volunteers to improve the immunogenicity of a DNA-based vaccine candidate was published by Vasan and colleagues [91]. This group used the Ichor Medical Systems TriGrid Intramuscular System to deliver ADVAX, a multigenic HIV-1 DNA vaccine candidate. EP was reported to be both safe and well-tolerated, and considered an acceptable procedure for a prophylactic vaccine by the recipients in a questionnaire. Importantly, EP delivery of ADVAX significantly augmented the HIV-1 specific cell mediate immunity by upto 70-fold over IM delivery alone. Robust CD4+ and CD8+ T cell responses were detected by IFN-γ ELISPOT.

Recently, an HIV pDNA plus interleukin-12 (IL-12) cytokine vaccine treatment strategy was performed in the clinic [27]. Kalams *et al.* used Inovio Pharmaceuticals' CELLECTRA®-5P device to deliver PENNVAX-B®, a HIV vaccine candidate consisting of a cocktail of three plasmids encoding HIV-1 clade B env, gag and pol, and pDNA encoding human IL-12 proteins p35 and p40. The vaccine delivery was IM. Authors reported the addition of EP immediately after the IM administration of the HIV pDNA vaccine had a significant dose-sparing effect that resulted in enhanced immunogenicity over delivery without EP [27]. Further information pertaining to the devolpment of prophylactic and therapeutic DNA vaccine and the utilization of the EP delivery platform to target HIV can be found in the review entitled "Therapeutic and prophylactic DNA vaccines for HIV" [92].

A recent phase I/IIa clinical trial tested the therapeutic potential of a HCV DNA-based vaccine candidate delivered by IM EP in 12 patients with chronic HCV infection [93]. Investigators showed that an IM immunization protocol with a codon-optimized HCV nonstructural (NS) 3/4A-expressing DNA-based vaccine in conjunction with EP along with standard-of-care (SOC) therapy resulted in an improvement of IFN-γ T cell responses during the first six weeks of therapy; it has previously been demonstrated that clearance of infections caused by HCV correlates with virus-specific T cell function. Importantly, the investigators observed a reduction in serum HCV RNA in five patients, and six of the eight patients that started SOC therapy within 1-30 months within the last vaccination were cured. This study was reported as the first human therapeutic HCV DNA vaccine study using EP delivery to show transient effects in patients with chronic HCV genotype 1 infection. The success of this phase I/IIa study led to a larger phase II trial being initiated. This study compared the clinical out come in terms of HCV RNA levels. A group of HCV 17 patients received the HCV DNA vaccine delived IM with EP along with SOC; another group received SOC alone. Unfortunately, interim analysis revealed no statistical difference between the two groups: 65% of the vaccinated groups were HCV RNA negative compared to 58% in the non-vaccinated group (ChronTech press release). Even though this study did not achieve its clinical efficacy end point target, further clinical studies will be initiated using a broader HCV vaccine candidate, INO-8000. This vaccine is coded to produce the NS antigens NS3/4A, NS4B and NS5A of HCV genotypes 1a and 1b. A rodent preclinical study revealed the induction of functional T cells in the liver after immunization with INO-8000 [94]. Table **3** outlines the current infectious disease DNA vaccine trials being performed using EP as a delivery enabling platform.

Table 3. ***In vivo*** **electroporation devices.**

Device Name	Manufacturer (website)	Target Tissue	References
Derma Vax™	Cyto Pulse Sciences, Inc (www.cytopulse.com)	Skin	El Kamary [41], Eriksson [75]
CELLECTRA®	Inovio Pharmaceuticals (www.inovio.com)	Muscle/Skin	Diehl [55], Bagarrazzi [25], Kalams [27]
TriGrid Intramuscular Delivery System	Ichor Medical Systems (www.ichorms.com)	Muscle	Vasan [91], Hooper [26]
Medpulser	Inovio Pharmaceuticals (www.inovio.com)	Muscle	Diaz [96], Weiland [93]
ELGEN 2000	Inovio Pharmaceuticals (www.inovio.com)	Muscle/skin	Chudley [76], Broderick [47]
CLINIPORATOR	Igea Medical (www.igeamedical.com)	Tumor	Quaglino [97], Denzi [98]

7. FUTURE PROSPECTS AND CHALLENGES

The marriage of DNA-based vaccine with delivery enhancing platforms such as electroporation has re-ignited the excitement that DNA-based immunization will become a successful strategy to tackle many unmet medical needs. There are currently 838 DNA vaccine trials listed on ClinicalTrials.gov, and 58 of these are using EP-enhanced delivery (ClinicalTrials.gov.). Due to promising data collected from completed and on-going clinical trials, the number of trials using EP as an enabling delivery technology has risen steadily over the last five years. The safety profile of DNA vaccination along with EP has been excellent, and the worry of integration of pDNA into the host genome is unfounded. A phase II study has now demonstrated that a DNA+EP vaccination protocol can generate impressive therapeutic efficacy in the clinic and as such is a massive milestone for the field. The clinical use of EP technologies to deliver DNA-based vaccines is still at an early stage and there are certain hurdles to overcome before it becomes a widely accepted treatment protocol in the delivery of vaccines. The first obvious drawback in the use of EP is the associated pain, which may be acceptable in some immunotherapeutic protocols, but is unlikely to be readily accepted in the prophylactic setting. Studies are ongoing to reduce the pain associated with these DNA-based vaccination protocols by optimizing the electrical parameters used so the least amount of discomfort is experienced by the patient, but without the loss of immunogenicity. Additionally, other less invasive (than muscle) delivery sites such as the skin or mucosal surface are being investigated [47, 95]. The first generation EP devices have generally been cumbersome, not easy to use for an untrained operator and not esthetically pleasing. Generally they have been more suitable to the laboratory setting than the clinic. There is currently a movement to redesign EP devise to become esthetically pleasing, easy to operate, compatible with low cost disposable electrode arrays and cost effective (Table **3**). The vaccination plus EP protocol has been a two component procedure. We and others in the medical device development field are now designing more compact "all-i--one" devices that possess the ability to inject the vaccine formulation and perform the EP. We believe the development of such devices to be essential for the widespread use of EP. Recently, the research and development field is working towards a device that would be able to perform needleless injection of the DNA-based vaccine and EP at the surface in a non-invasive manner. Such a device should fulfill the criteria that will result in the EP-enhanced DNA-based vaccine procedure being both needle-free and tolerable.

In summary, the authors believe the ever growing pre-clinical and clinical data being generated will rapidly increase our understanding of the process and quickly lead to optimized immunotherapeutic protocols.

CONFLICT OF INTEREST

The authors confirm that they have no conflict of interest to declare for this publication.

ACKNOWLEDGEMENTS

We would like to thank Laurent Humeau and Bernie Hertel for helpful comments and editorial assistance with the manuscript.

REFERENCES

[1] Neumann E, Schaefer-Ridder M, Wang Y, Hofschneider PH. Gene transfer into mouse lyoma cells by electroporation in high electric fields. EMBO J 1982; 1(7): 841-5.
[PMID: 6329708]

[2] Gothelf A, Mir LM, Gehl J. Electrochemotherapy: results of cancer treatment using enhanced delivery of bleomycin by electroporation. Cancer Treat Rev 2003; 29(5): 371-87. [http://dx.doi.org/10.1016/S0305-7372(03)00073-2] [PMID: 12972356]

[3] Miklavcic D, Davalos RV. Electrochemotherapy (ECT) and irreversible electroporation (IRE) - advanced techniques for treating deep-seated tumors based on electroporation. Biomed Eng Online 2015; 14 (Suppl. 3): I1. [http://dx.doi.org/10.1186/1475-925X-14-S3-I1] [PMID: 26355606]

[4] Gehl J. Electroporation for drug and gene delivery in the clinic: doctors go electric. Methods Mol Biol 2008; 423: 351-9. [http://dx.doi.org/10.1007/978-1-59745-194-9_27] [PMID: 18370213]

[5] Cai Y, Rodriguez S, Hebel H. DNA vaccine manufacture: scale and quality. Expert Rev Vaccines 2009; 8(9): 1277-91. [http://dx.doi.org/10.1586/erv.09.84] [PMID: 19722898]

[6] Sardesai NY, Weiner DB. Electroporation delivery of DNA vaccines: prospects for success. Curr Opin Immunol 2011; 23(3): 421-9. [http://dx.doi.org/10.1016/j.coi.2011.03.008] [PMID: 21530212]

[7] Wang B, Ugen KE, Srikantan V, *et al.* Gene inoculation generates immune responses against human immunodeficiency virus type 1. Proc Natl Acad Sci USA 1993; 90(9): 4156-60. [http://dx.doi.org/10.1073/pnas.90.9.4156] [PMID: 8483929]

[8] Tang DC, DeVit M, Johnston SA. Genetic immunization is a simple method for eliciting an immune response. Nature 1992; 356(6365): 152-4. [http://dx.doi.org/10.1038/356152a0] [PMID: 1545867]

[9] Ulmer JB, Donnelly JJ, Parker SE, *et al.* Heterologous protection against influenza by injection of DNA encoding a viral protein. Science 1993; 259(5102): 1745-9. [http://dx.doi.org/10.1126/science.8456302] [PMID: 8456302]

[10] Conry RM, LoBuglio AF, Loechel F, *et al.* A carcinoembryonic antigen polynucleotide vaccine has *in vivo* antitumor activity. Gene Ther 1995; 2(1): 59-65. [PMID: 7712333]

[11] Triozzi PL, Aldrich W, Allen KO, Carlisle RR, LoBuglio AF, Conry RM. Phase I study of a plasmid DNA vaccine encoding MART-1 in patients with resected melanoma at risk for relapse. J Immunother 2005; 28(4): 382-8. [http://dx.doi.org/10.1097/01.cji.0000162779.88687.4c] [PMID: 16000957]

[12] Weiner DB. DNA vaccines: crossing a line in the sand. Introduction to special issue. Vaccine 2008; 26(40): 5073-4. [http://dx.doi.org/10.1016/j.vaccine.2008.07.024] [PMID: 18652867]

[13] Liu MA. Immunologic basis of vaccine vectors. Immunity 2010; 33(4): 504-15. [http://dx.doi.org/10.1016/j.immuni.2010.10.004] [PMID: 21029961]

[14] Yang NS, Burkholder J, Roberts B, Martinell B, McCabe D. *In vivo* and *in vitro* gene transfer to mammalian somatic cells by particle bombardment. Proc Natl Acad Sci USA 1990; 87(24): 9568-72. [http://dx.doi.org/10.1073/pnas.87.24.9568] [PMID: 2175906]

[15] Klein RM, Wolf ED, Wu R, Sanford JC. High-velocity microprojectiles for delivering nucleic acids into living cells. 1987. Biotechnology 1992; 24: 384-6.
[PMID: 1422046]

[16] Wang C, Ge Q, Ting D, *et al.* Molecularly engineered poly(ortho ester) microspheres for enhanced delivery of DNA vaccines. Nat Mater 2004; 3(3): 190-6.
[http://dx.doi.org/10.1038/nmat1075] [PMID: 14991022]

[17] Yamashita Y, Shimada M, Tachibana K, *et al. In vivo* gene transfer into muscle *via* electro-sonoporation. Hum Gene Ther 2002; 13(17): 2079-84.
[http://dx.doi.org/10.1089/10430340260395929] [PMID: 12490002]

[18] Manome Y, Nakamura M, Ohno T, Furuhata H. Ultrasound facilitates transduction of naked plasmid DNA into colon carcinoma cells *in vitro* and *in vivo.* Hum Gene Ther 2000; 11(11): 1521-8.
[http://dx.doi.org/10.1089/10430340050083252] [PMID: 10945766]

[19] Huang LY, Wang KY, Xiao D, *et al.* Safety and immunogenicity of an oral DNA vaccine encoding Sip of Streptococcus agalactiae from Nile tilapia Oreochromis niloticus delivered by live attenuated Salmonella typhimurium. Fish Shellfish Immunol 2014; 38(1): 34-41.
[http://dx.doi.org/10.1016/j.fsi.2014.02.017] [PMID: 24631734]

[20] Laddy DJ, Yan J, Khan AS, *et al.* Electroporation of synthetic DNA antigens offers protection in nonhuman primates challenged with highly pathogenic avian influenza virus. J Virol 2009; 83(9): 4624-30.
[http://dx.doi.org/10.1128/JVI.02335-08] [PMID: 19211745]

[21] Nyström J, Chen A, Frelin L, *et al.* Improving on the ability of endogenous hepatitis B core antigen to prime cytotoxic T lymphocytes. J Infect Dis 2010; 201(12): 1867-79.
[http://dx.doi.org/10.1086/652808] [PMID: 20446851]

[22] Rosati M, Valentin A, Jalah R, *et al.* Increased immune responses in rhesus macaques by DNA vaccination combined with electroporation. Vaccine 2008; 26(40): 5223-9.
[http://dx.doi.org/10.1016/j.vaccine.2008.03.090] [PMID: 18468743]

[23] Livingston BD, Little SF, Luxembourg A, Ellefsen B, Hannaman D. Comparative performance of a licensed anthrax vaccine *versus* electroporation based delivery of a PA encoding DNA vaccine in rhesus macaques. Vaccine 2010; 28(4): 1056-61.
[http://dx.doi.org/10.1016/j.vaccine.2009.10.111] [PMID: 19896452]

[24] Laddy DJ, Yan J, Kutzler M, *et al.* Heterosubtypic protection against pathogenic human and avian influenza viruses *via in vivo* electroporation of synthetic consensus DNA antigens. PLoS One 2008; 3(6): e2517.
[http://dx.doi.org/10.1371/journal.pone.0002517] [PMID: 18575608]

[25] Bagarazzi ML, Yan J, Morrow MP, *et al.* Immunotherapy against HPV16/18 generates potent TH1 and cytotoxic cellular immune responses. Sci Transl Med 2012; 4(155): 155ra138.
[http://dx.doi.org/10.1126/scitranslmed.3004414] [PMID: 23052295]

[26] Hooper JW, Moon JE, Paolino KM, *et al.* A Phase 1 clinical trial of Hantaan virus and Puumala virus M-segment DNA vaccines for haemorrhagic fever with renal syndrome delivered by intramuscular electroporation. Clin Microbiol Infect 2014; 20(s5): 110-7.

[27] Kalams SA, Parker SD, Elizaga M, *et al.* Safety and comparative immunogenicity of an HIV-1 DNA vaccine in combination with plasmid interleukin 12 and impact of intramuscular electroporation for delivery. J Infect Dis 2013; 208(5): 818-29. [http://dx.doi.org/10.1093/infdis/jit236] [PMID: 23840043]

[28] Low L, Mander A, McCann K, *et al.* DNA vaccination with electroporation induces increased antibody responses in patients with prostate cancer. Hum Gene Ther 2009; 20(11): 1269-78. [http://dx.doi.org/10.1089/hum.2009.067] [PMID: 19619001]

[29] Khan AS, Broderick KE, Sardesai NY. Clinical development of intramuscular electroporation: providing a "boost" for DNA vaccines. Methods Mol Biol 2014; 1121: 279-89. [http://dx.doi.org/10.1007/978-1-4614-9632-8_25] [PMID: 24510832]

[30] Keane-Myers AM, Bell M, Hannaman D, Albrecht M. DNA electroporation of multi-agent vaccines conferring protection against select agent challenge: TriGrid delivery system. Methods Mol Biol 2014; 1121: 325-36. [http://dx.doi.org/10.1007/978-1-4614-9632-8_29] [PMID: 24510836]

[31] Somiari S, Glasspool-Malone J, Drabick JJ, *et al.* Theory and *in vivo* application of electroporative gene delivery. Mol Ther 2000; 2(3): 178-87.

[32] Breton M, Delemotte L, Silve A, Mir LM, Tarek M. Transport of siRNA through lipid membranes driven by nanosecond electric pulses: an experimental and computational study. J Am Chem Soc 2012; 134(34): 13938-41. [http://dx.doi.org/10.1021/ja3052365] [PMID: 22880891]

[33] Silk M, Tahour D, Srimathveeravalli G, Solomon SB, Thornton RH. The state of irreversible electroporation in interventional oncology. Semin Intervent Radiol 2014; 31(2): 111-7. [http://dx.doi.org/10.1055/s-0034-1373785] [PMID: 25053862]

[34] Satkauskas S, Bureau MF, Puc M, *et al.* Mechanisms of *in vivo* DNA electrotransfer: respective contributions of cell electropermeabilization and DNA electrophoresis. Mol Ther 2002; 5(2): 133-40.

[35] Mir LM, Bureau MF, Gehl J, *et al.* High-efficiency gene transfer into skeletal muscle mediated by electric pulses. Proc Natl Acad Sci USA 1999; 96(8): 4262-7. [http://dx.doi.org/10.1073/pnas.96.8.4262] [PMID: 10200250]

[36] Teissie J. Electropermeabilization of the cell membrane. Methods Mol Biol 2014; 1121: 25-46. [http://dx.doi.org/10.1007/978-1-4614-9632-8_2] [PMID: 24510809]

[37] Satkauskas S, André F, Bureau MF, Scherman D, Miklavcic D, Mir LM. Electrophoretic component of electric pulses determines the efficacy of *in vivo* DNA electrotransfer. Hum Gene Ther 2005; 16(10): 1194-201. [http://dx.doi.org/10.1089/hum.2005.16.1194] [PMID: 16218780]

[38] André FM, Gehl J, Sersa G, *et al.* Efficiency of high- and low-voltage pulse combinations for gene electrotransfer in muscle, liver, tumor, and skin. Hum Gene Ther 2008; 19(11): 1261-71. [http://dx.doi.org/10.1089/hum.2008.060] [PMID: 19866490]

[39] Hojman P, Gissel H, Andre FM, *et al.* Physiological effects of high- and low-voltage pulse combinations for gene electrotransfer in muscle. Hum Gene Ther 2008; 19(11): 1249-60. [http://dx.doi.org/10.1089/hum.2008.059] [PMID: 19866489]

[40] Wolff JA, Ludtke JJ, Acsadi G, Williams P, Jani A. Long-term persistence of plasmid DNA and foreign gene expression in mouse muscle. Hum Mol Genet 1992; 1(6): 363-9. [http://dx.doi.org/10.1093/hmg/1.6.363] [PMID: 1301910]

[41] El-Kamary SS, Billington M, Deitz S, *et al.* Safety and tolerability of the Easy Vax clinical epidermal electroporation system in healthy adults. Mol Ther 2012; 20(1): 214-20. [http://dx.doi.org/10.1038/mt.2011.235]

[42] Heller L, Pottinger C, Jaroszeski MJ, Gilbert R, Heller R. *In vivo* electroporation of plasmids encoding GM-CSF or interleukin-2 into existing B16 melanomas combined with electrochemotherapy induces long-term antitumour immunity. Melanoma Res 2000; 10(6): 577-83. [http://dx.doi.org/10.1097/00008390-200012000-00010] [PMID: 11198480]

[43] Tevaearai HT, Gazdhar A, Giraud MN, Flück M. *In vivo* electroporation-mediated gene delivery to the beating heart. Methods Mol Biol 2014; 1121: 223-9. [http://dx.doi.org/10.1007/978-1-4614-9632-8_19] [PMID: 24510826]

[44] Hao J, Li SK, Kao WW, Liu CY. Gene delivery to cornea. Brain Res Bull 2010; 81(2-3): 256-61. [http://dx.doi.org/10.1016/j.brainresbull.2009.06.011] [PMID: 19560524]

[45] Ding XF, Ma DL, Zhang Q, Peng W, Fan M, Suo WZ. Progress of *in vivo* electroporation in the rodent brain. Curr Gene Ther 2014; 14(3): 211-7. [http://dx.doi.org/10.2174/1566523214666140424145305] [PMID: 24766135]

[46] Banchereau J, Steinman RM. Dendritic cells and the control of immunity. Nature 1998; 392(6673): 245-52. [http://dx.doi.org/10.1038/32588] [PMID: 9521319]

[47] Broderick KE, Shen X, Soderholm J, *et al.* Prototype development and preclinical immunogenicity analysis of a novel minimally invasive electroporation device. Gene Ther 2011; 18(3): 258-65. [http://dx.doi.org/10.1038/gt.2010.137] [PMID: 20962869]

[48] Hirao LA, Draghia-Akli R, Prigge JT, *et al.* Multivalent smallpox DNA vaccine delivered by intradermal electroporation drives protective immunity in nonhuman primates against lethal monkeypox challenge. J Infect Dis 2011; 203(1): 95-102. [http://dx.doi.org/10.1093/infdis/jiq017] [PMID: 21148501]

[49] Adam L, Le Grand R, Martinon F. Electroporation-mediated intradermal delivery of DNA vaccines in nonhuman primates. Methods Mol Biol 2014; 1121: 309-13. [http://dx.doi.org/10.1007/978-1-4614-9632-8_27] [PMID: 24510834]

[50] Heller R, Cruz Y, Heller LC, Gilbert RA, Jaroszeski MJ. Electrically mediated delivery of plasmid DNA to the skin, using a multielectrode array. Hum Gene Ther 2010; 21(3): 357-62. [http://dx.doi.org/10.1089/hum.2009.065] [PMID: 19839722]

[51] Broderick KE, Kardos T, McCoy JR, Fons MP, Kemmerrer S, Sardesai NY. Piezoelectric permeabilization of mammalian dermal tissue for *in vivo* DNA delivery leads to enhanced protein expression and increased immunogenicity. Hum Vaccin 2011; 7 (Suppl.): 22-8. [http://dx.doi.org/10.4161/hv.7.0.14559] [PMID: 21263230]

[52] Connolly RJ, Rey JI, Lambert VM, Wegerif G, Jaroszeski MJ, Ugen KE. Enhancement of antigen specific humoral immune responses after delivery of a DNA plasmid based vaccine through a contact-

independent helium plasma. Vaccine 2011; 29(39): 6781-4.
[http://dx.doi.org/10.1016/j.vaccine.2010.12.054] [PMID: 21195804]

[53] Donate A, Coppola D, Cruz Y, Heller R. Evaluation of a novel non-penetrating electrode for use in DNA vaccination. PLoS One 2011; 6(4): e19181.
[http://dx.doi.org/10.1371/journal.pone.0019181] [PMID: 21559474]

[54] Roos AK, Moreno S, Leder C, Pavlenko M, King A, Pisa P. Enhancement of cellular immune response to a prostate cancer DNA vaccine by intradermal electroporation. Mol Ther 2006; 13(2): 320-7.
[http://dx.doi.org/10.1016/j.ymthe.2005.08.005]

[55] Diehl MC, Lee JC, Daniels SE, *et al.* Tolerability of intramuscular and intradermal delivery by CELLECTRA(®) adaptive constant current electroporation device in healthy volunteers. Hum Vaccin Immunother 2013; 9(10): 2246-52.
[http://dx.doi.org/10.4161/hv.24702] [PMID: 24051434]

[56] Mendoza JM, Amante DH, Kichaev G, *et al.* Elucidating the kinetics of expression and immune cell infiltration resulting from plasmid gene delivery enhanced by surface dermal electroporation. Vaccines (Basel) 2013; 1(3): 384-97.
[http://dx.doi.org/10.3390/vaccines1030384] [PMID: 26344120]

[57] Amante DH, Smith TR, Mendoza JM, *et al.* Skin transfection patterns and expression kinetics of electroporation-enhanced plasmid delivery using the CELLECTRA-3P, a portable next-generation dermal electroporation device. Hum Gene Ther Methods 2015; 26(4): 134-46.
[http://dx.doi.org/10.1089/hgtb.2015.020] [PMID: 26222896]

[58] Smith TR, Schultheis K, Kiosses WB, *et al.* DNA vaccination strategy targets epidermal dendritic cells, initiating their migration and induction of a host immune response. Mol Ther Methods Clin Dev 2014; 1: 14054.
[http://dx.doi.org/10.1038/mtm.2014.54] [PMID: 26052522]

[59] Steinman RM, Hawiger D, Nussenzweig MC. Tolerogenic dendritic cells. Annu Rev Immunol 2003; 21: 685-711.
[http://dx.doi.org/10.1146/annurev.immunol.21.120601.141040] [PMID: 12615891]

[60] Ishikawa H, Ma Z, Barber GN. STING regulates intracellular DNA-mediated, type I interferon-dependent innate immunity. Nature 2009; 461(7265): 788-92.
[http://dx.doi.org/10.1038/nature08476] [PMID: 19776740]

[61] Yuan TF. Vaccination by muscle electroporation: the injury helps. Vaccine 2008; 26(33): 4105-6.
[http://dx.doi.org/10.1016/j.vaccine.2008.05.078] [PMID: 18585829]

[62] Roos AK, Eriksson F, Timmons JA, *et al.* Skin electroporation: effects on transgene expression, DNA persistence and local tissue environment. PLoS One 2009; 4(9): e7226.
[http://dx.doi.org/10.1371/journal.pone.0007226] [PMID: 19789652]

[63] Dobaño C, Widera G, Rabussay D, Doolan DL. Enhancement of antibody and cellular immune responses to malaria DNA vaccines by *in vivo* electroporation. Vaccine 2007; 25(36): 6635-45.
[http://dx.doi.org/10.1016/j.vaccine.2007.06.036] [PMID: 17669562]

[64] Best SR, Peng S, Juang CM, *et al.* Administration of HPV DNA vaccine *via* electroporation elicits the

strongest CD8+ T cell immune responses compared to intramuscular injection and intradermal gene gun delivery. Vaccine 2009; 27(40): 5450-9.
[http://dx.doi.org/10.1016/j.vaccine.2009.07.005] [PMID: 19622402]

[65] Seo SH, Jin HT, Park SH, Youn JI, Sung YC. Optimal induction of HPV DNA vaccine-induced CD8+ T cell responses and therapeutic antitumor effect by antigen engineering and electroporation. Vaccine 2009; 27(42): 5906-12.
[http://dx.doi.org/10.1016/j.vaccine.2009.07.033] [PMID: 19651174]

[66] Hirao LA, Wu L, Satishchandran A, *et al.* Comparative analysis of immune responses induced by vaccination with SIV antigens by recombinant Ad5 vector or plasmid DNA in rhesus macaques. Mol Ther 2010; 18(8): 1568-76.
[http://dx.doi.org/10.1038/mt.2010.112]

[67] Topalian SL, Hodi FS, Brahmer JR, *et al.* Safety, activity, and immune correlates of anti-PD-1 antibody in cancer. N Engl J Med 2012; 366(26): 2443-54.
[http://dx.doi.org/10.1056/NEJMoa1200690] [PMID: 22658127]

[68] Hodi FS, O'Day SJ, McDermott DF, *et al.* Improved survival with ipilimumab in patients with metastatic melanoma. N Engl J Med 2010; 363(8): 711-23.
[http://dx.doi.org/10.1056/NEJMoa1003466] [PMID: 20525992]

[69] Brahmer JR, Tykodi SS, Chow LQ, *et al.* Safety and activity of anti-PD-L1 antibody in patients with advanced cancer. N Engl J Med 2012; 366(26): 2455-65.
[http://dx.doi.org/10.1056/NEJMoa1200694] [PMID: 22658128]

[70] Grupp SA, Kalos M, Barrett D, *et al.* Chimeric antigen receptor-modified T cells for acute lymphoid leukemia. N Engl J Med 2013; 368(16): 1509-18.
[http://dx.doi.org/10.1056/NEJMoa1215134] [PMID: 23527958]

[71] Gill S, June CH. Going viral: chimeric antigen receptor T-cell therapy for hematological malignancies. Immunol Rev 2015; 263(1): 68-89.
[http://dx.doi.org/10.1111/imr.12243] [PMID: 25510272]

[72] Sims RB. Development of sipuleucel-T: autologous cellular immunotherapy for the treatment of metastatic castrate resistant prostate cancer. Vaccine 2012; 30(29): 4394-7.
[http://dx.doi.org/10.1016/j.vaccine.2011.11.058] [PMID: 22122856]

[73] Kantoff PW, Higano CS, Shore ND, *et al.* Sipuleucel-T immunotherapy for castration-resistant prostate cancer. N Engl J Med 2010; 363(5): 411-22.
[http://dx.doi.org/10.1056/NEJMoa1001294] [PMID: 20818862]

[74] Rice J, Ottensmeier CH, Stevenson FK. DNA vaccines: precision tools for activating effective immunity against cancer. Nat Rev Cancer 2008; 8(2): 108-20.
[http://dx.doi.org/10.1038/nrc2326] [PMID: 18219306]

[75] Eriksson F, Tötterman T, Maltais AK, Pisa P, Yachnin J. DNA vaccine coding for the rhesus prostate specific antigen delivered by intradermal electroporation in patients with relapsed prostate cancer. Vaccine 2013; 31(37): 3843-8.
[http://dx.doi.org/10.1016/j.vaccine.2013.06.063] [PMID: 23831327]

[76] Chudley L, McCann K, Mander A, *et al.* DNA fusion-gene vaccination in patients with prostate cancer

induces high-frequency CD8(+) T-cell responses and increases PSA doubling time. Cancer Immunol Immunother 2012; 61(11): 2161-70.
[http://dx.doi.org/10.1007/s00262-012-1270-0] [PMID: 22729556]

[77] Yuan J, Ku GY, Adamow M, *et al.* Immunologic responses to xenogeneic tyrosinase DNA vaccine administered by electroporation in patients with malignant melanoma. J Immunother Cancer 2013; 1: 20.
[http://dx.doi.org/10.1186/2051-1426-1-20] [PMID: 24829756]

[78] Trimble CL, Morrow MP, Kraynyak KA, *et al.* Safety, efficacy, and immunogenicity of VGX-3100, a therapeutic synthetic DNA vaccine targeting human papillomavirus 16 and 18 E6 and E7 proteins for cervical intraepithelial neoplasia 2/3: a randomised, double-blind, placebo-controlled phase 2b trial. Lancet 2015; 386(10008): 2078-88.
[http://dx.doi.org/10.1016/S0140-6736(15)00239-1] [PMID: 26386540]

[79] Kim TJ, Jin HT, Hur SY, *et al.* Clearance of persistent HPV infection and cervical lesion by therapeutic DNA vaccine in CIN3 patients. Nat Commun 2014; 5: 5317.
[http://dx.doi.org/10.1038/ncomms6317] [PMID: 25354725]

[80] Rutgeerts P, Van Assche G, Vermeire S. Optimizing anti-TNF treatment in inflammatory bowel disease. Gastroenterology 2004; 126(6): 1593-610.
[http://dx.doi.org/10.1053/j.gastro.2004.02.070] [PMID: 15168370]

[81] Feldmann M, Maini RN. Lasker Clinical Medical Research Award. TNF defined as a therapeutic target for rheumatoid arthritis and other autoimmune diseases. Nat Med 2003; 9(10): 1245-50.
[http://dx.doi.org/10.1038/nm939] [PMID: 14520364]

[82] Yan J, Corbitt N, Pankhong P, *et al.* Immunogenicity of a novel engineered HIV-1 clade C synthetic consensus-based envelope DNA vaccine. Vaccine 2011; 29(41): 7173-81.
[http://dx.doi.org/10.1016/j.vaccine.2011.05.076] [PMID: 21651948]

[83] Bråve A, Gudmundsdotter L, Sandström E, *et al.* Biodistribution, persistence and lack of integration of a multigene HIV vaccine delivered by needle-free intradermal injection and electroporation. Vaccine 2010; 28(51): 8203-9.
[http://dx.doi.org/10.1016/j.vaccine.2010.08.108] [PMID: 20951666]

[84] Chakrabarti BK, Feng Y, Sharma SK, *et al.* Robust neutralizing antibodies elicited by HIV-1 JRFL envelope glycoprotein trimers in nonhuman primates. J Virol 2013; 87(24): 13239-51.
[http://dx.doi.org/10.1128/JVI.01247-13] [PMID: 24067980]

[85] Kulkarni V, Jalah R, Ganneru B, *et al.* Comparison of immune responses generated by optimized DNA vaccination against SIV antigens in mice and macaques. Vaccine 2011; 29(39): 6742-54.
[http://dx.doi.org/10.1016/j.vaccine.2010.12.056] [PMID: 21195080]

[86] Latimer B, Toporovski R, Yan J, *et al.* Strong HCV NS3/4a, NS4b, NS5a, NS5b-specific cellular immune responses induced in Rhesus macaques by a novel HCV genotype 1a/1b consensus DNA vaccine. Hum Vaccin Immunother 2014; 10(8): 2357-65.
[http://dx.doi.org/10.4161/hv.29590] [PMID: 25424943]

[87] Zhao YG, Peng B, Deng H, *et al.* Anti-HBV immune responses in rhesus macaques elicited by electroporation mediated DNA vaccination. Vaccine 2006; 24(7): 897-903.
[http://dx.doi.org/10.1016/j.vaccine.2005.08.093] [PMID: 16253404]

[88] Ferraro B, Talbott KT, Balakrishnan A, *et al.* Inducing humoral and cellular responses to multiple sporozoite and liver-stage malaria antigens using exogenous plasmid DNA. Infect Immun 2013; 81(10): 3709-20.
[http://dx.doi.org/10.1128/IAI.00180-13] [PMID: 23897618]

[89] Grant-Klein RJ, Van Deusen NM, Badger CV, Hannaman D, Dupuy LC, Schmaljohn CS. A multiagent filovirus DNA vaccine delivered by intramuscular electroporation completely protects mice from ebola and Marburg virus challenge. Hum Vaccin Immunother 2012; 8(11): 1703-6.
[http://dx.doi.org/10.4161/hv.21873] [PMID: 22922764]

[90] Shedlock DJ, Aviles J, Talbott KT, *et al.* Induction of broad cytotoxic T cells by protective DNA vaccination against Marburg and Ebola. Mol Ther 2013; 21(7): 1432-44.
[http://dx.doi.org/10.1038/mt.2013.61]

[91] Vasan S, Hurley A, Schlesinger SJ, *et al. In vivo* electroporation enhances the immunogenicity of an HIV-1 DNA vaccine candidate in healthy volunteers. PLoS One 2011; 6(5): e19252.
[http://dx.doi.org/10.1371/journal.pone.0019252] [PMID: 21603651]

[92] Ramirez LA, Arango T, Boyer J. Therapeutic and prophylactic DNA vaccines for HIV-1. Expert Opin Biol Ther 2013; 13(4): 563-73.
[http://dx.doi.org/10.1517/14712598.2013.758709] [PMID: 23477730]

[93] Weiland O, Ahlen G, Diepolder H, *et al.* Therapeutic DNA vaccination using *in vivo* electroporation followed by standard of care therapy in patients with genotype 1 chronic hepatitis C. Mol Ther 2013; 21(9): 1796-805.

[94] Lang Kuhs KA, Ginsberg AA, Yan J, *et al.* Hepatitis C virus NS3/NS4A DNA vaccine induces multiepitope T cell responses in rhesus macaques mimicking human immune responses [corrected]. Mol Ther 2012; 20(3): 669-78. [corrected].
[http://dx.doi.org/10.1038/mt.2011.188] [PMID: 21952169]

[95] Kichaev G, Mendoza JM, Amante D, *et al.* Electroporation mediated DNA vaccination directly to a mucosal surface results in improved immune responses. Hum Vaccin Immunother 2013; 9(10): 2041-8.
[http://dx.doi.org/10.4161/hv.25272] [PMID: 23954979]

[96] Diaz CM, Chiappori A, Aurisicchio L, *et al.* Phase 1 studies of the safety and immunogenicity of electroporated HER2/CEA DNA vaccine followed by adenoviral boost immunization in patients with solid tumors. J Transl Med 2013; 11: 62.
[http://dx.doi.org/10.1186/1479-5876-11-62] [PMID: 23497415]

[97] Quaglino E, Riccardo F, Macagno M, *et al.* Chimeric DNA Vaccines against ErbB2+ Carcinomas: From Mice to Humans. Cancers (Basel) 2011; 3(3): 3225-41.
[http://dx.doi.org/10.3390/cancers3033225] [PMID: 24212954]

[98] Denzi A, Strigari L, Di Filippo F, *et al.* Modeling the positioning of single needle electrodes for the treatment of breast cancer in a clinical case. Biomed Eng Online 2015; 14 (Suppl. 3): S1.
[http://dx.doi.org/10.1186/1475-925X-14-S3-S1] [PMID: 26355703]

CHAPTER 4

Sonophoresis: Therapeutical Uses and Devices

José Juan Escobar-Chávez*, Pablo Serrano Castañeda, Omar Rodrigo Guadarrama-Escobar, Alma Lidia Aguiñaga-Mireles, Miriam López-Cervantes, Clara Luisa Domínguez-Delgado and **Jessica Martínez-Hernández**

Unidad de Investigación Multidisciplinaria. Laboratorio 12: "Sistemas Transdérmicos y Nanomateriales", Facultad de Estudios Superiores Cuautitlán-Universidad Nacional Autónoma de México. Km 2.5 Carretera Cuautitlán–Teoloyucan, San Sebastián Xhala, Cuautitlán Izcalli, Estado de México, México

Abstract: The administration of drugs in the skin using ultrasound is recognized like sonophoresis. The ultrasound is dating back to the fifties for high frequency (HF) and low frequency (LF). It has been investigated over the past two decades. Clearly, the use of ultrasound to drug delivery (DD) recently gained importance, thereby increasing patents and new commercial devices.

This chapter shows the important findings in sonophoresis. Particular attention is focused into therapeutical applications including transdermal drug delivery (TDD), gene therapy, sport medicine and sonophoretic devices.

Keywords: Physical enhancers, Skin, Sonolysis, Sonophoresis, Sonophoretic devices, Sport medicine, Ultrasound.

1. INTRODUCTION

Applications of ultrasound were used as an imaging technique. In the decade of the twenties, ultrasound (US) showed that could generate modification in human's

* **Corresponding author José Juan Escobar-Chávez:** Unidad de Investigación Multidisciplinaria. Laboratorio 12: "Sistemas Transdérmicos y Nanomateriales", Facultad de Estudios Superiores Cuautitlán-Universidad Nacional Autónoma de México. Km 2.5 Carretera Cuautitlán–Teoloyucan, San Sebastián Xhala, Cuautitlán Izcalli, Estado de México, CP. 54714, México; Tel: + (52 55).56.23.19.99; Fax: + (52 55). 56.15.70.77;
E-mail: josejuanescobarchavez@gmail.com

organisms, thus began the US treatment [1].

The use of ultrasound in tissue generates heat thereof due to absorption of energy, allowing the use under different conditions. Recently it has been studied that the same benefit is obtained without thermal application by US.

US treatments could be divided as low and high frequency, LF covers the applications as phonophoresis, gene and physiotherapy, and last but not least important it can be used for bone healing.

The application of US has been used for many years in the medical field.

US have 3 different arrangement applications. These are shown in Table **1**.

Table 1. Set of US conditions based on frequency (F) range.

Ultrasound types (frequency ultrasound)	Range of frequencies (KHz)
Low	20-100
Medium	0.7-3.0
High	3.0-10.0

Table 2. Principal applications of US.

Relevant Applications of Ultrasound
(i) For diagnosis in medicine.
(ii) For physical therapy (0.1- 15 MHz) the application of higher frequencies restricts the action to more superficial layers in to the skin.
(iii) In sport medicine. It can reduce healing times in fresh fractures or injuries in almost 30 -38% (<0.1 W/cm^2).
(iv) For transdermal, ocular and ungual/transungual DD, ocular permeability enhance through changes in the structure of the cornea (20kHz).
(v) In surgery, practice patterns, traditional delegation of use and involving procedures (5-10 MgHz).
(vi) In gene therapy increases plasmid transfection through the formation of short pores in the plasma membrane.
(vii) For the treatment of tumors. US is used to treat a variety of solid tumors with the advantage that this technique have a fewer complications after treatment.

The principal medical applications of US are shown in Table **2**. Initially US was investigated for the treatment of skin conditions [2, 3] and swelling of joints [4]. Lately is of interest to use it for TDD [5] and gene therapy [6].

In recent years, reviews with important information on a lot of aspects of sonophoresis have been published [7 - 15]. This chapter displays a well-run view of therapeutic, pharmaceutical applications of US and sonophoretic devices. This Approach is justified because of the information available by US uses.

2. THE US

US is an energy that spreads [16,17]. Path propagation is parallel to oscillation direction as observed in Fig. (**1**).

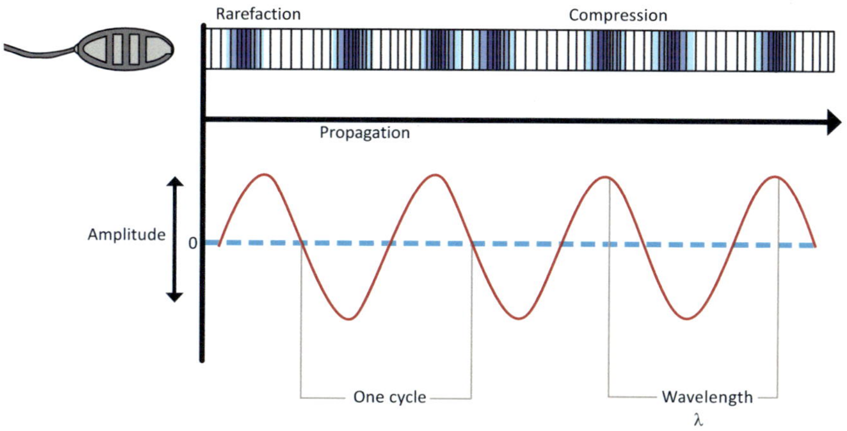

Fig. (1). Representation of sound wave propagation.

The concentration of energy within a specific area in an US ray is called intensity (I). The intensity is decreasingly when US pass into the body, this is called attenuation. Tissue attenuation occurs for the absorption and sound force that are converted to warmth and scattered [13, 18] (Fig. **2**).

Other experimental variables [17] that are important in sonophoresis are shown in Table **3**.

Duty cycles are common at 10%, 25%, 50% or continuous application [19 - 28]. US is frequently used in pulsating as it lowers the effects of warming related by US. Various horn-to-skin spaces are utilized in sonophoresis studies, ranging from placing the US horn skin contact about 4 cm [28, 29]. Treatments vary over time, from a few seconds [30 - 33] minutes [34] or even hours [35]. The medium is vital in sonophoresis because their properties can determine the degree of permeability as a result of treatment. In addition coupling medium may contain drug with a chemical promoter [36].

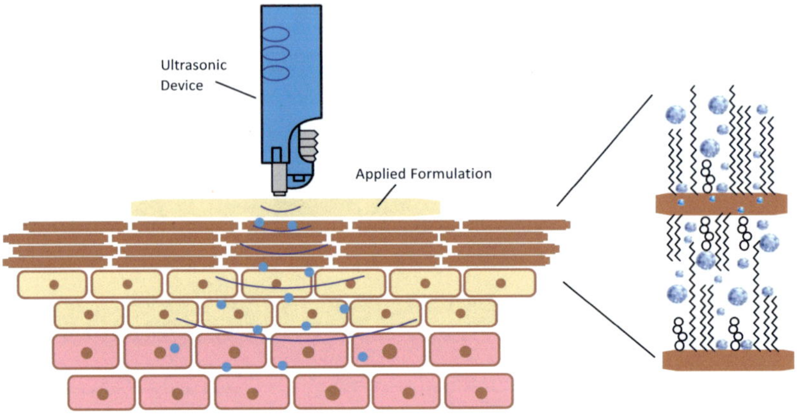

Fig. (2). Disruption of stratum corneum (SC) by ultrasound to increase skin permeability.

Table 3. Most important experimental variables in sonophoretic studies.

Important Experimental Variables in Sonophoresis
(i) US duty cycle in range of 25%, 50% allow to reduce the possibility of damage from excess of heat or other effects.
(ii) Distance between US horn and the skin conductivity enhancement is affected directly by the distance between the skin and horn, this increase with the decreasing distance of the horn from the skin.
(iii) Treatment time, applied pre-treatment US and a prolonged time of exposure enhance the permeability of the skin.
(iv) Composition of the US coupling medium coupling agents must have certain characteristics for application in US therapies, within the most used and best result are water and gels, that's because they present the best acoustic features.

3. ADVANTAGES AND DISADVANTAGES OF SONOPHORESIS

Sonophoresis can have different therapeutic applications and a large number of drugs can be delivered by topical and transdermal routes and to others non-conventional routes like ocular and nail DD. It is a physical penetration enhancer which is not as invasive whereby intact skin is maintained and therefore does not generate an immunological sensitization, when it is applied, disrupts the lipid barrier of the skin by increasing the passage of drugs through it. The continuous or pulsatile US can increase the diffusion of drugs applied topically or transdermally allowing control the rate of penetration and thus reducing fluctuation in plasma drug concentrations. However, requires time to be administered, in addition the energy of US absorbed by the tissues ends turning into heat and raises the temperature of the area because molecules and tissues are subjected to HF vibrations and consequently the energy is transformed into heat. The main advantages and disadvantages of sonophoresis [37] are summarized in Table **4**.

Table 4. Summary of the benefits and drawbacks of using sonophoresis.

Advantages	***Disadvantages***
Low risk of infection because the skin remains intact [1]	
Greater diffusion of substance *vs* passive transport	Could consume more time
It lets you control the penetration velocity	Irritation, tingling or burns maybe occur but is easily to eliminated only adjusting the US [38]) An intact skin for a better penetration [13, 36]
Reduction of fluctuation in plasma level of drugs [1]	
Enables fast ending of DD by US [13]	
Allows both local and systemic effects [1]	
Intact skin: consequently uninfected and not immunological sensitizing	
It causes less anxiety compared with injections	
Greater patient satisfaction [36]	
Absorption is not as fast as an injectable in case of adverse reaction [36]	
Useful for gene therapy [13]	
It has been utilized in physiotherapy [36]	
Helpful to disintegration of blood clots	

4. ULTRASOUND THERAPEUTICAL APPLICATIONS

4.1. Drug Delivery

4.1.1. Topical/Transdermal Drug Delivery

Sonophoresis is a good physical promoter for transdermal [39 - 78], ungual/ transungual [79 - 81], and ocular [82] delivery of drugs and besides of other important applications (tumors, kelloids, wound healing, *etc.*) [83 - 91]. In Tables **5** and **6** we are able to read the condensed investigations on US and many experimental conditions.

4.1.2. Ocular Drug Delivery

US gives us the opportunity provide an excellent technique for eye release [79].

Zderic *et al.* [80] demonstrated that US improve by up to 10 times the permeability of the cornea by beta-blockers and fluorescein. Enhancement of sodium fluorescein, in corneas of rabbit was obtained by means of US at a F of 880 kHz. Another study Zderic *et al.* [81] investigated the application of a US standard pulsation I of 14 W/cm^2, for improving corneal permeability of atenolol, carteolol, timolol and betaxolol for treating glaucoma. All corneal cases increased the permeability by different amounts for an hour after contact US *in vitro*.

Table 5. Investigations on uses of sonophoresis using different drugs.

Topical /Transdermal Drug Delivery			
Anaesthetics			
Research	**Results**	**Author(s)**	**Ref.**
Lidocaine skin penetration	Topical application of US increased the concentration of lidocaine in an animal model (rabbit)	Wells *et al.*	[39]
Double blind trial in healthy volunteers for lidocaine cream	Not increasing absorption of lidocaine in cream by using US	McEnlay *et al.*	[40]
Trial in healthy volunteers for lidocaine oil	It was found that the variation in concentrations of lidocaine induce differences in US frequencies	Novak *et al.*	[41]

(Table 5) contd.....

Topical /Transdermal Drug Delivery			
Lidocaine skin penetration	Increase the penetration of lidocaine at 250 kHz	Griffin and Touchstone.	[42]
Impact of lidocaine by use of US	Combining US with local applied solution of lidocaine increase drug efficacy in the mice	Tachibana *et al.*	[43]
Topical sonophoresis of benzocaine and dibucaine	The increased penetration of the anaesthetic was not detectable	Williams *et al.*	[44]
Transdermal lidocaine dispensation with US.	It was used US 0.5 MHz to promote the penetration of lidocaine hydrochloride, which showed it was more effective to 1 MHz and this F is most commonly used in clinical situations	Kim *et al.*	[45]
Procaine hydrochloride permeation by US.	Rate of permeation (procaine hydrochloride) through MDCK could be monitored.	Hehn *et al.*	[46]
Painkillers and Drugs for Inflammation			
Research	**Results**	**Author(s)**	**Ref.**
Permeation of non-steroidal drugs for inflammation throughout skin	The synergistic effect on the transport of NSAIDs by modifying the parameters of temperature and US function was demonstrated	Meshali *et al.*	[47]
US penetration of indomethacin from an ointment in rats	In the case of indomethacin it was observed that the duration (10 minutes) at I (0.75 W/cm^2) play an important role for sonophoretic delivery of the drug	Miyazaki *et al.*	[48]
The impact of US on ketorolac tromethamine penetration *in vitro* throughout skin	Significant increase in the concentration of ketorolac applied in rat skin after being treated with ultrasound 3 W/cm^2 compared with permeation at 1 and 2 W/cm^2 was observed	Tiwari *et al.*	[49]
Permeation of ketorolac tromethamine (KT) gel by US.	The effect of gel contained KT for transdermal application had significant anti-inflammatory effects when is combined with sonophoresis	Yang *et al.*	[50]
US (ibuprofen nurofen gel at 5%) in humans	There is an efficiency of 5% Nurofen when applied transdermally to treat osteoarthrosis	Serikov *et al.*	[51]
Examination of therapeutic effects of sonophoresis with ketoprofen gel	When a ketoprofen gel is used with US, positive and significant results were obtained in objective assessments (clinical examination) and subjective (the interview)	Cabak *et al.*	[52]
To deliver ketoprofen into and across the skin by testing LF sonophoresis at 20 kHz.	Transdermal and topical administration of ketoprofen improves considerably when using LF sonophoresis once the parameters are optimized US	Herwadkar *et al.*	[53]
Using US for sodium diclofenac	Before applied US enhances the percutaneous penetration of diclofenac in gel (topical use), while the mechanism is unclear	Rosim *et al.*	[54]

(Table 5) contd.....

Topical /Transdermal Drug Delivery			
In vitro/in vivo effect of flufenamic with US.	Using *in vitro* pattern, allows to correlate with *in vivo* transdermal administration of flufenamic	Hippius *et al.*	[55]
Antibiotics			
Research	**Results**	**Author(s)**	**Ref.**
US release of topically applied amphotericin B.	The skin Amphotericin B quantity was higher using US	Rornanenko and Araviiskii.	[56]
Sonophoresis and electrophoresis tetracycline application in rabbits	Increased tissue levels of tetracycline administered with electro and sonophoresis.	Ragelis *et al.*	[57]
Immunosuppressives			
Topical Cyclosporin A transportation by means of LF of US	The accumulation of cyclosporin A in the skin caused by the application of a LF of US in conjunction with chemical enhancers could significantly help the penetration of the drug without observing an increase in adverse reactions.	Liu *et al.*	[58]
LF sonophoresis for treatment of alopecia areata, melasma and solar lentigo.	Results of LF with US increased penetration of topical agents generated an effect at skin.	Santoianni *et al.*	[59]
Antitumor Drugs			
Nanobubbles and US for cancer and gene therapy.	A drastic reduction of tumour dimension was observed.	Aoi *et al.*	[60]
Carry of 5-fluorouracil through skin by using US	It was shown that ultrasonication causes a reduction of drug diffusion transdermally	Meidan *et al.*	[61]
Insulin			
Glucose reduction in hyperglycemic rabbits.	Levels of glucose decreased faster and to a level of -200.8±5.9 mg/dL after 90 minutes	Luis *et al.*	[62]
US transdermal delivery (TD) of insulin *in vivo* using rabbits.	For the group that was tested US-insulin it was found that the glucose level decreased after 60 minutes at levels -132.6 ± 35.7 mg/dL	Lee *et al.*	[63]
Release of insulin with the use of a cymbal transducer US.	A cohort was exposed 60 minutes to US, the glucose levels were in the parameters of - -267.5 ± 61.9 mg/dL in an hour, on the other hand the group that used insulin was exposed for 20 min at the same conditions with similar results	Smith *et al.*	[64]
Corticosteroids			
US effect on dexamethasone through the skin	By applying dexamethasone in the skin and combined with sonophoresis, the sonophoretic effect was observed	Saliba *et al.*	[65]

(Table 5) contd.....

Topical /Transdermal Drug Delivery			
US increases the flow of transdermal corticosteroids.	When using US in combination with dexamethasone could measure in terms of the reduction of collagen in the deep layers of the skin	Byl *et al.*	[66]
Use of sonophoresis and iontophoresis in administration of dexamethasone for recovering knee osteoarthritis	Important improvement in total WOMAC scores was analysed in improvement rate of knee osteoarthritis by using phonophoresis and iontophoresis.	Akinbo *et al.*	67]
Design of a sonophoretic arrangement (DSS) to improve permeation of triamcinolone	Use of US at LF, continuous mode and high intensity, increased the permeation of triamcinolone	Yang *et al.*	[68]
Cardiotonics			
Research	**Results**	**Author(s)**	**Ref.**
US *in vitro* mouse and human skin permeation of digoxin	US is not increasing digoxin skin penetration	Machet *et al.*	[69]
Vasodilators			
Percutaneous diffusion of methyl nicotinate in in good physical shape patients.	US previously applied improve the percutaneous absorption of methyl nicotinate.	McEnlay *et al.*	[70]
Hormones			
Use of chemical enhancers, lipid microparticles (SLM), LF and HF US for testosterone skin penetration.	Use of chemical enhancers has not increased permeation of testosterone in comparison of LF US and HF US. The use of SLM gives an extra skin defence.	El-Kamel *et al.*	[71]
Cicatrizants			
US efficacy of hyaluronan using an *in vivo* osteoarthritis pattern.	Fluoresce microscopy analysis of synovial fluid showed that absorption of HA1000 and HA3000 was increased.	Park *et al.*	[72]
Calcein			
Calcein and-labelled dextran's penetration across the skin under the influence of US.	Excellent correlations were showed for all dextran's evaluated.	Morimoto *et al.*	[73]
Oligonucleotides			
Assessment of the potential of LF US to release of oligonucleotides.	Heterogeneous diffusion into the skin was revealed with microscopic evaluations	Tezel *et al.*	[74]
Stimulants			
Use of LF US for fentanyl and caffeine throughout two kind of skins (rat and human)	Is more effective the discontinuous US mode in fentanyl transdermal diffusion. On the contrary, for caffeine the pulse mode is preferred.	Boucaud *et al.*	[75]

(Table 5) contd.....

Topical /Transdermal Drug Delivery			
To optimize US protocol for studying *in vitro* transdermal DD of caffeine	The best conditions for the skin permeation of caffeine were: current 5 minutes, 10% working pulse and an I of 0.37 W/cm^2	Sarheed & Abdul Rasool.	[76]
Calcium			
Research	**Results**	**Author(s)**	**Ref.**
Manipulation of the Ca^{2+} by phonophoresis by using mouse stratum corneum.	The barrier function with 15 MHz is not altered by using US	Menon *et al.*	[77]
Panax Notoginseng			
Effect of a therapeutic US coupled with a Panax notoginseng gel to mend rat ligaments.	An excellent effect in ligaments was observed.	Ng *et al.*	[78]
Ocular Drug Delivery			
To demonstrate that US enhances sodium fluoresceine corneal permeability in rabbit.	Corneal permeability for compounds like fluorescein and beta blockers increases 10 times with US	Zderic *et al.*	[80]
Enhancement of corneal permeability of different drugs for treatment of glaucoma.	The permeability *in vitro* of rabbit cornea increase in different orders for glaucoma drugs behind sixty minutes with ultrasound.	Zderic *et al.*	[81]
Transcleral delivery of dyes (Rhodamine 6 G)	HF US (1.1 MHz, with application time of 10-50 milliseconds in porcine sclera) can augment the penetration depth of bicinchoninic acid and Rhodamine fluorescence by two times in opposition to passive diffusion.	Murugappan & Zhou.	[82]
LF US for transferring macromolecules to the eye.	LF US (40 kHz in continuous mode) considerably improved the permeation of dextrans by transscleral route in New Zealand rabbits. There were not undesirable effects.	Suen *et al.*	[83]
Nail Drug Delivery			
Design of a novel US-mediated drug delivery system (DDS) for treatment of onychomycosis	Use of US may be a promising alternative for the treatment of onychomycosis	Abadi & Zderic.	[84]
Other Important Therapeutic Applications in Addition to Drug Delivery			
(i) Diffusion mechanisms owing to ultrasound across the skin			
Use of calcein and US to study skin perviousness across transport skin regions.	Calcein permitted to study the way of penetration of substances throughout the skin.	Kushner IV *et al.*	[85]
LF US increases skin penetration.	Under application of LF US lipids in SC (30%) were detached for the duration of process	Alvarez-Roman *et al.*	[86]

(Table 5) contd.....

Topical /Transdermal Drug Delivery			
Analysis of short periods of US	A short time of appliance of US increased transport of fluorescein through the skin for a factor (2–9)	Cancel *et al.*	[87]
Utilization of LF US and quantum dots as display technique in different kind of microscopies.	US augmented flow in lacunar spaces in skin. Lacunar spaces were increased by using lauryl sulfate in combination with LF US.	Paliwal *et al.*	[88]
(ii) Scarfs			
US treatment by means of a hydrogel.	Absolute smashing of scarfs using US by 4 minutes.	Walker.	[89]
(iii) Tumors			
Optimization of US for *in vivo* bleomycin release.	Antitumor result has been shown in tumors in human cell lines and murine	Larkin *et al.*	[90]
Use of HF US on tumors.	HUS enhanced tumor uptake at short times.	Khaibullina *et al.*	[91]
(iv) To treat Injuries			
Handling purulent wounds by using US.	The use of US and ethylenediaminetetra acetic acid and quinoxaline antibiotic showed to be efficient to accelerate disinfection and elimination of necrotic tissues	Levenets.	[92]
Treatment of suppurated wounds with US.	The use of papain (1% solution) with dimethyl sulfoxide using US resulted in a very interesting way to treat suppurated wounds	Matinian *et al.*	[93]

Table 6. Experimental conditions for different researchers to study transdermal, ungual and ocular delivery of drugs by sonophoresis.

Drug	Experimental Conditions Used by Different Researchers for Topical Transdermal Drug Delivery	Ref.
Lidocaine	▪ Healthy volunteers ▪ Rabbit skin ▪ Different drug concentrations and frequencies (250-100kHz)	[39 - 45]
Procaine hydrochloride	▪ Cultured epithelial cell ▪ Continuous irradiation of 1.0 W/cm^2	[46]
Piroxicam	▪ Membranes ▪ 0.5 - 3.0 W/cm^2	[47]
Ibuprofen	▪ Membranes ▪ 0.5 - 3.0 W/cm^2	[47]
Sodium diclofenac	▪ Membranes ▪ 0.5 - 3.0 W/cm^2 ▪ Humans	[47, 54]

(Table 6) contd.....

Drug	Experimental Conditions Used by Different Researchers for Topical Transdermal Drug Delivery	Ref.
Indomethacin	▪ Rat skin ▪ I (0.25 - 1 W/cm^2), Time 5-20min.	[48]
Ketorolac tromethamine	▪ Rat skin ▪ Continuous mode, I 1-3 W/cm^2 and a F of 1 MHz for 30 minutes.	[49, 50]
Ketoprofen	▪ Humans ▪ Pulsation manner of US with I of 0.8 W/cm^2 ▪ Hairless rat skin ▪ F of 20kHz	[52, 53]
Flufenamic acid	▪ Human skin ▪ Range of intensities (up to 1.5W/cm^2) Time US energy between 5 and 30 min	[55]
Amphotericin B	▪ Guinea pigs ▪ Dimethyl sulfoxide as a chemical penetration enhancer	[56]
Tetracycline	▪ Healthy rabbits ▪ Galvanization apparatus "Potok-1"	[57]
Ciclosporin A	▪ Rat skin ▪ Using chemical promoters (Azone® and sodium lauryl sulfate) ▪ 3 treatment with Azone®+US + electroporation	[58]
Methyl prednisolone	▪ Human patients affected with alopecia ▪ F 25kHz	[59]
Ganciclovir	▪ Mice bearing subcutaneous tumors ▪ US and nano/microbubbles ▪ Low-intensity pulsed US (1 MHz; 3 W/cm^2)	[60]
5- Fluorouracil	▪ Whole rat skin ▪ heat-alone and Azone® enhancement	[61]
Insulin	▪ Hyperglycemic rabbits and New Zealand white rabbits ▪ 3x1 rectangular cymbal array ▪ 50 mWcm^{-2} ▪ Rats ▪ US exposure for 60 min (100 mW/cm^2)	[62 - 64]
Hydrocortisone acetate and Dexamethasone	▪ Yucatan pigs ▪ 1.5 W/cm^2, 1 MHz, 5 minutes	[66]
Dexamethasone sodium phosphate	▪ Patients with knee joint osteoarthritis ▪ F of 1 MHz for 5 minutes	[67]
Triamcinolone acetonide	▪ Mouse skin ▪ F (1.0, 3.0 MHz), I (1.0, 2.5 W/cm^2), and (constant and pulsation mode)	[68]

(Table 6) contd.....

Drug	Experimental Conditions Used by Different Researchers for Topical Transdermal Drug Delivery	Ref.
Digoxin	▪ Human and hairless mouse skin ▪ Continuous mode, I of 1, 3 W/cm^2 and F of 3.3 MHz for ten minutes	[69]
Methyl nicotinate	▪ Healthy human volunteers ▪ 3.0 MHz, 1.0 W/cm^2 nonstop manner for 5 min	[70]
Testosterone	▪ Abdominal rat skin ▪ Use of transdermal penetration enhancers (1% oleic acid or 1% dodecylamine)	[71]
Hyaluronan	▪ An animal model of osteoarthritis (knee rabbits) ▪ 1 MHz, 400 mW/cm^2 applied by ten minutes	[72]
Calcein	▪ Hairless rat skin ▪ 41 kHz, 60-300 mW/cm^2	[73]
Oligonucleotids	▪ Human skin ▪ 20 kHz, 2.4 W/cm^2	[74]
Fentanyl and Caffeine	▪ Human and hairless rat skin ▪ 20 kHz US constant or alternating mode, I of 2.5 W/cm^2	[75]
Caffeine	▪ Porcine skin ▪ F of 20kHz at different (5seconds-10 minutes) by means of three different modes (10%, 33% or 100% duty cycles) and two different sonication actions	[76]
Calcium	▪ Hairless mouse SC ▪ 15 MHz	[77]
Panax notoginseng	▪ Rats with injured ligaments by surgery. ▪ Duration of treatment: 2 weeks ▪ Four minutes of pulsate ultrasound (1 MHz) at I of 0.5W/cm^2	[78]
Drug	**Experimental Conditions Used by Different Researchers for Ocular Drug Delivery**	Ref.
Sodium fluoresceine	▪ Rabbit cornea ▪ F of 880kHz with I of 0.19-0.56 W/cm^2 and duration of five min.	[80]
Atenolol, carteolol, timolol and betaxolol	▪ Rabbit cornea ▪ 20 kHz US	[81]
Dye (Rodhamine 6G)	▪ Porcine sclera ▪ 1.1 MHz, pulse duration of 10-50	[82]
Macromolecules (Dextrans)	▪ New Zealand rabbit's sclera ▪ I: 0.12 W/cm^2, 40 kHz and continuous mode	[83]
Drug	**Experimental Conditions Used by Different Researchers for Nail Drug Delivery**	Ref.
Drugs for onychomycosis	▪ Canine nails ▪ Three different energy modes.	[84]

Murugapan and Zhou [82] have good results by using high intensity focused US instead of LF US for trans sclera DD in *ex vivo* porcine sclera. The conditions of the experiments were 100 HF US pulses with a F of 1.1 MHz and a duration of pulses of 10-50 ms. Penetration of Rodamine 6G dye by using passive diffusion and US was evaluated. They found that HF US increased penetration dye depth by 2.0 folds with no morphological sclera changes for the use of US.

Suen *et al.* [83] on the other hand, have evaluated the use of LF US (Intensity of 0.12 W/cm^2, F of 40 kHz and 90 seconds in continuous mode) in the permeation of macromolecules by transscleral route throughout New Zealand rabbit's sclera. LF US considerably enhanced the dextran eye penetration, with no adverse effects after two weeks of US appliance.

4.1.3. Application in Nail by US

Treatment for diseases in nails is complex due to low permeability of the nail. Currently Abadi and Zderic [84] have designed a DDS using US for the treatment of onychomycosis which allows increasing the permeability of the nails. *In vitro* tests dog nails were put through to three modes of energy (1.2 W for 30, 60 and 120 sec). Showing all statistical difference compared with control ($p < 0.05$) with a permeability factor of 1.3, 1.3 and 1.5 times at 30 sec, 60 sec and 120 sec. This US device is a promising alternative for administering drugs through nail.

4.2. Gene Delivery

Gene therapy is a procedure wherein a gene that is functional is introduced into a patient's cells to correct a genetic defect or provide the cells new function (Fig. **3**).

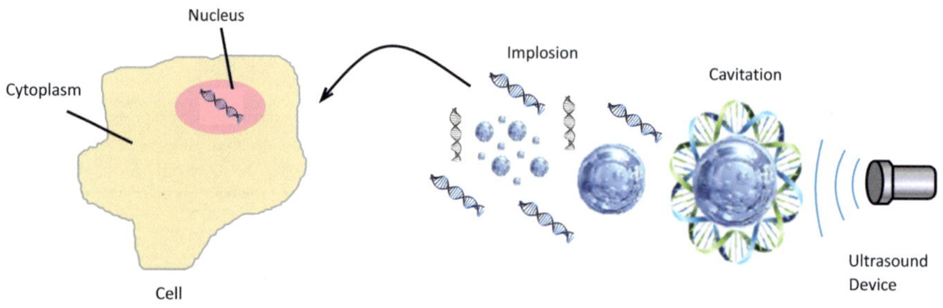

Fig. (3). Ultrasound gene therapy.

Such therapies are performed by viral gene, but can also be done by non-viral methods. The non-viral gene transfer has highlighted some important features [94]. Gene delivery methods are applied *in vivo*, they are simple and direct, the therapeutic agents are generally inexpensive and easy to manufacture, non-viral agents can be mixed and coupled in different combinations, giving flexibility to a desired therapeutic goal [95], the non-viral agent can be administered in repeated doses over time, non-viral vectors can be used for immunization due to dendritic cells and antigen presenting cells of Langerhans located in the skin.

Initial attempts of *in vitro* transfection dates back to 1987 when Fechheimer *et al.* [96] reported a low level of transfected murine fibroblasts using 3 half-second pulses with an intensity of 20 kHz with a sonicator used to homogenize tissues. All these techniques were improved and currently transfections are performed in a variety of eukaryotic cells. The US increases the permeability of the cell membrane and hence can be administered plasmids and genetic material. This technique is usually performed by injection of DNA plasmids and subsequently applying ultrasonic waves to assist the migration and penetration of the material into cells to be treated. The combination of microbubbles with US has been shown to increase the penetration of genetic material considerably [97]. To date, this methodology was applied in combination with microbubbles and ultrasonic irradiation in vascular cells, muscle and mouse fetuses [98].

The effectiveness of the sonoporation may depend on the cellular cycle phase wherein the cells are sonoporated, since these have different viscoelastic membrane properties depending on the stage in the cycle in which they are [99]. Also when changing the membrane permeability of small blood vessels due to US by the generation of microbubbles, can cause leakage of particles into the interstitial space [100, 101].

The approximations of non-viral gene therapy in skin results in a transient gene expression and variation of gene expression levels due to rapid replacement and renewal of epithelial cells [102], in addition, are up to 1000 times less efficient than viral therapies, as well as cause cellular acute toxicity and cell death in many cases.

4.3. Sports Medicine

US in sports have shown that this technique has no adverse effects within the range considered therapeutic (1-3 MHz F, I of 1-2 W/cm^2, lasting 5-10 minutes, continuous or pulsed mode) [103, 104]. Its therapeutic effectiveness was confirmed in tissue damaged and other conditions found in sport medicine [105 - 133].

There are other important uses of sonophoresis like sonothrombolysis for intra-cerebral hemorrhage [134 - 138], in physiotherapy primarily on the management of lesions, for increasing healing of lesion, reduction of edema and to make the damaged tissue stronger and more elastic [139 - 147].

5. SONOPHORETIC DEVICES

Sonophoretic equipment produces waves based on a power unit, wherein the energy is transformed into mechanic power by distortion of a piezoelectric material, and the waves are conveyed by molecular swings [148, 149].

Design and production of new and more efficient portable devices makes an interesting research area in sonophoresis. An example of this was the generation of a miniature transducer used in US studies [150]. The use of US by new transducers for improving transfer of insulin through skin was investigated. A cymbal transducer was used and set up for releasing insulin *via* transdermal route [151]. A sonophoresis device (weighs only 73.3 g) with dual flat flextensional US transducers with an acoustic I is higher than a solo US transducer has already been developed [152].

A lot of sonophoresis devices have been developed to the present days. It was proved that it is feasible to use short US exposure times to noninvasively release dosage of insulin to diminish the levels of glucose in blood, using a dish mold [153]. Similar results were found using a circular cymbal US array to deliver insulin in different animal models (pigs, rabbits and rats) [62 - 64, 153]. Efficiency of DD was improved using rectangular cymbal design [62]. Feasibility of a lightweight US cymbal transducer array for delivering transdermal insulin across the skin in animal model was assessed [154]. Results indicated that with a short exposure time US is sufficient to administer a dose of insulin capable of lowering blood glucose levels.

5.1. Sonophoretic Systems Available in the Market

5.1.1. Patch-Cap™, U-strip™, U-Wand™ and A-Wand™ Devices

Dermisonics® (USA) is a therapeutic apparatus company which develops and commercializes a transdermal patch system (TP) for releasing high molecular weight substances inside systemic circulation. Company patented the ultrasonic Patch-Cap™ device in June 2005, which represents a film system for TDD (mainly for applying antiseptic solutions to cuts, scrapes and lacerations) *via* US (Fig. **4**). The Patch-Cap™ device has the drug in a reservoir without adhesives.

The Medi-Cap is another device patented by Dermisonics Inc., USA that replaces conventional TP, U-Strip™ ultrasound TD apparatus (Dermisonics Inc, USA). It has a reservoir of therapeutic ingredient with US equipment (Fig. **5**) [155, 156]. U-strip™ machinery enables TD of insulin and could be promising to deliver other drugs that not have an effectively release across the skin [155].

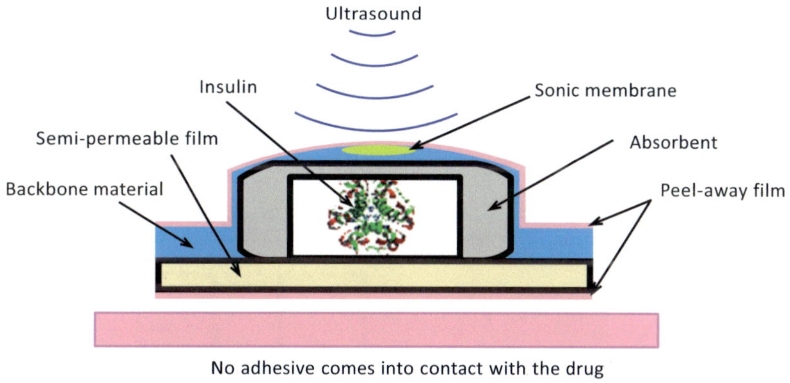

Fig. (4). Ultrasonic patch-cap.

The U-Strip™ system is a noninvasiveness drug release that uses sonophoresis [79]. Hence, the device is an ultrasound release method that utilizes discontinuous sonic conduction to affect dilation skin pores and put down high molecular weight drugs into the skin. U-Strip™ produces a discontinuous US wave (Fig. **6**). Signal alternation decreases the warmth, which can affect the drug in a TP DS [157]. Dermisonics Inc., USA has produced a mold system, which is able to make their own production of transducers (Redding Generation-5 transducers-last name of his inventor) [158].

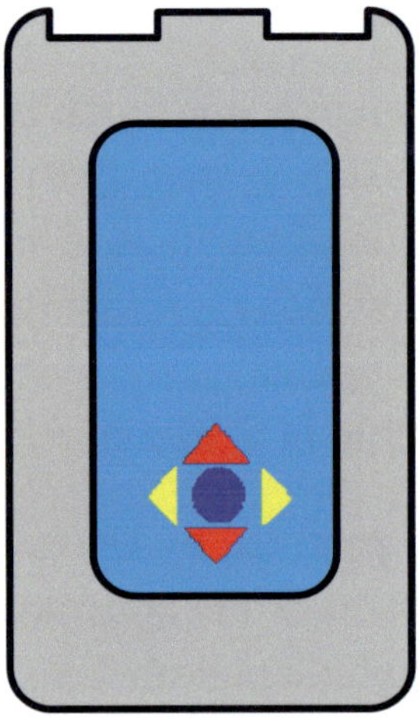

Fig. (5). Medi-Cap device.

Dermisonics Inc. (USA) has developed portable ultrasound systems as U-Wand™ with application in skin care and A-Wand ™ for medical purposes. The A-Wand can be applied for antiseptic solutions, cuts or lesions. U-Wand ™ can also be used for cosmetic products.

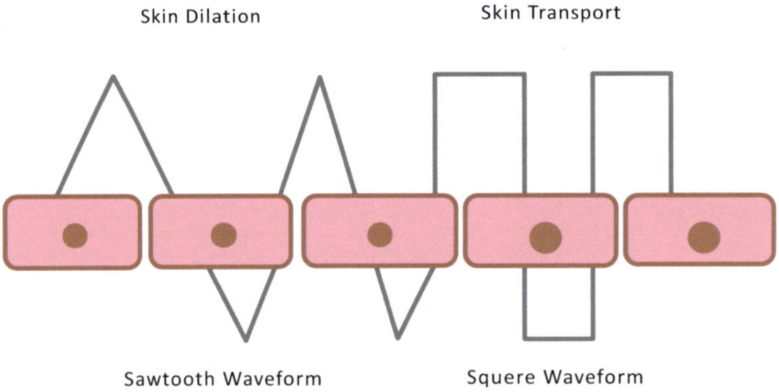

Fig. (6). The alternating signal.

5.1.2. Sonoderm Technology

Another interesting sonophoretic device is Sonoderm®, that is manufactured by BioMedical Electronics (France) is an Anti-Aging Company, which integrates a set of additional technologies which brings a personalized answer to slimming and cellulite issues (Fig. **7**) [159].

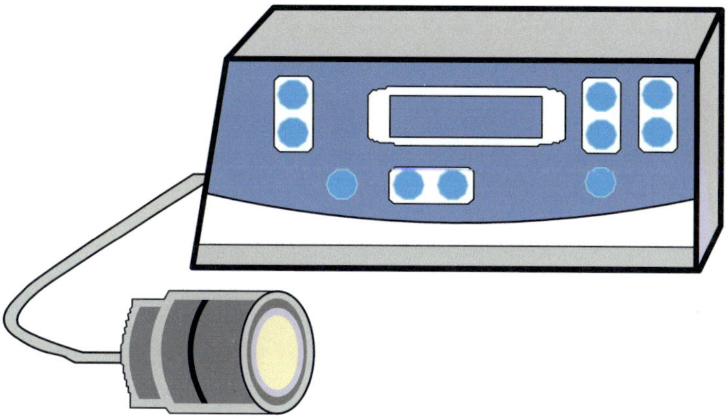

Fig. (7). Sonophoretic device (Sonoderm®).

The Sonoderm™ is a generator of US, when is applied directly in the skin has a decongestant action of adipose tissue, improving the appearance of orange peel skin. The device has a movable transducer which allows to be used comfortably in all areas of the body, thus allowing cellular exchanges into fibrosis areas [160, 161]. For large molecules or drugs may be useful for assisted transdermal transport [14].

5.1.3. SonoLysis

In early 2008, ImaRx Therapeutics, Inc., USA developed an US-enhanced transdermal drug DS called SonoLysis. It includes the administration of their microbubble-based agent MRX-801 and US with or without a thrombolytic drug to disintegrate thrombus. MRX-801microbubles are a proprietary encapsulating formulation in an inert gas through a lipid envelope [162]. These microbubbles involves intravenous injection of a contrast solution containing microbubbles of a gas called perfluten [138], covered by a lipid membrane that circulate through the blood, which when in contact with US explode and release energy. This released energy within clogged cerebral artery by a blood clot, accelerates disintegration of it for better recovery of patient because shortens the time of recanalization (unclogging cerebral artery).

ImaRx Therapeutics, Inc. performed its TUCSON (Transcranial Ultrasound in Clinical SONoLysis) United States Food and Drug Administration (US FDA) clinical pilot with 35 patients. Randomized, placebo controlled clinical pilot to evaluate, tolerability, therapeutic effectiveness of application of MRX-801 and US energy (*i.e.*, Sonolysis™) as an adjunctive therapy (tPA) management in patients with severe ischemic stroke, however, in 2008, 3 patients enrolled in the TUCSON trial had brain hemorrhages and the product (Sonolysis™) was recalled because it needed to pass security tests. So, ImaRx Therapeutics, Inc. suspended their further enrollment in the trial.

More lately the results from the TUCSON trial were again analyzed and showed at the Statistical analysis revealed that 67% of patients who received tPA with MR X-801 (1.4 ml) 67% had clean arteries after 36 hours compared with 46% of those who received tPA with MRX -801 (2.8 ml) and 33% who received only tPA. Patients who had blockages and received Sonolysis therapy 30 min their arteries had been cleaned, compared to patients who received tPA alone (control group). After 90 days around of 75% of patients who received the dose of MRX-801 (1.4 ml) had progress in their disability scores compared to the control group with 36%. Here, researchers suggested that investigations with SonoLysis should continue for the treatment of two different groups of patients with acute ischemic stroke [163].

Group 1 included 18 patients that received either a single vial (1.8mL) of MRX-801 (n=12) or placebo (n=6). Group 2 included 17 patients, where 11 patients received two vials (2.8mL) of MRX-801 and 6 patients received no treatment. Preliminary safety data indicated that in group 2 more intracranial hemorrhages occurred in patients that received study drug (tPA) compared to controls. The Company suspended the enrollment again. A researcher of ImaRx Therapeutics, Inc. noted that there is a known association between tPA and the risk of intracranial hemorrhage. It was suggested to conduct SONoLysis clinical trials without using tPA [164].

5.1.4. ClotBust-ER™

Cerevast Therapeutics, Inc., (USA, 2009) acquired the assets of ImaRx Therapeutics, Inc., with main importance in the area of SonoLysis for the treatment of acute ischemic stroke and other vascular disorders. This non-invasive treatment called the ClotBust-ER™, is a device to securely administer the US energy for SonoLysis treatment (Fig. **8**) [165].

Clinical studies have shown that applying conventional US for tPA intravenous thrombolytic therapy, dissolve blood clots in ischemic brain regions and restore blood flow [137, 166 - 169]. When the tissue containing fluid (such as blood), US energy is transformed into kinetic energy of the fluid. This is called acoustic flow, which is the main means of fibrinolysis US-potentiated in which additional fibrin binding sites are exposed to plasmin at the site of the clot [170].

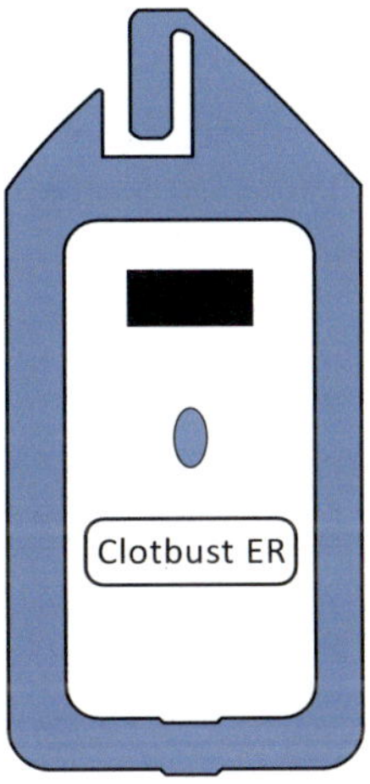

Fig. (8). ClotBust-ER™ device.

ClotBust ER™ device works with multiple transducers operating at 2 MHz. These transducers are on an adjustable head structure, which allows the transducers to be posted on the site where they will be given the US in the main regions of occlusion that occur in the brain. Thus, the device applies the energy needed to achieve therapeutic acoustic streaming, enhancing clot lysis within the occluded vessel of the brain without the need for a trained sonographer.

5.1.4.1. Future Applications with Clotbuster

5.1.4.1.1. Spectral Doppler Add-on Module

Monitoring the blood flow in the brain with conventional devices is difficult to perform because it requires trained personnel. Having the ability to monitor the intracranial blood flow during treatment with SonoLysis is an attractive feature because it gives the clinician the ability to assess the recanalization of the occluded vessel in real time. Magnetic resonance nuclear imaging only provides an assessment of a point in time "snapshot" of blood flow. It is believed that the unique configuration of Clotbuster™ has the potential to simplify the procedure and provides clinicians with the ability to not only manage US energy to stroke patients, also allow recanalization simultaneously [165].

5.1.4.1.2. Microspheres

Studies conducted in humans with stroke by using US - tPA combined with microspheres as intravenous thrombolytic therapy [171 - 174]. The studies have provided results showing that the microspheres have ability to increase the therapeutic effect of Clot Buster for the treatment of ischemic stroke. These microspheres have an average diameter of 1.2 microns; small enough to penetrate into the fibrin of blood clots that cavitation (expansion and contraction) when subjected to the correct energy levels US, improving the acoustic streaming effect related with only US, thus enhancing dissolution of the clot.

5.1.5. EkoSonic® Endovascular System, EkoSonic® Endovascular System with MACH4e and EkoSonic® SV (Small Vessel) Endovascular System

The EKOS Company has developed devices for clinical-medical drugs administration by using ultrasound, with its first system (the Microlysis device) for vascular thrombosis in 2005. The devices EKOS generally hurry the diffusion of thrombolytic mediators in the thrombus, giving excellent stages of performance and security in lysis. In 2008, the company introduced 2nd-generation ITS EkoSonic® with quick pulsate variation for disbanding of vascular blood coagulates. EkoSonic® can transfer microsonic power, active substances and it is safe in removing clots. The EkoSonic Endovascular System® is endorsed by the FDA and other international agencies [175].

EkoSonic® MACH4e was introduced at 2009 and it was approved by the FDA for precise and specific application of medical solutions. Presently is utilized to treat arterial occlusion and others applications are being investigated [176]. The difference with its original generation of MicroSonic™ equipment is the rate, which raised the bar with MACH4. Nowadays the system of MACH4e is forty percent faster than EkoSonic® MACH4. The use of equipment shows no sign of hemolysis, dissolution thrombus time short that implies a lower dosage of the drug and lower risk of complications [177, 178].

Advantages of using the EkoSonic® Endovascular System with MACH4e:

- Penetrates thrombus in difficult places to access [179].
- Less lytic drug about 50-70% [179].
- No thrombus breakage, decreasing the danger of distal embolism [180].
- The thrombus can absorb more drug [180].
- It does not cause damage to the endothelium [178].
- It does not cause hemolysis [178].
- It becomes more permeable the vessel and eliminates completely thrombus [181].

Indications to use the EkoSonic® Endovascular System with MACH4e

- Outlying vasculature: EkoSonic™ and EkoSonic SV™ are designed for controlling and infusing medical solutions with drugs.
- Pulmonic blood vessel: EkoSonic™ is indicated for controlling infusion of thrombolytic medical solutions in outlying vasculature. Endovascular EkoSonic™ also is used in infusion solutions in the pulmonary arteries.

The company EKOS participate in the ATTRACT trial, to assess the advantages of US in dissolution of blood clots [176].

The EkoSonic® SV Endovascular System consists of the 3F microcatheter, 150 cm working length, central lumen, and the US element at tip. EkoSonic SV incorporates the technology ultrasonic that accelerated thrombolysis. Acoustical technologies increase the clots capacity to absorb the lytic, resulting in the speeding up of lysis. The design allows a level of flexibility that allows easily be used in small vessels inside the body [176].

Indications to use the EkoSonic SV Endovascular System

- Neuro Vasculature: This system is designed for the infusion of contrast materials into neurovasculature. But studies are needed to ensure thrombolytic therapy in neurovasculature and avoid adverse effects such as intracranial hemorrhage.
- *Coronary Vasculature:* The equipment is designed for managing specific fluids to the coronary vasculature. But the clot disruptions have not been established [176].

5.1.6. SonoPrep® Skin Permeation System

SonoPrep® (Fig. **9**), represents a non-invasive and painless technology used to enhance skin permeability for therapeutic and diagnostic purpose. SonoPrep® technology can be used for:

- Enhancement of transdermal permeation of drugs
- Needle free DD
- Continued glucose monitoring
- Analyte extraction

Advantages of the SonoPrep® device:

- Non-invasive,
- Painless,
- Not irritating,
- Needle free
- Safe,
- Easy to use,

- Cost-effective skin permeation process,
- Patient comfort, compliance and acceptable results.

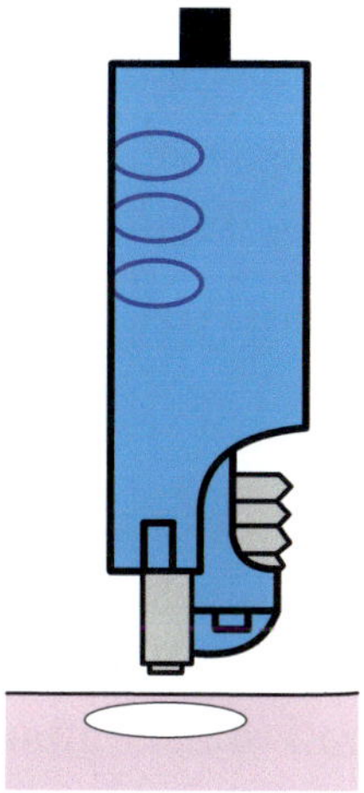

Fig. (9). Schematic representation of Sonoprep® device.

SonoPrep® is a device accepted by FDA, which is based on a program and an electric system among skin and the reference electrode to control conductance in actual moment and accomplish most favorable skin permeability. Short focal US can be used to momentarily diminish skin barrier [182]. The use of US increase the flow of glucose compared to the use of electrical current (iontophoresis) [6]. However, *Prelude SkinPrep System*™ which is intended to replace Sonoprep™ device has a not reusable end driven and an electric engine. The US uses a mechanical means to remove SC [183] using same mechanism of SonoPrep conductance. Both use the Symphony™ tCGM System (Echo Therapeutics), which contains a sensitive biosensor that can get in touch with skin using a hydrogel and an enzyme as chemical detector [184]. In addition, it has alarms for excessively high and low glucose levels [185].

Studies have shown that Prelude SkinPrep™ exhibited equal functions to SonoPrep™ for tCGM use. tCGM arrangement is an ideal therapeutic apparatus for diabetes treatment [186].

Simphony™ tCGM system is a noninvasive system that allows continuous glucose monitoring, providing real-time data monitoring and cost effectively to analyze glucose. Every one of FDA approved continuous glucose monitoring systems use needles, which leads to risk of infection. The system not uses needles and therefore does not give rise to the risk related with needles.

It is important to mention that Prelude® SkinPrep system is currently used as the first topical application of lidocaine, and it is intended that other drugs are incorporated into this system for the treatment of other conditions.

6. COMBINATION OF SONOPHORETIC SYSTEMS WITH OTHER ENHANCING TECHNOLOGIES

Studies show that LF US enhances drug permeation into the skin. However, combinations with additional techniques have shown to be more effective compared to only US. In particular, LF US (20 kHz-100 kHz) has been shown to synergistically enhance skin penetration in combination with chemical penetration promoters, iontophoresis and microneedles.

6.1. US and Chemical Penetration Enhancers

Chemical enhancers increase TD either by increasing the fluency of the lipids of stratum corneum otherwise changing the organization of lipids [187] or increasing diffusion coefficient of skin [188, 189]. Combination of US and surface active agents (*e.g.* sodium-lauryl-sulfate) augment the transfer [190]. However, the properties of the skin prevent that surfactants can spread easily and change our skin. It is thought that synergism between sonophoresis and surfactants is due to the skill of sonophoresis to augment concentration and spreading of surface active agents in SC, as a result of the increase in drug transport through the skin [191]. Chemical promoters make the skin permeable by making soluble or taking out skin lipids and this fact is enhanced with the use of US [192, 193]. Johnson *et al.*; did investigations about synergism of chemical promoters with US, with various combination of chemical promoters by using sonophoresis, they observed and interesting increasing in *in vitro* skin permeability [194]. The main result was that corticosterone in combination with ethanol/linoleic acid, at same magnitude increase permeability of skin by 8.7 and the flow of drug by 903. Nevertheless, when is combined with sonophoresis (1 MHz and 1.4 W/cm^2), permeation increase by 14.4 and flow in over 13 000 [194]. The authors explained that sonophoresis and linoleic acid enhancement is caused by the augment in fluency of lipid field in SC. Oleic acid (OA) is a penetration enhancer very useful in pharmaceutical products [195]. As additional example, the application of sodium luaryl sulphate lonely and US (20 kHz) lonely, improved skin permeation of mannitol by 3 and 8 units of magnitude, respectively. Yet the combination of US and 1% sodium lauryl sulfate amplify skin permeation of mannitol. In addition, without surface active agents the power of US to produce a flow of drug was 141 J/cm^2, while the combination of both decreased at 18 J/cm^2 [191].

Another study demonstrated the synergism between 1.1 and 3.3 MHz HF ultrasound and chemical enhancer laurocapram for delivering hydrocortisone through rat skin *in vitro* [196]. The penetration was accelerated by US thermal effects. Nonetheless, LF sonophoresis (20 kHz) using rat skin with Azone® or sodium lauryl sulfate enhanced synergistically topical release of cyclosporine A [6]. Others research showing synergism between US and chemical enhancers that include: 1) HF sonophoresis and d-limonene/ethanol on skin penetration of ketorolac-tromethamine across *in vitro* rat skin [48, 49], 2) HF sonophoresis and thiazone or glycerol to rise skin optical clearing [197 - 200], 3) HF sonophoresis (0.8MHz) and Azone®, oleic acid, or 2- propanediol on the *in vitro* release of sinomenine-hydrochloride across rat skin [28], 4) HF sonophoresis (0.8 MHz) and ethanol-with aqueous gels on the release of ibuprofen across *in vitro* and *in vivo* skin´s rabbit [201], 5) LF sonophoresis (20 kHz) and capsaicin or nonivamide on the transdermal flow of indomethacin throughout mouse skin *in vitro* [202],6) LF sonophoresis (20 kHz) and 14 diverse chemical promoters on *in vitro* transdermal penetration of tizanidine-hydrochloride throughout mouse skin [203], and vii) LF sonophoresis (20 kHz) and both liposomes and solid lipid structures to transport antigens across rat skin *in vitro* and *in vivo* [204], *etc.*

6.2. US and Iontophoresis

The physical enhancers that have been studied combined with LF sonophoresis and iontophoresis, increase the skin penetration with low electrical current. As an example, US (20 KHz, intensity of 7.4 W/cm^2 in a pulse mode) was applied once to each piece of skin (1% dodecyl pyridinium chloride solution as chemical penetration enhancer) for 10 min previous to application of iontophoresis. The current used in iontophoresis can modify skin penetration because change the organization lipids [205]. In the small period of time that skin barrier changes due to electrical current application, drugs or peptides of great molecular weight are able to pass the skin [206]. Heparin flux is improved because of the combination of US with iontophoresis as treatment was 56-fold, the result was higher than the sum of those obtained with iontophoresis or US both alone (3 and 15-fold respectively) [207]. In another study it was also found that LF sonophoresis (20 kHz) using iontophoresis (0.5 mA/cm^2) synergistically raised *in vitro* penetration of sodium nonivamide acetate through skin´s nude mouse [208]. Recently, it was used an intermediate US F (270 kHz) with the application of iontophoresis (20 V and 0.45–1.0 mA), It was observed insignificant improving when they are used apart, however used together augment release of antipyrine and sodiumsalicylate by ten-fold [209].

Another study found that in the case of non-ionized drugs with a molecular weight of 1000 Daltons or more, US and iontophoresis synergistically enhanced the drug permeation, while ionized drugs showed similar permeation profiles compared with only iontophoretic treatment. It was concluded, that the synergism between US-iontophoresis occurred due to the increased skin diffusivity followed by increased electroosmosis induced by cavitation and by an electroosmotic water flow) [210].

A synergistic effect was observed by using LF sonophoresis (SonoPrep® device, Echo Therapeutics, Franklin, MA), followed by 2 min of low-voltage iontophoresis (Phoresor PM700® device, Iomed Incorporated), to release local anesthetic Iontocaine® (Abbot Laboratories) [33]. In a similar study it was found that with higher US frequencies (1 MHz) and iontophoresis (5 mA) the delivery of cortisol was effective and it decreased the subjective pain complaints of patients with mild to intermediate stages of carpal tunnel syndrome [211].

6.3. US and Microneedles

Recently a study showed the existence of an array of microneedles with US (AMUS). The AMUS method enhanced greatly TD rates of calcein (623 Da) and bovine serum albumin (BSA) (66,430 Da). More importantly, the TDD of macromolecules can be performed. Using microneedles, the drug is released in epidermis with no bleeding or pain. The LF US produces little spaces into epidermis, enhancing transdermal transport of drugs. The scheme and the device are shown in Fig. (**10**).

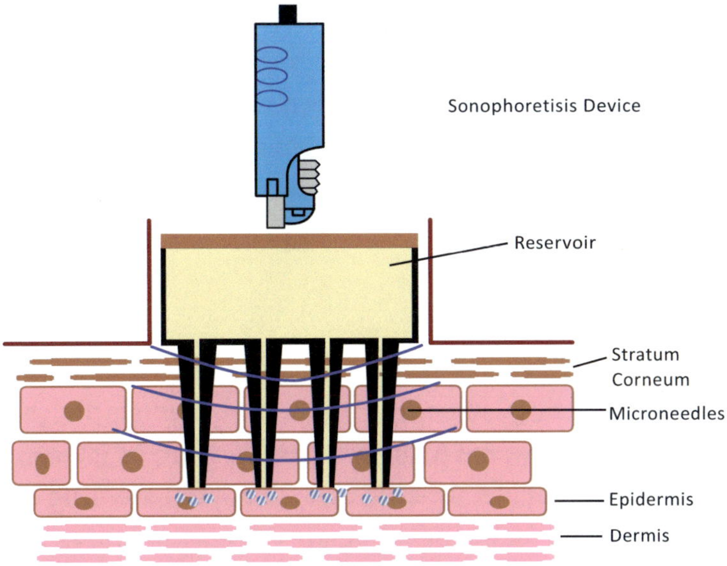

Fig. (10). The AMUS device applied in skin for transdermal DD.

The device is composed for two parts (empty microneedles and ultrasound transmitter). Microneedles are made with microfabrication technology and ultrasound transmitter with commercial available piezoelectric ceramic membrane. The piezoelectric have a pair of holes in its ultrasonic membrane and reservoir with drug [64].

Tested hydrophilic particles that calcein is not be able to spread into the skin by passive diffusion. Skin penetrability was increased 5 fold by microneedles compared to passive diffusion, 7 times increased by the use of sonophoresis and 9 fold by utilizing AMUS. Analogous outcomes were gotten with bovine albumin using microneedles increased 7 times, 8.5 fold with ultrasound and 12 fold with AMUS, compared to passive diffusion without microneedles. It was found that the bovine albumin was not being able to diffuse across skin with no enhancer due to its big size. Results show a great release of calcein (623 Da) and bovine serum albumin (BSA) (66,430 Da) [212]. Penetration doubles compared with the microneedles. Because the cavitation effect increases the permeability

Another study, shows that the combination of different enhancers like sonophoresis, microneedles and electroporation increase the total cumulative amount of hydrophilic macromolecular compound fluorescein isothiocyanate-dextran that is permeated on porcine skin using three methods in combination (sonophoresis, microneedles and electroporation) was better than among using a single method or two combinations (sonophoresis-microneedleso or other combination). These results suggest that combination of 3 techniques could help as a possible effective combination strategy to transdermally delivers of numerous hydrophilic macromolecules without skin harm or causing structural changes [213].

6.4. US and Nanocarriers Systems

DD investigations by using micelles and solid nanoparticles (polymeric, nanotubes and fullerenes, liposome nanoparticles, *etc.*) are of interest today [214]. In particular nanocarriers that can provide elevated cytotoxic drug concentrations in tissues selectively, thus reducing adverse effects in body. US is used in diagnostics, it is noninvasive and it is able to target the nanocarriers with drugs in an specific tissue [215].

Ultrasound delivery of drug from micelles typically employs polyether-bloc--copolymers and it has shown to be successful to treat tumors *in vivo*. US delivers the drug from micelles possibly by tension and tremor waves. Solid lipid nanoparticles and liquid emulsions are utilized with US to deliver genes *in vitro* and *in vivo*. This type of ultrasound has potential use for many drugs and genes and gives us the possibility of administering drugs by non-invasive means [214].

Actually there are reports mentioning that US can efficiently delivers different kind of substances for medical and pharmaceutical interest Marxer *et al.* [216] generated novel carriers of drugs with oil preparations. Related with SonoVue™, their carriers systems have adaptable and good characteristics as are their biocompatibility and high loading capacity. Becker *et al.* [217] studied the US and the antithrombotic effects of oil dispersals with SonoVue®. The particle size of dispersion of lipids was of 200 nm. Lipidic dispersion has good results for thrombolysis with US.

Additionally, it has been shown, that US and microbubbles improve cellular uptake of drugs inside kidneys. The microbubbles can induce changes in selectivity of the kidney allowing drugs to enter compartments which previously could not access. Microbubbles efficiency depends on the injection into the renal artery combining the drug and the microbubbles. Through this technique and conjugation of antibodies, when is injected it can also be used as a technique for diagnostic imaging US in the kidney or DD [218, 219].

CONCLUSION

Current evidence [9, 13, 15, 17, 36] suggests that sonophoresis is a potential method which improves the delivery of drugs, peptides and proteins by topical/transdermal route as well as ocular [80 - 83] and nail routes [84] (see Tables **5** and **6**).

US can also be administered in conjunction with enhancers such as chemical promoters [191, 196], electrical methods (iontophoresis and electroporation) [193, 210, 211, 220, 221], microneedles [64, 212, 222] and nanocarrier systems [214, 215, 223, 224] or combination of these, with the purpose to make more efficient the administration of drugs, peptides and proteins.

The use of US for other non-pharmaceutical applications is ultimately a very powerful tool, since it takes advantage of properties of US in tissue, such as tendons, muscles and bones. Physicochemical properties of US such as cavitation, tissue heating or the effect of the shock wave per se, mean that this physical enhancer can be used for physical therapy, sport medicine, to break up clots and preventing strokes, as well as their use in non-viral gene therapy, angiogenesis of jaws [225], and as an adjuvant in vaccines [226].

In summary, the use of sonic therapy in various areas has become a very important, noninvasive and economical option. In future, US will have more applications in many other areas for its versatility and safety.

CONFLICT OF INTEREST

The authors confirm that they have no conflict of interest to declare for this publication.

ACKNOWLEDGEMENTS

José Juan Escobar-Chávez wishes to acknowledge PAPIIT IT 200115, Cátedra PIAPI 1619 and PAPIME PE 200414.

REFERENCES

[1] Wood RW, Loomis AL. The physical and biological effects of high frequency sound waves of great intensity. Philos Mag 1927; 4: 417-36. [http://dx.doi.org/10.1080/14786440908564348]

[2] Benwell AD, Bly SH. Sources and applications of ultrasound. In: Repacholi MH, Grandolfo M, Rindi A, Eds. Ultrasound: Medical application, biological effects and hazard potentials. New York: Plenum Press 1987; pp. 29-47. [http://dx.doi.org/10.1007/978-1-4613-1811-8_3]

[3] Skauen DM, Zentner GM. Phonophoresis. Int J Pharm 1984; 20: 235-45. [http://dx.doi.org/10.1016/0378-5173(84)90171-6]

[4] McElnay JC, Matthews MP, Harland R, McCafferty DF. The effect of ultrasound on the percutaneous absorption of lignocaine. Br J Clin Pharmacol 1985; 20(4): 421-4. [http://dx.doi.org/10.1111/j.1365-2125.1985.tb05089.x] [PMID: 4074611]

[5] Mitragotri S, Blankschtein D, Langer R. Transdermal drug delivery using low-frequency sonophoresis. Pharm Res 1996; 13(3): 411-20. [http://dx.doi.org/10.1023/A:1016096626810] [PMID: 8692734]

[6] Kost J, Mitragotri S, Gabbay RA, Pishko M, Langer R. Transdermal monitoring of glucose and other analytes using ultrasound. Nat Med 2000; 6(3): 347-50. [http://dx.doi.org/10.1038/73213] [PMID: 10700240]

[7] Joshi A, Raje J. Sonicated transdermal drug transport. J Control Release 2002; 83(1): 13-22. [http://dx.doi.org/10.1016/S0168-3659(02)00200-6] [PMID: 12220834]

[8] Kushner J IV, Blankschtein D, Langer R. Heterogeneity in skin treated with low-frequency ultrasound. J Pharm Sci 2008; 97(10): 4119-28. [http://dx.doi.org/10.1002/jps.21308] [PMID: 18240305]

[9] ter Haar G. Therapeutic applications of ultrasound. Prog Biophys Mol Biol 2007; 93(1-3): 111-29. [http://dx.doi.org/10.1016/j.pbiomolbio.2006.07.005] [PMID: 16930682]

[10] Lavon I, Kost J. Ultrasound and transdermal drug delivery. Drug Discov Today 2004; 9(15): 670-6. [http://dx.doi.org/10.1016/S1359-6446(04)03170-8] [PMID: 15279850]

[11] Machet L, Boucaud A. Phonophoresis: efficiency, mechanisms and skin tolerance. Int J Pharm 2002; 243(1-2): 1-15. [http://dx.doi.org/10.1016/S0378-5173(02)00299-5] [PMID: 12176291]

[12] Merino G, Kalia YN, Guy RH. Ultrasound-enhanced transdermal transport. J Pharm Sci 2003; 92(6): 1125-37. [http://dx.doi.org/10.1002/jps.10369] [PMID: 12761802]

[13] Escobar-Chávez JJ, Bonilla-Martínez D, Villegas-González MA, Rodríguez-Cruz IM, Domínguez-Delgado CL. The use of sonophoresis in the administration of drugs throughout the skin. J Pharm Pharm Sci 2009; 12(1): 88-115. [http://dx.doi.org/10.18433/J3C30D] [PMID: 19470295]

[14] Saroha K, Sharma B. Yadav Bhavna. Sonophoresis: An advanced tool in transdermal drug delivery system. Int J Current Pharm Res 2011; 3(3): 89-97.

[15] Modi SB, Pokiya AB, Dhandhalya MC. A review on sonophoresis mediated transdermal drug delivery system. Am J Pharm Tech Res 2012; 2(3): 257-77.

[16] Zagzebski JA. Physics of diagnostic ultrasound. In: Lading DE, Potts L, Eds. Essentials of ultrasound physics. St. Louis, MO: Mosby-Year Book 1996; pp. 1-19.

[17] Polat BE, Hart D, Langer R, Blankschtein D. Ultrasound-mediated transdermal drug delivery: mechanisms, scope, and emerging trends. J Control Release 2011; 152(3): 330-48. [http://dx.doi.org/10.1016/j.jconrel.2011.01.006] [PMID: 21238514]

[18] Weyman AE. Physical principles of ultrasound. In: Weyman AE, Ed. Principles and practice of echocardiography. Philadelphia: Lea and Febiger 1991; pp. 3-28.

[19] Mitragotri S, Blankschtein D, Langer R. Ultrasound-mediated transdermal protein delivery. Science 1995; 269(5225): 850-3. [http://dx.doi.org/10.1126/science.7638603] [PMID: 7638603]

[20] Mitragotri S, Blankschtein D, Langer R. Transdermal drug delivery using low-frequency sonophoresis. Pharm Res 1996; 13(3): 411-20. [http://dx.doi.org/10.1023/A:1016096626810] [PMID: 8692734]

[21] Mitragotri S, Ray D, Farrell J, *et al.* Synergistic effect of low-frequency ultrasound and sodium lauryl sulfate on transdermal transport. J Pharm Sci 2000; 89(7): 892-900. [http://dx.doi.org/10.1002/1520-6017(200007)89:7<892::AID-JPS6>3.0.CO;2-V] [PMID: 10861590]

[22] Boucaud A, Montharu J, Machet L, *et al.* Clinical, histologic, and electron microscopy study of skin exposed to low-frequency ultrasound. Anat Rec 2001; 264(1): 114-9. [http://dx.doi.org/10.1002/ar.1122] [PMID: 11505377]

[23] Tang H, Mitragotri S, Blankschtein D, Langer R. Theoretical description of transdermal transport of hydrophilic permeants: application to low-frequency sonophoresis. J Pharm Sci 2001; 90(5): 545-68. [http://dx.doi.org/10.1002/1520-6017(200105)90:5<545::AID-JPS1012>3.0.CO;2-H] [PMID: 11288100]

[24] Tang H, Wang CC, Blankschtein D, Langer R. An investigation of the role of cavitation in low-frequency ultrasound-mediated transdermal drug transport. Pharm Res 2002; 19(8): 1160-9. [http://dx.doi.org/10.1023/A:1019898109793] [PMID: 12240942]

[25] Alvarez-Román R, Merino G, Kalia YN, Naik A, Guy RH. Skin permeability enhancement by low frequency sonophoresis: lipid extraction and transport pathways. J Pharm Sci 2003; 92(6): 1138-46. [http://dx.doi.org/10.1002/jps.10370] [PMID: 12761803]

[26] Kushner J IV, Kim D, So PT, Blankschtein D, Langer RS. Dual-channel two-photon microscopy study of transdermal transport in skin treated with low-frequency ultrasound and a chemical enhancer. J Invest Dermatol 2007; 127(12): 2832-46.

[http://dx.doi.org/10.1038/sj.jid.5700908] [PMID: 17554365]

[27] Polat BE, Figueroa PL, Blankschtein D, Langer R. Transport pathways and enhancement mechanisms within localized and non-localized transport regions in skin treated with low-frequency sonophoresis and sodium lauryl sulfate. J Pharm Sci 2011; 100(2): 512-29. [http://dx.doi.org/10.1002/jps.22280] [PMID: 20740667]

[28] Lee SE, Choi KJ, Menon GK, *et al.* Penetration pathways induced by low-frequency sonophoresis with physical and chemical enhancers: iron oxide nanoparticles *versus* lanthanum nitrates. J Invest Dermatol 2010; 130(4): 1063-72. [http://dx.doi.org/10.1038/jid.2009.361] [PMID: 19940858]

[29] Terahara T, Mitragotri S, Kost J, Langer R. Dependence of low-frequency sonophoresis on ultrasound parameters; distance of the horn and intensity. Int J Pharm 2002; 235(1-2): 35-42. [http://dx.doi.org/10.1016/S0378-5173(01)00981-4] [PMID: 11879737]

[30] Katz NP, Shapiro DE, Herrmann TE, Kost J, Custer LM. Rapid onset of cutaneous anesthesia with EMLA cream after pretreatment with a new ultrasound-emitting device. Anesth Analg 2004; 98(2): 371-6. [http://dx.doi.org/10.1213/01.ANE.0000099716.02783.C4] [PMID: 14742372]

[31] Becker BM, Helfrich S, Baker E, Lovgren K, Minugh PA, Machan JT. Ultrasound with topical anesthetic rapidly decreases pain of intravenous cannulation. Acad Emerg Med 2005; 12(4): 289-95. [http://dx.doi.org/10.1111/j.1553-2712.2005.tb01942.x] [PMID: 15805318]

[32] Brown MB, Martin GP, Jones SA, Akomeah FK. Dermal and transdermal drug delivery systems: current and future prospects. Drug Deliv 2006; 13(3): 175-87. [http://dx.doi.org/10.1080/10717540500455975] [PMID: 16556569]

[33] Spierings EL, Brevard JA, Katz NP. Two-minute skin anesthesia through ultrasound pretreatment and iontophoretic delivery of a topical anesthetic: a feasibility study. Pain Med 2008; 9(1): 55-9. [http://dx.doi.org/10.1111/j.1526-4637.2007.00281.x] [PMID: 18254767]

[34] Seto JE, Polat BE, Lopez RF, Blankschtein D, Langer R. Effects of ultrasound and sodium lauryl sulfate on the transdermal delivery of hydrophilic permeants: Comparative *in vitro* studies with full-thickness and split-thickness pig and human skin. J Control Release 2010; 145(1): 26-32. [http://dx.doi.org/10.1016/j.jconrel.2010.03.013] [PMID: 20346994]

[35] Tang H, Blankschtein D, Langer R. Prediction of steady-state skin permeabilities of polar and nonpolar permeants across excised pig skin based on measurements of transient diffusion: characterization of hydration effects on the skin porous pathway. J Pharm Sci 2002; 91(8): 1891-907. [http://dx.doi.org/10.1002/jps.10177] [PMID: 12115816]

[36] Escobar-Chávez JJ, Bonilla-Martínez D, Villegas-González MA. Sonophoresis: A valuable physical enhancer to increase transdermal drug delivery. In: Escobar-Chávez JJ, Merino V, Eds. Current Technologies to Increase the Transdermal Delivery of Drugs. Bentham Science Publishers 2010; Vol. 1: pp. 53-76.

[37] Kassan DG, Lynch AM, Stiller MJ. Physical enhancement of dermatologic drug delivery: iontophoresis and phonophoresis. J Am Acad Dermatol 1996; 34(4): 657-66. [http://dx.doi.org/10.1016/S0190-9622(96)80069-7] [PMID: 8601657]

[38] Maloney JM, Bezzant JL, Stephen RL, Petelenz TJ. Iontophoretic administration of lidocaine anesthesia in office practice. An appraisal. J Dermatol Surg Oncol 1992; 18(11): 937-40. [http://dx.doi.org/10.1111/j.1524-4725.1992.tb02764.x] [PMID: 1430549]

[39] Wells PN. Biomedical ultrasonics. New York: Academic Press 1997.

[40] McElnay JC, Matthews MP, Harland R, McCafferty DF. The effect of ultrasound on the percutaneous absorption of lignocaine. Br J Clin Pharmacol 1985; 20(4): 421-4. [http://dx.doi.org/10.1111/j.1365-2125.1985.tb05089.x] [PMID: 4074611]

[41] Novak EJ. Experirnental wansmission of lidocalne through intact skin by ultrasound. Arch Phys Med Rehabil 1964; 45: 231-2. [PMID: 14146780]

[42] Griffin JE, Touchstone JC. Effects of ultrasound frequency on cortisone into swine tissue. Am J Phys Med 1972; 51: 62-78. [PMID: 5021935]

[43] Tachibana K, Tachibana S. Use of ultrasound to enhance the local anesthetic effect of topically applied aqueous lidocaine. Anesthesiology 1993; 78(6): 1091-6. [http://dx.doi.org/10.1097/00000542-199306000-00011] [PMID: 8512102]

[44] Williams AR. Phonophoresis: an *in vivo* evaluation using three topical anaesthetic preparations. Ultrasonics 1990; 28(3): 137-41. [http://dx.doi.org/10.1016/0041-624X(90)90075-Y] [PMID: 2339470]

[45] Kim TY, Jung DI, Kim YI, Yang JH, Shin SC. Anesthetic effects of lidocaine hydrochloride gel using low frequency ultrasound of 0.5 MHz. J Pharm Pharm Sci 2007; 10(1): 1-8. [PMID: 17498388]

[46] Hehn B, Moll F. Phonophoretic permeation of procaine hydrochloride through an MDCK cell monolayer. Pharmazie 1996; 51(5): 341-5. [PMID: 8710957]

[47] Meshali MM, Abdel-Aleem HM, Sakr FM, Nazzal S, El-Malah Y. *In vitro* phonophoresis: effect of ultrasound intensity and mode at high frequency on NSAIDs transport across cellulose and rabbit skin membranes. Pharmazie 2008; 63(1): 49-53. [PMID: 18271303]

[48] Miyazaki S, Mizuoka H, Kohata Y, Takada M. External control of drug release and penetration. VI. Enhancing effect of ultrasound on the transdermal absorption of indomethacin from an ointment in rats. Chem Pharm Bull (Tokyo) 1992; 40(10): 2826-30. [http://dx.doi.org/10.1248/cpb.40.2826] [PMID: 1464116]

[49] Tiwari SB, Pai RM, Udupa N. Influence of ultrasound on the percutaneous absorption of ketorolac tromethamine *in vitro* across rat skin. Drug Deliv 2004; 11(1): 47-51. [http://dx.doi.org/10.1080/10717540490265261] [PMID: 15168791]

[50] Yang JH, Kim TY, Lee JH, Yoon SW, Yang KH, Shin SC. Anti-hyperalgesic and anti-inflammatory effects of ketorolac tromethamine gel using pulsed ultrasound in inflamed rats. Arch Pharm Res 2008; 31(4): 511-7. [http://dx.doi.org/10.1007/s12272-001-1186-5] [PMID: 18449510]

[51] Serikov NP. Efficacy of ibuprofen (nurofen gel) ultraphonophoresis for pain relief in osteoarthrosis. Ter Arkh 2007; 79(5): 79-81.
[PMID: 17672081]

[52] Cabak A, Maczewska M, Lyp M, Dobosz J, Gasiorowska U. The effectiveness of phonophoresis with ketoprofen in the treatment of epicondylopathy. Ortop Traumatol Rehabil 2005; 7(6): 660-5.
[PMID: 17611432]

[53] Herwadkar A, Sachdeva V, Taylor LF, Silver H, Banga AK. Low frequency sonophoresis mediated transdermal and intradermal delivery of ketoprofen. Int J Pharm 2012; 423(2): 289-96.
[http://dx.doi.org/10.1016/j.ijpharm.2011.11.041] [PMID: 22172289]

[54] Rosim GC, Barbieri CH, Lanças FM, Mazzer N. Diclofenac phonophoresis in human volunteers. Ultrasound Med Biol 2005; 31(3): 337-43.
[http://dx.doi.org/10.1016/j.ultrasmedbio.2004.11.012] [PMID: 15749556]

[55] Hippius M, Uhlemann C, Smolenski U, Schreiber U, Reissig S, Hoffmann A. *In vitro* investigations of drug release and penetration--enhancing effect of ultrasound on transmembrane transport of flufenamic acid. Int J Clin Pharmacol Ther 1998; 36(2): 107-11.
[PMID: 9520159]

[56] Rornanenko IM, Araviiskii RA. Comparative levels of amphoteficin B in the skin and subcutaneous fatty tissue after cutaneous application of amphotericin ointment by phonophoresis and with preliminary treatment by dimethyl sulfoxide. Antibiot Khimioter 1991; 36: 29-31.

[57] Ragelis SIu. Tetracycline penetration into tissue by modified electro- and phonophoretic methods. Antibiotiki 1981; 26(9): 699-703.
[PMID: 7294763]

[58] Liu H, Li S, Pan W, Wang Y, Han F, Yao H. Investigation into the potential of low-frequency ultrasound facilitated topical delivery of Cyclosporin A. Int J Pharm 2006; 326(1-2): 32-8.
[http://dx.doi.org/10.1016/j.ijpharm.2006.07.022] [PMID: 16949776]

[59] Santoianni P, Nino M, Calabro G. Intradermal drug delivery by low-frequency sonophoresis (25 kHz). Dermatol Online J 2004; 10(2): 24-33.
[PMID: 15530314]

[60] Aoi A, Watanabe Y, Mori S, Takahashi M, Vassaux G, Kodama T. Herpes simplex virus thymidine kinase-mediated suicide gene therapy using nano/microbubbles and ultrasound. Ultrasound Med Biol 2008; 34(3): 425-34.
[http://dx.doi.org/10.1016/j.ultrasmedbio.2007.09.004] [PMID: 18096302]

[61] Meidan VM, Walmsley AD, Docker MF, Irwin WJ. Ultrasound-enhanced diffusion into coupling gel during phonophoresis of 5-fluorouracil. Int J Pharm 1999; 185(2): 205-13.
[http://dx.doi.org/10.1016/S0378-5173(99)00168-4] [PMID: 10460916]

[62] Luis J, Park EJ, Meyer RJ, Smith NB. Rectangular cymbal arrays for improved ultrasonic transdermal insulin delivery. J Acoust Soc Am 2007; 122(4): 2022-30.
[http://dx.doi.org/10.1121/1.2769980] [PMID: 17902839]

[63] Lee S, Snyder B, Newnham RE, Smith NB. Noninvasive ultrasonic transdermal insulin delivery in rabbits using the light-weight cymbal array. Diabetes Technol Ther 2004; 6(6): 808-15.

[http://dx.doi.org/10.1089/dia.2004.6.808] [PMID: 15684633]

[64] Smith NB, Lee S, Shung KK. Ultrasound-mediated transdermal *in vivo* transport of insulin with low-profile cymbal arrays. Ultrasound Med Biol 2003; 29(8): 1205-10. [http://dx.doi.org/10.1016/S0301-5629(03)00908-6] [PMID: 12946523]

[65] Saliba S, Mistry DJ, Perrin DH, Gieck J, Weltman A. Phonophoresis and the absorption of dexamethasone in the presence of an occlusive dressing. J Athl Train 2007; 42(3): 349-54. [PMID: 18059989]

[66] Byl NN, McKenzie A, Halliday B, Wong T, O'Connell J. The effects of phonophoresis with corticosteroids: a controlled pilot study. J Orthop Sports Phys Ther 1993; 18(5): 590-600. [http://dx.doi.org/10.2519/jospt.1993.18.5.590] [PMID: 8268961]

[67] Akinbo SR, Aiyejusunle CB, Akinyemi OA, Adesegun SA, Danesi MA. Comparison of the therapeutic efficacy of phonophoresis and iontophoresis using dexamethasone sodium phosphate in the management of patients with knee osteoarthritis. Niger Postgrad Med J 2007; 14(3): 190-4. [PMID: 17767200]

[68] Yang JH, Kim DK, Yun MY, Kim TY, Shin SC. Transdermal delivery system of triamcinolone acetonide from a gel using phonophoresis. Arch Pharm Res 2006; 29(5): 412-7. [http://dx.doi.org/10.1007/BF02968592] [PMID: 16756087]

[69] Machet L, Pinton J, Patat F, *et al. In vitro* phonophoresis of digoxin across hairless mice and human skin: thermal effect of ultrasound. Int J Pharm 1996; 133: 39-45. [http://dx.doi.org/10.1016/0378-5173(96)04447-X]

[70] McElnay JC, Benson HA, Harland R, Hadgraft J. Phonophoresis of methyl nicotinate: a preliminary study to elucidate the mechanism of action. Pharm Res 1993; 10(12): 1726-31. [http://dx.doi.org/10.1023/A:1018918013489] [PMID: 8302758]

[71] El-Kamel AH, Al-Fagih IM, Alsarra IA. Effect of sonophoresis and chemical enhancers on testosterone transdermal delivery from solid lipid microparticles: an *in vitro* study. Curr Drug Deliv 2008; 5(1): 20-6. [http://dx.doi.org/10.2174/156720108783331014] [PMID: 18220547]

[72] Park SR, Jang KW, Park S-H, *et al.* The effect of sonication on simulated osteoarthritis. Part I: effects of 1 MHz ultrasound on uptake of hyaluronan into the rabbit synovium. Ultrasound Med Biol 2005; 31(11): 1551-8. [http://dx.doi.org/10.1016/j.ultrasmedbio.2005.07.002] [PMID: 16286032]

[73] Morimoto Y, Mutoh M, Ueda H, *et al.* Elucidation of the transport pathway in hairless rat skin enhanced by low-frequency sonophoresis based on the solute-water transport relationship and confocal microscopy. J Control Release 2005; 103(3): 587-97. [http://dx.doi.org/10.1016/j.jconrel.2005.01.005] [PMID: 15820406]

[74] Tezel A, Dokka S, Kelly S, Hardee GE, Mitragotri S. Topical delivery of anti-sense oligonucleotides using low-frequency sonophoresis. Pharm Res 2004; 21(12): 2219-25. [http://dx.doi.org/10.1007/s11095-004-7674-6] [PMID: 15648253]

[75] Boucaud A, Machet L, Arbeille B, *et al. In vitro* study of low-frequency ultrasound-enhanced transdermal transport of fentanyl and caffeine across human and hairless rat skin. Int J Pharm 2001;

228(1-2): 69-77.
[http://dx.doi.org/10.1016/S0378-5173(01)00820-1] [PMID: 11576769]

[76] Sarheed O, Rasool BK. Development of an optimised application protocol for sonophoretic transdermal delivery of a model hydrophilic drug. Open Biomed Eng J 2011; 5: 14-24.
[http://dx.doi.org/10.2174/1874120701105010014] [PMID: 21629673]

[77] Menon GK, Price LF, Bommannan B, Elias PM, Feingold KR. Selective obliteration of the epidermal calcium gradient leads to enhanced lamellar body secretion. J Invest Dermatol 1994; 102(5): 789-95.
[http://dx.doi.org/10.1111/1523-1747.ep12377921] [PMID: 8176264]

[78] Ng GY, Wong RY. Ultrasound phonophoresis of panax notoginseng improves the strength of repairing ligament: a rat model. Ultrasound Med Biol 2008; 34(12): 1919-23.
[http://dx.doi.org/10.1016/j.ultrasmedbio.2008.04.017] [PMID: 18692299]

[79] Rao R, Nanda S. Sonophoresis: recent advancements and future trends. J Pharm Pharmacol 2009; 61(6): 689-705.
[http://dx.doi.org/10.1211/jpp.61.06.0001] [PMID: 19505359]

[80] Zderic V, Clark JI, Martin RW, Vaezy S. Ultrasound-enhanced transcorneal drug delivery. Cornea 2004; 23(8): 804-11.
[http://dx.doi.org/10.1097/01.ico.0000134189.33549.cc] [PMID: 15502482]

[81] Zderic V, Clark JI, Vaezy S. Drug delivery into the eye with the use of ultrasound. J Ultrasound Med 2004; 23(10): 1349-59.
[PMID: 15448325]

[82] Murugappan SK, Zhou Y. Transscleral drug delivery by pulsed high-intensity focused ultrasound (HIFU): an *ex vivo* study. Curr Eye Res 2015; 40(11): 1172-80.
[http://dx.doi.org/10.3109/02713683.2014.980006] [PMID: 25380302]

[83] Suen WL, Wong HS, Yu Y, Lau LC, Lo AC, Chau Y. Ultrasound-mediated transscleral delivery of macromolecules to the posterior segment of rabbit eye *in vivo*. Invest Ophthalmol Vis Sci 2013; 26;54(6): 4358-65.

[84] Abadi D, Zderic V. Ultrasound-mediated nail drug delivery system. J Ultrasound Med 2011; 30(12): 1723-30.
[PMID: 22124008]

[85] Kushner J IV, Blankschtein D, Langer R. Experimental demonstration of the existence of highly permeable localized transport regions in low-frequency sonophoresis. J Pharm Sci 2004; 93(11): 2733-45.
[http://dx.doi.org/10.1002/jps.20173] [PMID: 15389675]

[86] Alvarez-Román R, Merino G, Kalia YN, Naik A, Guy RH. Skin permeability enhancement by low frequency sonophoresis: lipid extraction and transport pathways. J Pharm Sci 2003; 92(6): 1138-46.
[http://dx.doi.org/10.1002/jps.10370] [PMID: 12761803]

[87] Cancel LM, Tarbell JM, Ben-Jebria A. Fluorescein permeability and electrical resistance of human skin during low frequency ultrasound application. J Pharm Pharmacol 2004; 56(9): 1109-18.
[http://dx.doi.org/10.1211/0022357044193] [PMID: 15324479]

[88] Paliwal S, Menon GK, Mitragotri S. Low-frequency sonophoresis: ultrastructural basis for stratum

corneum permeability assessed using quantum dots. J Invest Dermatol 2006; 126(5): 1095-101. [http://dx.doi.org/10.1038/sj.jid.5700248] [PMID: 16528354]

[89] Walker JJ. Ultrasound therapy for keloids. S Afr Med J 1983; 64(8): 270. [PMID: 6879382]

[90] Larkin JO, Casey GD, Tangney M, *et al.* Effective tumor treatment using optimized ultrasound-mediated delivery of bleomycin. Ultrasound Med Biol 2008; 34(3): 406-13. [http://dx.doi.org/10.1016/j.ultrasmedbio.2007.09.005] [PMID: 17988788]

[91] Khaibullina A, Jang BS, Sun H, *et al.* Pulsed high-intensity focused ultrasound enhances uptake of radiolabeled monoclonal antibody to human epidermoid tumor in nude mice. J Nucl Med 2008; 49(2): 295-302. [http://dx.doi.org/10.2967/jnumed.107.046888] [PMID: 18199622]

[92] Levenets AA, Shuvalov SM, Poliakov AV. The effect of the disodium salt of ethylenediaminetetraacetate on the healing of experimental suppurative wounds. Stomatologia (Mosk) 1989; 68(5): 14-6. [PMID: 2511646]

[93] Matinian LA, Nagapetian KhO, Amirian SS, Mkrtchian SR, Mirzoian VS, Voskanian RM. Papain phonophoresis in the treatment of suppurative wounds and inflammatory processes. Khirurgiia (Mosk) 1990; 9(9): 74-6. [PMID: 2273855]

[94] Newman CM, Lawrie A, Brisken AF, Cumberland DC. Ultrasound gene therapy: on the road from concept to reality. Echocardiography 2001; 18(4): 339-47. [http://dx.doi.org/10.1046/j.1540-8175.2001.00339.x] [PMID: 11415507]

[95] Taniyama Y, Tachibana K, Hiraoka K, *et al.* Development of safe and efficient novel nonviral gene transfer using ultrasound: enhancement of transfection efficiency of naked plasmid DNA in skeletal muscle. Gene Ther 2002; 9(6): 372-80. [http://dx.doi.org/10.1038/sj.gt.3301678] [PMID: 11960313]

[96] Fechheimer M, Boylan JF, Parker S, Sisken JE, Patel GL, Zimmer SG. Transfection of mammalian cells with plasmid DNA by scrape loading and sonication loading. Proc Natl Acad Sci USA 1987; 84(23): 8463-7. [http://dx.doi.org/10.1073/pnas.84.23.8463] [PMID: 2446324]

[97] Lawrie A, Brisken AF, Francis SE, Cumberland DC, Crossman DC, Newman CM. Microbubble-enhanced ultrasound for vascular gene delivery. Gene Ther 2000; 7(23): 2023-7. [http://dx.doi.org/10.1038/sj.gt.3301339] [PMID: 11175314]

[98] Niidome T, Huang L. Gene therapy progress and prospects: nonviral vectors. Gene Ther 2002; 9(24): 1647-52. [http://dx.doi.org/10.1038/sj.gt.3301923] [PMID: 12457277]

[99] Karshafian R, Bevan PD, Williams R, Samac S, Burns PN. Sonoporation by ultrasound-activated microbubble contrast agents: effect of acoustic exposure parameters on cell membrane permeability and cell viability. Ultrasound Med Biol 2009; 35(5): 847-60. [http://dx.doi.org/10.1016/j.ultrasmedbio.2008.10.013] [PMID: 19110370]

[100] Skyba DM, Price RJ, Linka AZ, Skalak TC, Kaul S. Direct *in vivo* visualization of intravascular destruction of microbubbles by ultrasound and its local effects on tissue. Circulation 1998; 98(4): 290-3.
[http://dx.doi.org/10.1161/01.CIR.98.4.290] [PMID: 9711932]

[101] Juffermans LJ, Kamp O, Dijkmans PA, Visser CA, Musters RJ. Low-intensity ultrasound-exposed microbubbles provoke local hyperpolarization of the cell membrane *via* activation of BK(Ca) channels. Ultrasound Med Biol 2008; 34(3): 502-8.
[http://dx.doi.org/10.1016/j.ultrasmedbio.2007.09.010] [PMID: 17993242]

[102] Pouton CW, Seymour LW. Key issues in non-viral gene delivery. Adv Drug Deliv Rev 1998; 34(1): 3-19.
[http://dx.doi.org/10.1016/S0169-409X(98)00048-9] [PMID: 10837667]

[103] Machet L, Boucaud A. Phonophoresis: efficiency, mechanisms and skin tolerance. Int J Pharm 2002; 243(1-2): 1-15.
[http://dx.doi.org/10.1016/S0378-5173(02)00299-5] [PMID: 12176291]

[104] Byl NN. The use of ultrasound as an enhancer for transcutaneous drug delivery: phonophoresis. Phys Ther 1995; 75(6): 539-53.
[PMID: 7770499]

[105] Kumagai K, Takeuchi R, Ishikawa H, *et al.* Low-intensity pulsed ultrasound accelerates fracture healing by stimulation of recruitment of both local and circulating osteogenic progenitors. J Orthop Res 2012; 30(9): 1516-21.
[http://dx.doi.org/10.1002/jor.22103] [PMID: 22419401]

[106] Watanabe Y, Matsushita T, Bhandari M, Zdero R, Schemitsch EH. Ultrasound for fracture healing: current evidence. J Orthop Trauma 2010; 24 (Suppl. 1): S56-61.
[http://dx.doi.org/10.1097/BOT.0b013e3181d2efaf] [PMID: 20182238]

[107] Warden SJ. A new direction for ultrasound therapy in sports medicine. Sports Med 2003; 33(2): 95-107.
[http://dx.doi.org/10.2165/00007256-200333020-00002] [PMID: 12617689]

[108] Ebenbichler GR, Erdogmus CB, Resch KL, *et al.* Ultrasound therapy for calcific tendinitis of the shoulder. N Engl J Med 1999; 340(20): 1533-8.
[http://dx.doi.org/10.1056/NEJM199905203402002] [PMID: 10332014]

[109] Rutten S, Nolte PA, Korstjens CM, van Duin MA, Klein-Nulend J. Low-intensity pulsed ultrasound increases bone volume, osteoid thickness and mineral apposition rate in the area of fracture healing in patients with a delayed union of the osteotomized fibula. Bone 2008; 43(2): 348-54.
[http://dx.doi.org/10.1016/j.bone.2008.04.010] [PMID: 18538648]

[110] Naruse K, Sekiya H, Harada Y, *et al.* Prolonged endochondral bone healing in senescence is shortened by low-intensity pulsed ultrasound in a manner dependent on COX-2. Ultrasound Med Biol 2010; 36(7): 1098-108.
[http://dx.doi.org/10.1016/j.ultrasmedbio.2010.04.011] [PMID: 20620697]

[111] Seo YK, Kim UK, Park SJ, *et al.* Effect of low-intensity pulsed ultrasound on bone healing around titanium implant in tibia of diabetes mellitus induced rats. Journal of Korean Association of

Maxillofacial Plastic and Reconstructive Surgeons 2012; 34(3): 163-72.

[112] Lu H, Qin L, Cheung W, Lee K, Wong W, Leung K. Low-intensity pulsed ultrasound accelerated bone-tendon junction healing through regulation of vascular endothelial growth factor expression and cartilage formation. Ultrasound Med Biol 2008; 34(8): 1248-60. [http://dx.doi.org/10.1016/j.ultrasmedbio.2008.01.009] [PMID: 18378382]

[113] Rohrbach D, Hesse B, Preininger B, *et al.* Assessment of soft and mineralized tissue formation in a rat bone healing model using quantitative ultrasound (QUS). J Acoust Soc Am 2012; 131(4): 3458. [http://dx.doi.org/10.1121/1.4709031]

[114] Fujihara S, Kataura T, Nakamura T, *et al.* The effect of low-intensity pulsed ultrasound on maxillofacial bone healing. 89th IADR 2011.

[115] Gurney AB, Wascher D, Schenck R, *et al.* Absorption of hydrocortisone acetate in human connective tissue using phonophoresis. Sports Health: A Multidisciplinary Approach 2011; 3(4): 346-51. [http://dx.doi.org/10.1177/1941738111405970]

[116] Clijsen R, Baeyens JP, Barel AO, Clarys P. Influence of the timing of ultrasound application on the penetration of corticosteroids. Skin Res Technol 2013; 19(1): e279-82. [http://dx.doi.org/10.1111/j.1600-0846.2012.00639.x] [PMID: 22712560]

[117] Ebrahimi S, Abbasnia K, Motealleh A, Kooroshfard N, Kamali F, Ghaffarinezhad F. Effect of lidocaine phonophoresis on sensory blockade: pulsed or continuous mode of therapeutic ultrasound? Physiotherapy 2012; 98(1): 57-63. [http://dx.doi.org/10.1016/j.physio.2011.01.009] [PMID: 22265386]

[118] Miller DL, Smith NB, Bailey MR, Czarnota GJ, Hynynen K, Makin IR. Overview of therapeutic ultrasound applications and safety considerations. J Ultrasound Med 2012; 31(4): 623-34. [PMID: 22441920]

[119] Kelly MJ, Andres B, Briggs L, *et al.* Ultrasound-guided placement of a localization wire for arthroscopic treatment of calcific tendonitis. Tech Shoulder Elbow Surg 2012; 13(3): 134-7. [http://dx.doi.org/10.1097/BTE.0b013e31824f6192]

[120] Otadi K, Hadian MR, Olyaei G, Jalaie S. The beneficial effects of adding low level laser to ultrasound and exercise in Iranian women with shoulder tendonitis: a randomized clinical trial. J Back Musculoskeletal Rehabil 2012; 25(1): 13-9. [PMID: 22398262]

[121] Adahan HM, Sharon H, Siev-Ner I. A sound solution to tendonitis: healing tendon tears with a novel low-intensity, low-frequency surface acoustic ultrasound patch. PM R 2010; 2(7): 685-7. [http://dx.doi.org/10.1016/j.pmrj.2010.04.028] [PMID: 20659726]

[122] Tsai WC, Tang ST, Liang FC. Effect of therapeutic ultrasound on tendons. Am J Phys Med Rehabil 2011; 90(12): 1068-73. [http://dx.doi.org/10.1097/PHM.0b013e31821a70be] [PMID: 21552108]

[123] Brosseau L, Casimiro L, Milne S, *et al.* Deep transverse friction massage for treating tendinitis. Cochrane Database Syst Rev 2002; 4(4): CD003528. [PMID: 12519601]

[124] Chester R, Costa ML, Shepstone L, Cooper A, Donell ST. Eccentric calf muscle training compared

with therapeutic ultrasound for chronic Achilles tendon pain--a pilot study. Man Ther 2008; 13(6): 484-91.
[http://dx.doi.org/10.1016/j.math.2007.05.014] [PMID: 17662639]

[125] Ng GY. Comparing therapeutic ultrasound with microamperage stimulation therapy for improving the strength of Achilles tendon repair. Connect Tissue Res 2011; 52(3): 178-82.
[http://dx.doi.org/10.3109/03008207.2010.500752] [PMID: 20672987]

[126] Draper DO, Edvalson CG, Knight KL, Eggett D, Shurtz J. Temperature increases in the human Achilles tendon during ultrasound treatments with commercial ultrasound gel and full-thickness and half-thickness gel pads. J Athl Train 2010; 45(4): 333-7.
[http://dx.doi.org/10.4085/1062-6050-45.4.333] [PMID: 20617906]

[127] Deans VM, Miller A, Ramos J. A prospective series of patients with chronic Achilles tendinopathy treated with autologous-conditioned plasma injections combined with exercise and therapeutic ultrasonography. J Foot Ankle Surg 2012; 51(6): 706-10.
[http://dx.doi.org/10.1053/j.jfas.2012.06.009] [PMID: 22824319]

[128] Kosaka T, Masaoka T, Yamamoto K. Possible molecular mechanism of promotion of repair of acute Achilles tendon rupture by low intensity-pulsed ultrasound treatment in a rat model. West Indian Med J 2011; 60(3): 263-8.
[PMID: 22224336]

[129] van den Bekerom MP, van der Windt DA, Ter Riet G, van der Heijden GJ, Bouter LM. Therapeutic ultrasound for acute ankle sprains. Eur J Phys Rehabil Med 2012; 48(2): 325-34.
[PMID: 22614893]

[130] Cullum NA, Al-Kurdi D, Bell-Syer SE. Therapeutic ultrasound for venous leg ulcers. Cochrane Database Syst Rev 2010; (6): CD001180.
[PMID: 20556749]

[131] Ebadi S, Ansari NN, Henschke N, Naghdi S, van Tulder MW. The effect of continuous ultrasound on chronic low back pain: protocol of a randomized controlled trial. BMC Musculoskelet Disord 2011; 12(1): 59.
[http://dx.doi.org/10.1186/1471-2474-12-59] [PMID: 21406117]

[132] Cetin N, Aytar A, Atalay A, Akman MN. Comparing hot pack, short-wave diathermy, ultrasound, and TENS on isokinetic strength, pain, and functional status of women with osteoarthritic knees: a single-blind, randomized, controlled trial. Am J Phys Med Rehabil 2008; 87(6): 443-51.
[http://dx.doi.org/10.1097/PHM.0b013e318174e467] [PMID: 18496246]

[133] Dogru H, Basaran S, Sarpel T. Effectiveness of therapeutic ultrasound in adhesive capsulitis. Joint Bone Spine 2008; 75(4): 445-50.
[http://dx.doi.org/10.1016/j.jbspin.2007.07.016] [PMID: 18455944]

[134] Öhberg L, Alfredson H. Ultrasound guided sclerosis of neovessels in painful chronic Achilles tendinosis: pilot study of a new treatment. Br J Sports Med 2002; 36(3): 173-5.
[http://dx.doi.org/10.1136/bjsm.36.3.173] [PMID: 12055110]

[135] Qureshi AI, Mendelow AD, Hanley DF. Intracerebral haemorrhage. Lancet 2009; 373(9675): 1632-44.
[http://dx.doi.org/10.1016/S0140-6736(09)60371-8] [PMID: 19427958]

[136] Eggers J, Seidel G, Koch B, König IR. Sonothrombolysis in acute ischemic stroke for patients ineligible for rt-PA. Neurology 2005; 64(6): 1052-4. [http://dx.doi.org/10.1212/01.WNL.0000154599.45969.D6] [PMID: 15781825]

[137] Alexandrov AV, Molina CA, Grotta JC, *et al.* Ultrasound-enhanced systemic thrombolysis for acute ischemic stroke. N Engl J Med 2004; 351(21): 2170-8. [http://dx.doi.org/10.1056/NEJMoa041175] [PMID: 15548777]

[138] Kuliha M, Roubec M, Fadrná T, *et al.* Endovascular sono-lysis using EKOS system in acute stroke patients with a main cerebral artery occlusion–A pilot study. Perspectives in Medicine 2012; 1(1-12): 65-72.

[139] Mason TJ. Therapeutic ultrasound an overview. Ultrason Sonochem 2011; 18(4): 847-52. [http://dx.doi.org/10.1016/j.ultsonch.2011.01.004] [PMID: 21316286]

[140] Green S, Buchbinder R, Hetrick S. Physiotherapy interventions for shoulder pain. Cochrane Database Syst Rev 2003; 2(2): CD004258. [review]. [PMID: 12804509]

[141] Watson T. Ultrasound in contemporary physiotherapy practice. Ultrasonics 2008; 48(4): 321-9. [http://dx.doi.org/10.1016/j.ultras.2008.02.004] [PMID: 18466945]

[142] Khanna A, Nelmes RT, Gougoulias N, Maffulli N, Gray J. The effects of LIPUS on soft-tissue healing: a review of literature. Br Med Bull 2009; 89(1): 169-82. [http://dx.doi.org/10.1093/bmb/ldn040] [PMID: 19011263]

[143] Corradi M, Johnson S, Prout L. Therapeutic Ultrasound with Wound Healing| A Systematic Literature Review. Thesis, The college of St. Scholastica. 2009.

[144] van der Windt DA, van der Heijden GJ, van den Berg SG, ter Riet G, de Winter AF, Bouter LM. Ultrasound therapy for musculoskeletal disorders: a systematic review. Pain 1999; 81(3): 257-71. [http://dx.doi.org/10.1016/S0304-3959(99)00016-0] [PMID: 10431713]

[145] ter Haar G. Therapeutic ultrasound. Eur J Ultrasound 1999; 9(1): 3-9. [http://dx.doi.org/10.1016/S0929-8266(99)00013-0] [PMID: 10099161]

[146] Robertson VJ. Dosage and treatment response in randomized clinical trials of therapeutic ultrasound. Phys Ther Sport 2002; 3(3): 124-33. [http://dx.doi.org/10.1016/S1466-853X(02)90107-0]

[147] Kavros SJ, Schenck EC. Use of noncontact low-frequency ultrasound in the treatment of chronic foot and leg ulcerations: a 51-patient analysis. J Am Podiatr Med Assoc 2007; 97(2): 95-101. [http://dx.doi.org/10.7547/0970095] [PMID: 17369314]

[148] Meidan VM, Docker M, Walmsley AD, Irwin WJ. Low intensity ultrasound as a probe to elucidate the relative follicular contribution to total transdermal absorption. Pharm Res 1998; 15(1): 85-92. [http://dx.doi.org/10.1023/A:1011956905388] [PMID: 9487552]

[149] Talish RJ, Winder AA. Ultrasound bandages. US Patent 7211060, 2007.

[150] Maione E, Shung KK, Meyer RJ Jr, Hughes JW, Newnham RE, Smith NB. Transducer design for a portable ultrasound enhanced transdermal drug-delivery system. IEEE Trans Ultrason Ferroelectr Freq Control 2002; 49(10): 1430-6.

[http://dx.doi.org/10.1109/TUFFC.2002.1041084] [PMID: 12403144]

[151] Smith NB, Lee S, Maione E, Roy RB, McElligott S, Shung KK. Ultrasound-mediated transdermal transport of insulin in vitro through human skin using novel transducer designs. Ultrasound Med Biol 2003; 29(2): 311-7.
[http://dx.doi.org/10.1016/S0301-5629(02)00706-8] [PMID: 12659919]

[152] Yeo SH, Zhang HY. Development of a novel sonophoresis micro-device. Biomed Microdevices 2003; 5: 201-6.
[http://dx.doi.org/10.1023/A:1025756108574]

[153] Lee S, Newnham RE, Smith NB. Short ultrasound exposure times for noninvasive insulin delivery in rats using the lightweight cymbal array. IEEE Trans Ultrason Ferroelectr Freq Control 2004; 51(2): 176-80.
[http://dx.doi.org/10.1109/TUFFC.2004.1320765] [PMID: 15055807]

[154] Park EJ, Werner J, Smith NB. Ultrasound mediated transdermal insulin delivery in pigs using a lightweight transducer. Pharm Res 2007; 24(7): 1396-401.
[http://dx.doi.org/10.1007/s11095-007-9306-4] [PMID: 17443398]

[155] Redding J, Bruce K. Substance delivery device. Dermisonics, Inc US Patent 6908448, 2005.

[156] California: PR Newswire Association LLC. (2015) Available from: http://www.prnewswire.com /news-relea-ses/dermisonics-inc-prepares-u-striptm-ultrasonic-transducer-device-for-mass-production-56759392.html

[157] investing.businessweek.com. (2015) Available from: http://investing.businessweek.com/research/ stocks/snap-shot/snapshot.asp?ticker=DMSI

[158] Lyon: Reportlinker. (2012) Available from: http://www.reportlinker.com/p0894213-summary/ Dermisonics-Inc-DMSI-Strategic-SWOT-Analysis-Review.html

[159] bme-electronics.com. (2012) Available from: http://www.bme-electronics.com/fr/pdf/sonoderm _4_gb.pdf

[160] bme-electronics.com. (2012) Available from: http://www.bme-electronics.com/site/en_product _sonoderm.html

[161] bme-electronics.com. (2012) Available from: http://www.bme-electronics.com/documents/produits/ sonoderm_en_LD.pdf

[162] Unger EC, Matsunaga TO, Yellowhair D. Gas and gaseous precursor filled microspheres as topical and subcutaneous delivery vehicles. US Patent 5733572, 1998.

[163] United States: Sonoworld. (2015) Available from: http://www.sonoworld.com/Client/ ModuleContent/ModuleContent.aspx?ModuleId=5&ContentId=1947

[164] United States: Sonoworld. (2015) Available from: http://www.sonoworld.com/Client/ModuleContent/ ModuleContent.aspx?ModuleId=5&ContentId=1795

[165] Washington: Cerevast™. (2015) Available from: http://www.cerevast.com/sonolysis/

[166] Wu J, Nyborg WL. Ultrasound, cavitation bubbles and their interaction with cells. Adv Drug Deliv Rev 2008; 60(10): 1103-16.
[http://dx.doi.org/10.1016/j.addr.2008.03.009] [PMID: 18468716]

[167] Alexandrov AV, Demchuk AM, Burgin WS, Robinson DJ, Grotta JC. Ultrasound-enhanced thrombolysis for acute ischemic stroke: phase I. Findings of the CLOTBUST trial. J Neuroimaging 2004; 14(2): 113-7. [http://dx.doi.org/10.1111/j.1552-6569.2004.tb00226.x] [PMID: 15095555]

[168] Sharma VK, Rathakrishnan R, Ong BK, Chan BP. Ultrasound assisted thrombolysis in acute ischaemic stroke: preliminary experience in Singapore. Ann Acad Med Singapore 2008; 37(9): 778-82. [PMID: 18989495]

[169] Sharma VK, Tsivgoulis G, Nguyen HT, *et al.* Temporal profile of recanalization after ultrasound enhanced thrombolysis in acute basilar artery occlusion. Cerebrovasc Dis 2008; 26(1): 1-18. [PMID: 18511865]

[170] Sakharov DV, Rijken DC. Effect of flow on lysis of plasma clots in a plasma environment thromb haemost 2000; 83(3): 469-74.

[171] Molina CA, Ribo M, Rubiera M, *et al.* Microbubble administration accelerates clot lysis during continuous 2-MHz ultrasound monitoring in stroke patients treated with intravenous tissue plasminogen activator. Stroke 2006; 37(2): 425-9. [http://dx.doi.org/10.1161/01.STR.0000199064.94588.39] [PMID: 16373632]

[172] Alexandrov AV, Mikulik R, Ribo M, *et al.* A pilot randomized clinical safety study of sonothrombolysis augmentation with ultrasound-activated perflutren-lipid microspheres for acute ischemic stroke. Stroke 2008; 39(5): 1464-9. [http://dx.doi.org/10.1161/STROKEAHA.107.505727] [PMID: 18356546]

[173] Larrue V, Viguier A, Arnaud C, *et al.* Transcranial Ultrasound Combined with Intravenous Microbubbles and Tissue Plasminogen Activator for Acute Ischemic Stroke: a Randomized Controlled Study. Stroke 2007; 38: 472.

[174] Molina CA, Barreto AD, Tsivgoulis G, *et al.* Transcranial ultrasound in clinical sonothrombolysis (TUCSON) trial. Ann Neurol 2009; 66(1): 28-38. [http://dx.doi.org/10.1002/ana.21723] [PMID: 19670432]

[175] England: BioPortfolio Limited. Available from: http://www.bioportfolio.com/corporate/company/15-76/Ekos-corporation.html 2015.

[176] Interventional Medicine BTG. Available from: http://www.ekoscorp.com 2015.

[177] Braaten JV, Goss RA, Francis CW. Ultrasound reversibly disaggregates fibrin fibers. Thromb Haemost 1997; 78(3): 1063-8. [PMID: 9308755]

[178] Soltani A, Singhal R, García JL, Raju NR. Absence of biological damage from prolonged exposure to intravascular ultrasound: a swine model. Ultrasonics 2007; 46(1): 60-7. [http://dx.doi.org/10.1016/j.ultras.2006.10.004] [PMID: 17175000]

[179] Parikh S, Motarjeme A, McNamara T, *et al.* Ultrasound-accelerated thrombolysis for the treatment of deep vein thrombosis: initial clinical experience. J Vasc Interv Radiol 2008; 19(4): 521-8. [http://dx.doi.org/10.1016/j.jvir.2007.11.023] [PMID: 18375296]

[180] Francis CW, Blinc A, Lee S, Cox C. Ultrasound accelerates transport of recombinant tissue plasminogen activator into clots. Ultrasound Med Biol 1995; 21(3): 419-24.

[http://dx.doi.org/10.1016/0301-5629(94)00119-X] [PMID: 7645133]

[181] Soltani A, Volz KR, Hansmann DR. Effect of modulated ultrasound parameters on ultrasound-induced thrombolysis. Phys Med Biol 2008; 53(23): 6837-47.
[http://dx.doi.org/10.1088/0031-9155/53/23/012] [PMID: 19001697]

[182] Tezel A, Sens A, Mitragotri S. Investigations of the role of cavitation in low-frequency sonophoresis using acoustic spectroscopy. J Pharm Sci 2002; 91(2): 444-53.
[http://dx.doi.org/10.1002/jps.10024] [PMID: 11835204]

[183] Domínguez-Delgado CL, Rodríguez-Cruz IM, López-Cervantes M. The Skin: A valuable route for administration of drugs. In: Escobar-Chávez JJ, Merino V, Eds. Current technologies to increase the transdermal delivery of drugs. Bussum: Bentham Science Publishers Ltd 2010; pp. 1-22.

[184] Kellogg SC, Chuang H, Barman S, *et al.* Echo Therapeutics Inc. Assignee. System and method for continuous non-invasive glucose monitoring. US patent USSN 11/275,038, 2005.

[185] Echo Therapeutics,Inc. Available from: http://www.echotx.com/ 2015.

[186] Chuang H, Trieu MQ, Hurley J, Taylor EJ, England MR, Nasraway SA Jr. Pilot studies of transdermal continuous glucose measurement in outpatient diabetic patients and in patients during and after cardiac surgery. J Diabetes Sci Technol 2008; 2(4): 595-602.
[http://dx.doi.org/10.1177/193229680800200410] [PMID: 19885235]

[187] Golden GM, McKie JE, Potts RO. Role of stratum corneum lipid fluidity in transdermal drug flux. J Pharm Sci 1987; 76(1): 25-8.
[http://dx.doi.org/10.1002/jps.2600760108] [PMID: 3585718]

[188] Yu B, Dong CY, So PT, Blankschtein D, Langer R. *In vitro* visualization and quantification of oleic acid induced changes in transdermal transport using two-photon fluorescence microscopy. J Invest Dermatol 2001; 117(1): 16-25.
[http://dx.doi.org/10.1046/j.0022-202x.2001.01353.x] [PMID: 11442745]

[189] Yu B, Kim KH, So PT, Blankschtein D, Langer R. Visualization of oleic acid-induced transdermal diffusion pathways using two-photon fluorescence microscopy. J Invest Dermatol 2003; 120(3): 448-55.
[http://dx.doi.org/10.1046/j.1523-1747.2003.12061.x] [PMID: 12603859]

[190] Nino M, Calabrò G, Santoianni P. Topical delivery of active principles: the field of dermatological research. Dermatol Online J 2010; 16(1): 4.
[PMID: 20137746]

[191] Ueda H, Sugibayashi K, Morimoto Y. Skin penetration enhancing effects of drugs by phonophoresis. J Control Release 1995; 37: 291-7.
[http://dx.doi.org/10.1016/0168-3659(95)00087-9]

[192] Prausnitz MR, Mitragotri S, Langer R. Current status and future potential of transdermal drug delivery. Nat Rev Drug Discov 2004; 3(2): 115-24.
[http://dx.doi.org/10.1038/nrd1304] [PMID: 15040576]

[193] Escobar-Chávez JJ, Rodríguez Cruz IM, Domínguez-Delgado CL. Chemical and Physical enhancers for transdermal drug delivery. In: Gallelli L, Ed. Pharmacology. InTech Rijeka, Croatia 2012; pp. 397-434.

[194] Johnson ME, Mitragotri S, Patel A, Blankschtein D, Langer R. Synergistic effects of chemical enhancers and therapeutic ultrasound on transdermal drug delivery. J Pharm Sci 1996; 85(7): 670-9. [http://dx.doi.org/10.1021/js960079z] [PMID: 8818988]

[195] Srisuk P, Thongnopnua P, Raktanonchai U, Kanokpanont S. Physico-chemical characteristics of methotrexate-entrapped oleic acid-containing deformable liposomes for *in vitro* transepidermal delivery targeting psoriasis treatment. Int J Pharm 2012; 427(2): 426-34. [http://dx.doi.org/10.1016/j.ijpharm.2012.01.045] [PMID: 22310459]

[196] Meidan V, Docker M, Walmsley A, *et al.* Phonophoresis of hydrocortisone with enhancers: an acoustically defined model. Int J Pharm 1998; 170(2): 157-68. [http://dx.doi.org/10.1016/S0378-5173(98)00140-9]

[197] Xu X, Zhu Q, Sun C. Combined effect of ultrasound-SLS on skin optical clearing. IEEE Photonics Technol Lett 2008; 20(24): 2117-9. [http://dx.doi.org/10.1109/LPT.2008.2006987]

[198] Xu X, Zhu Q, Sun C. Assessment of the effects of ultrasound-mediated alcohols on skin optical clearing. J Biomed Opt 2009; 14(3): 034042. [http://dx.doi.org/10.1117/1.3156827] [PMID: 19566334]

[199] Zhong H, Guo Z, Wei H, *et al.* Synergistic effect of ultrasound and thiazone-PEG 400 on human skin optical clearing *in vivo*. Photochem Photobiol 2010; 86(3): 732-7. [http://dx.doi.org/10.1111/j.1751-1097.2010.00710.x] [PMID: 20202160]

[200] Zhong H, Guo Z, Wei H, *et al. In vitro* study of ultrasound and different-concentration glycerol-induced changes in human skin optical attenuation assessed with optical coherence tomography. J Biomed Opt 2010; 15(3): 036012. [http://dx.doi.org/10.1117/1.3432750] [PMID: 20615014]

[201] Meshali M, Abdel-Aleem H, Sakr F, Nazzal S, El-Malah Y. Effect of gel composition and phonophoresis on the transdermal delivery of ibuprofen: *in vitro* and *in vivo* evaluation. Pharm Dev Technol 2011; 16(2): 93-101. [http://dx.doi.org/10.3109/10837450903499358] [PMID: 20100032]

[202] Fang JY, Fang CL, Hong CT, Chen HY, Lin TY, Wei HM. Capsaicin and nonivamide as novel skin permeation enhancers for indomethacin. Eur J Pharm Sci 2001; 12(3): 195-203. [http://dx.doi.org/10.1016/S0928-0987(00)00118-4] [PMID: 11113638]

[203] Mutalik S, Parekh HS, Davies NM, Udupa N. A combined approach of chemical enhancers and sonophoresis for the transdermal delivery of tizanidine hydrochloride. Drug Deliv 2009; 16(2): 82-91. [http://dx.doi.org/10.1080/10717540802605053] [PMID: 19267299]

[204] Dahlan A, Alpar HO, Murdan S. An investigation into the combination of low frequency ultrasound and liposomes on skin permeability. Int J Pharm 2009; 379(1): 139-42. [http://dx.doi.org/10.1016/j.ijpharm.2009.06.011] [PMID: 19539736]

[205] Kassan DG, Lynch AM, Stiller MJ. Physical enhancement of dermatologic drug delivery: iontophoresis and phonophoresis. J Am Acad Dermatol 1996; 34(4): 657-66. [http://dx.doi.org/10.1016/S0190-9622(96)80069-7] [PMID: 8601657]

[206] Wong TW, Zhao YL, Sen A, Hui SW. Pilot study of topical delivery of methotrexate by

electroporation. Br J Dermatol 2005; 152(3): 524-30.
[http://dx.doi.org/10.1111/j.1365-2133.2005.06455.x] [PMID: 15787822]

[207] Le L, Kost J, Mitragotri S. Combined effect of low-frequency ultrasound and iontophoresis: applications for transdermal heparin delivery. Pharm Res 2000; 17(9): 1151-4.
[http://dx.doi.org/10.1023/A:1026426317413] [PMID: 11087051]

[208] Fang JY, Hwang TL, Huang YB, Tsai YH. Transdermal iontophoresis of sodium nonivamide acetate. V. Combined effect of physical enhancement methods. Int J Pharm 2002; 235(1-2): 95-105.
[http://dx.doi.org/10.1016/S0378-5173(01)00972-3] [PMID: 11879744]

[209] Watanabe S, Takagi S, Ga K, *et al.* Enhanced transdermal drug penetration by the simultaneous application of iontophoresis and sonophoresis. J Drug Deliv Sci Technol 2009; 19(3): 185-9.
[http://dx.doi.org/10.1016/S1773-2247(09)50034-2]

[210] Hikima T, Ohsumi S, Shirouzu K, Tojo K. Mechanisms of synergistic skin penetration by sonophoresis and iontophoresis. Biol Pharm Bull 2009; 32(5): 905-9.
[http://dx.doi.org/10.1248/bpb.32.905] [PMID: 19420762]

[211] Dakowicz A, Latosiewicz R. The value of iontophoresis combined with ultrasound in patients with the carpal tunnel syndrome. Rocz Akad Med Bialymst 2005; 50(1) (Suppl. 1): 196-8.
[PMID: 16119664]

[212] Chen B, Wei J, Iliescu C. Sonophoretic enhanced microneedles array (SEMA)—improving the efficiency of transdermal drug delivery. Sens Actuators B Chem 2010; 145(1): 54-60.
[http://dx.doi.org/10.1016/j.snb.2009.11.013]

[213] Petchsangsai M, Rojanarata T, Opanasopit P, Ngawhirunpat T. The combination of microneedles with electroporation and sonophoresis to enhance hydrophilic macromolecule skin penetration. Biol Pharm Bull 2014; 37(8): 1373-82.
[http://dx.doi.org/10.1248/bpb.b14-00321] [PMID: 24931312]

[214] Domínguez-Delgado CL, Rodríguez-Cruz IM, Escobar-Chávez JJ, Calderón-Lojero IO, Quintanar-Guerrero D, Ganem A. Preparation and characterization of triclosan nanoparticles intended to be used for the treatment of acne. Eur J Pharm Biopharm 2011; 79(1): 102-7.
[http://dx.doi.org/10.1016/j.ejpb.2011.01.017] [PMID: 21295142]

[215] Husseini GA, Pitt WG. Micelles and nanoparticles for ultrasonic drug and gene delivery. Adv Drug Deliv Rev 2008; 60(10): 1137-52.
[http://dx.doi.org/10.1016/j.addr.2008.03.008] [PMID: 18486269]

[216] Marxer EE, Brüssler J, Becker A, *et al.* Development and characterization of new nanoscaled ultrasound active lipid dispersions as contrast agents. Eur J Pharm Biopharm 2011; 77(3): 430-7.
[http://dx.doi.org/10.1016/j.ejpb.2010.12.007] [PMID: 21147221]

[217] Becker A, Marxer E, Brüssler J, *et al.* Ultrasound active nanoscaled lipid formulations for thrombus lysis. Eur J Pharm Biopharm 2011; 77(3): 424-9.
[http://dx.doi.org/10.1016/j.ejpb.2010.12.003] [PMID: 21168485]

[218] Deelman LE, Declèves AE, Rychak JJ, Sharma K. Targeted renal therapies through microbubbles and ultrasound. Adv Drug Deliv Rev 2010; 62(14): 1369-77.
[http://dx.doi.org/10.1016/j.addr.2010.10.002] [PMID: 20946925]

[219] Zhou Q, Chen Z, Wang Y, Yang F, Lin Y, Liao Y. Ultrasound-mediated local drug and gene delivery using nanocarriers. Biomed Res Int 2014; 1-13.

[220] Escobar-Chávez JJ, Bonilla-Martínez D, Villegas-González MA, Revilla-Vázquez AL. Electroporation as an efficient physical enhancer for skin drug delivery. J Clin Pharmacol 2009; 49(11): 1262-83. [http://dx.doi.org/10.1177/0091270009344984] [PMID: 19717723]

[221] Escobar-Chávez JJ, Merino-Sanjuán V, López-Cervantes M, *et al.* The use of iontophoresis in the administration of drugs through the skin for smoking cessation. Curr Drug Discov Technol 2009; 6(3): 171-85. [http://dx.doi.org/10.2174/157016309789054924] [PMID: 19496753]

[222] Escobar-Chávez JJ, Bonilla-Martínez D, Villegas-González MA, Molina-Trinidad E, Casas-Alancaster N, Revilla-Vázquez AL. Microneedles: a valuable physical enhancer to increase transdermal drug delivery. J Clin Pharmacol 2011; 51(7): 964-77. [http://dx.doi.org/10.1177/0091270010378859] [PMID: 21148047]

[223] Escobar-Chávez JJ, Rodríguez Cruz IM, Domínguez-Delgado CL, *et al.* Nanocarrier systems for transdermal drug delivery. Rijeka, Croatia: INTECH Open Access Publisher 2012; pp. 201-40.

[224] Escobar Chávez JJ, Díaz-Torres R, Rodríguez Cruz IM, *et al.* Nanocarriers for transdermal drug delivery. Research and Reports in Transdermal Drug Delivery 2012; 1: 3-17. [http://dx.doi.org/10.2147/RRTD.S32621]

[225] Zhou Z, Fan W, Lang M, Wang Y. Transdermal Drug Delivery. Transdermal bFGF delivery using low-frequency sonophoresis: An innovative potential therapy for osteoradionecrosis of jaws. JMHI 2012; 9: 9-12.

[226] Cobo Labarca C, Makhutu M, Lumsdon AE, *et al.* The adjuvant effect of low frequency ultrasound when applied with an inactivated Aeromonas salmonicida vaccine to rainbow trout (Oncorhynchus mykiss). Vaccine 2015; 33(11): 1369-74. [http://dx.doi.org/10.1016/j.vaccine.2015.01.027] [PMID: 25613719]

CHAPTER 5

Radiofrequency as Physical Approach for Transdermal Penetration Enhancement, Non-Surgical Skin Procedures, Orthopedics and Chronic Pain

Jennyfer Cázares Delgadillo*

R&I, L'Oreal, 188-200 rue Paul-Hochart, 94550 Chevilly-Larue, France

Abstract: This review provides a summary of studies on the use of radiofrequency to overcome the skin barrier in order to evaluate its therapeutic potential, primarily in the fields of drug delivery and gene therapy. Other applications in non-surgical dermatologic procedures, orthopedics and treatment of chronic pain are also addressed. Additionally, this chapter includes a description of common devices used in some of the fields described and information of risks, safety and cost of treatments in the area of medical skin procedures.

Keywords: Chronic pain, Dermatology, Drug delivery, Gene therapy, Non-contact, Non-invasive, Non-surgical, Orthopedics, Radiofrequency, Therapeutics.

1. INTRODUCTION

Radiofrequency (RF) is a versatile technology commonly employed to generate therapeutic intensities of heat in order to produce structural and biological responses. RF ablation methods were first introduced as a minimally-invasive procedure in the field of neurology, and it has been expanded to other domains to treat tumors in the lung, some types of ventricular arrhythmias, varicose veins,

* **Corresponding author Jennyfer Cázares Delgadillo:** R&I, L'Oreal, 188-200 rue Paul-Hochart, 94550 Chevilly-Larue, France; E-mail: jennyfer.cazares@gmail.com

José Juan Escobar-Chávez (Ed.)

endovenous ablation, treatment for Barret's esophagus, uterine fibroids, healing of bone tissue and skin lesions [1]. It is recently used as promising non-invasive strategy for transdermal penetration and gene delivery enhancement, orthopedics, sleep apnea and chronic pain [2 - 5]. The term non-invasive refers to non-surgical methods and does not involve penetrating the body as by incision or injection.

The principle mechanism of RF is electroconductive heating, also referred as ohmic heating or resistive heating. This term is defined as the passage of electrical current (either DC or alternating current) through a material which functions as an electrical resistance in which heat is generated.

One of the biggest challenges in drug delivery is the ability to transport the therapeutic agents into the body safely and reliably. Skin, the largest soft membrane tissue covering the body is an ideal target for certain treatments including gene therapy. However, the stratum corneum (SC), the outermost layer of the epidermis forms a barrier to protect underlying tissue, impeding the passage of therapeutic molecules. There are several penetration enhancement strategies that would increase the number of drugs available for transdermal administration without having safety issues. Vehicle-based drug which does not change the SC properties such as vesicles and particles [6], pro-drugs [7], and synergistic system [8, 9], or chemical penetration enhancers, representing a good strategy as absorption accelerants [10]. Another interesting approach is physical and electrical methods that temporarily diminish the barrier of the skin by accelerating the absorption of molecules to enhance either drug flux or gene expression [11]. Those may include iontophoresis [12, 13], electroporation [14], microneedles [15], laser techniques [16] and radiofrequency [2, 17, 18]. RF technology assists the percutaneous penetration of actives (including peptides and gens) by removal of the outermost layer of the skin by using an alternating electrical current preferably from 100 to 500 KHz. The flow of this current through the tissue produces ions to collide one another which results primarily in localized heat creating transitory micro-pathways across the SC and epidermis, increasing the passage of hydrophilic compounds across the skin. The risk of discomfort or painful sensation is minimal as the microchannels created do not reach ending nerves [19].

Non-contact RF is shown to be an effective alternative in the field of dermatology and cosmetics. It is called non-contact RF because the active electrode does not touch directly the tissue surface. Only few scientific data on the relevancy of this technique regarding its impact on structural changes of skin tissues has been communicated. Many clinical studies considering the RF procedures as safe, tolerable, of rapid recovery and effective for skin treatments have been carried out. However, such trials are commonly obtained from non-randomized and non-comparative data using subjective means of evaluation, showing modest results [20, 21].

Non-contact RF has also been employed in orthopedics as an effective tool for controlled heating of tissues (above physiological temperature) to generate structural and biological effects. Tendon diseases for instance represent an important (30%) proportion of rheumatologic consultations in day-to-day consultations [22]. RF energy works to shrink and tense ligaments and articular capsule tissue in a controlled manner [23]. Actually, hydrogen bonds of collagen molecules may break at supraphysiologic temperatures, which collapse the molecule allowing connective soft tissue to shrink. Some symptoms of tendinopathies coming from irritation of nociceptors may be treated by bipolar RF by inducing degeneration of nerve, and delay of newly developed sensitive afferent fibers into treated tissues [24]. RF energy applied above supraphysiologic temperatures may also induce an anticipated response, similar in time and nature of the wound healing responses of thermal and surgical damages, following a predictable sequence of events that contributes to inflammation [23].

This chapter presents experimental and clinical data of therapeutic applications of non-invasive RF to enhance primarily transdermal drug delivery. Furthermore, the effectiveness of this technique in cutaneous gene delivery, as well as in areas such as non-surgical dermatology, orthopedics and chronic pain is also discussed. To conclude, the description of devices used in the mentioned fields and the relationship between cost, risks and safety of different dermatological procedures is described.

2. DEFINITION AND THEORETICAL BASIS

The term RF refers to electromagnetic energy consisting of waves that oscillates in the range of 3 kHz to 300 GHz. Microwaves are a subset of radio waves that have frequencies ranging from 300 MHz to 3 GHz. Due to the combination of electrical and magnetic components, the RF at a given location can be expressed in volts per meter" (V/m) to define the strength of the electrical field and "amperes per meter" (A/m) to measure the strength of the magnetic field. RF field can be also defined by power per unit area, power density, which is expressed in milliwatts or microwatts per square centimeter (mW or μW //cm^2). RF and microwave energy do not cause ionization (extraction of ions from atoms) that may produce molecular changes and damage in the genetic material such as x-radiation or gamma radiation. However, the exposure to high levels of RF radiation may produce rapidly heating of biological tissues, referred as thermal effects.

RF in this chapter may be defined as application of oscillating electric current in the range of high frequency 100-1,200 kHz that produces collisions between ions and charged molecules, which are then transformed into heat. Due to the relatively high electrical resistance of tissue (1000 ohm cm or greater), there is a significant agitation of the ions present in the tissue that creates friction within the body and, thus heat. This may cause denaturation of proteins, resulting in different tissue effects such as coagulation, dehydration, *etc.* (Fig. **1**) [25].

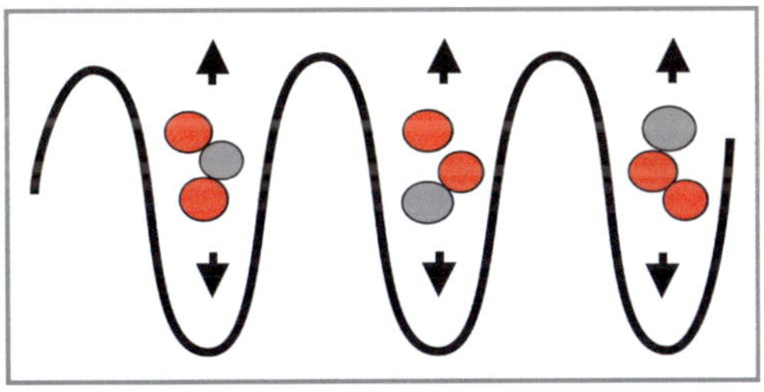

Fig. (1). Ionic agitation by alternating electric current (Adapted by permission from Rhim *et al.* Essential Techniques for Successful Radiofrequency Thermal Ablation of Malignant Hepatic Tumors, RadioGraphics 2001; 21:S17-S39 Copyright RSNA. 2001).

The heat generated can be tightly controlled through modulation of the amount of RF energy deposited.

The heating of tissue due to the power dissipated into the tissue can be expressed as follows:

$$P = pVI_d \tag{1}$$

Where P is the power in watts (W), ρ is the resistivity of the tissue in Ohm-metres (Ω-m), V is the tissue volume in cubic metres (m^3), and I_d is the current density in amperes per square metre (A/m^2).

3. MECHANISM OF ACTION

RF field therapies can be classified in two general categories based on their mechanism of action: non-thermal [26] and thermal [27].

Non thermal mechanisms are mostly associated to some interactions produced into the tissue by the RF field and not directly related with the magnitude of temperature increase. Normal cell membranes show a potential difference (70mV) as a result of the relative concentration of different ions (sodium, potassium, calcium, chloride, sodium bicarbonate) [28]. The altered potential disturbs ion transport across the membrane, and the ionic difference results in the variation of cellular osmotic pressures. The application of pulsed radiofrequency seems to reestablish the cell membrane potential and thus, the membrane passage and ionic balance. The mechanism of action suggests a direct transport or a stimulation of sodium/potassium pumps caused by the pulse energy; intercellular effects may be stimulated or enhanced by the energy that is absorbed in the membrane *via* a mechanism of signal transduction [28].

Therapeutic uses of non-thermal RF (at a carrier frequency of 13-27 MHz) are currently being employed to treat bone repair, edema, and chronic wounds.

Thermal mechanisms are principally associated to the absorption of the RF energy resulting from the resistance, and thus the electrical conductivity of most biological tissues.

RF energy field creates a fluctuating current, which leads to a fast transfer of energy into the molecular motion resulting in an increase in the local temperature [29]. This may produce modifications in biochemical reactions since those are affected by a change in temperature at some degree. The other main contribution concerns the hindered rotation of water [30]. The water molecule has an asymmetric distribution of charge and a permanent dipole moment that is randomly aligned in the absence of an applied electric field. The water dipoles tend to follow a motion but need to overcome viscosity of water, the field has to exert a work to produce a rotation of the dipoles, resulting in energy transfer in the liquid by heat [29].

Low-level RF radiation causes predominantly non-thermal effect because the intensity is not high enough to importantly modify tissue temperature; however, there is a very small thermal variation during the generation of each pulse (Fig. **2**) [28].

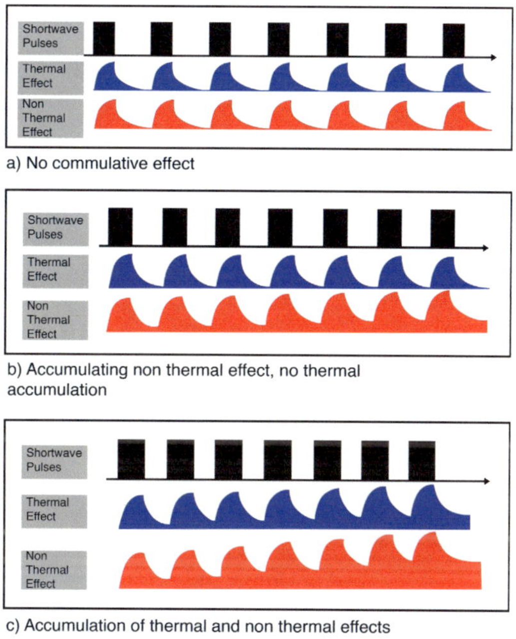

Fig. (2). Components of pulsed radiofrequency energy therapy; (**a**) no accumulation of either thermal or non-thermal effects; the pulse rate is sufficiently spaced to avoid thermal build up; (**b**) the pulses are sufficiently close to generate an accumulative non-thermal effect, and (**c**) there is an accumulation of both thermal and non-thermal effects. (Adapted by permission from Tim Watson, Copyright Prof. Tim Watson 1995-2014).

The potential thermal effect of pulsed short wave is specified in terms of: a) pulse repetition rate (pulses per second); b) pulse duration (width; microseconds), and c) power (peak and mean).

3.1. RF Waveforms and Power Modes

1. Non-modulated sinusoidal waveform: achieves a high average power without extensive thermal damage (Fig. **3**).

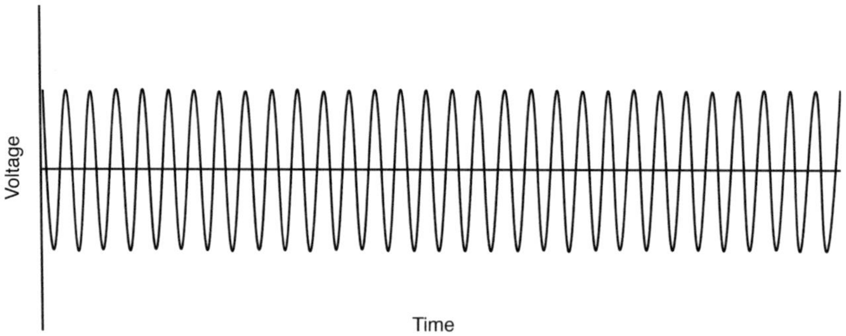

Fig. (3). Non-modulated sinusoïdal waveform.

2. Damped sine waves of high peak voltages (Fig. **4**): usually employed for the coagulation of bleeding vessels. These waves produce temperatures increased tissue temperatures, and significant thermal destruction.

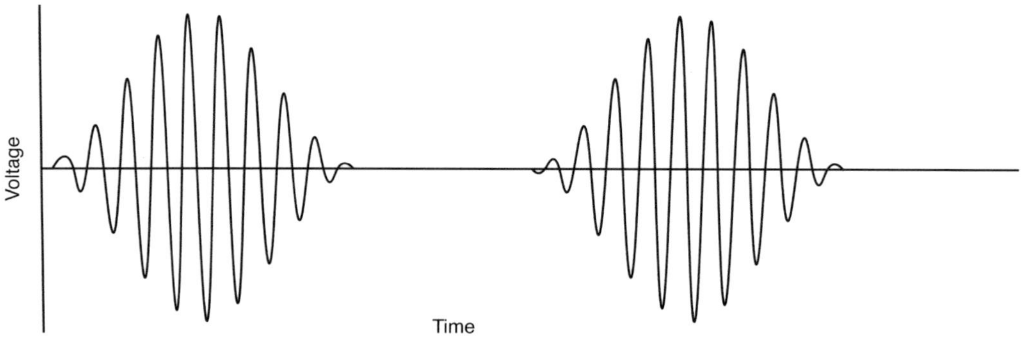

Fig. (4). Intermittent bursts of high voltage current.

3. Lower frequency, higher amplitude sine wave with the sine wave producing a higher peak-to-peak voltage: intermittent bursts containing a lower average power than a pure sinusoidal waveform due to the duty cycle (Fig. **5**).

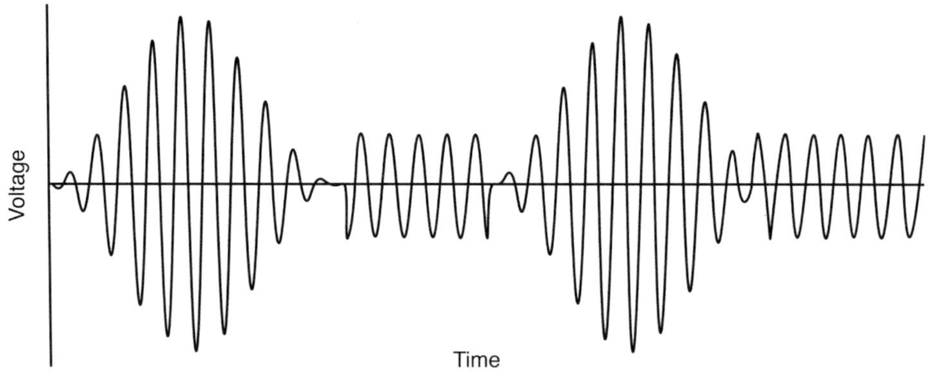

Fig. (5). Combination of a modulated lower frequency sine wave with a sine wave at low power.

3.1.1. Monopolar Mode

Use a single electrode with a distant ground pad or plate connected to the patient.

3.1.2. Unipolar Mode

The term unipolar is used to describe only one electrode of the dipole at the site of application and a grounding pad, wherein current is driven solely by the voltage difference between the electrode and the organic tissue. Both electrodes are connected to the patient to form a circuit. The current is conducted from the active electrode to the ground electrode and back to the generator, completing the circuit.

3.1.3. Bipolar Mode

Bipolar RF employs two electrodes, positive and negative, of equal size to create a dipole circuit. The depth of tissue heated is determined by the distance of electrodes in relation to one another. The loss of energy generated is evenly dispersed between the electrodes, providing more controlled distribution of energy and less pain.

3.2. RF Tissue Effects

The creation of lesion caused by RF heating is mainly dependent on tissue temperature achieved and the duration of heating [31] (Fig. **6**). When temperature is augmented to 42°C, tissue cells become to be exposed. Temperature above 45°C for several hours produces irreversible cellular injury [32]. When heating temperatures are increased from 60°C to 100°C, a coagulum formation and thus irreversible damage to mitochondrial and cytosolic enzymes of the cells is observed. At more than 100°-110°C, tissue carbonizes and vaporizes [31].

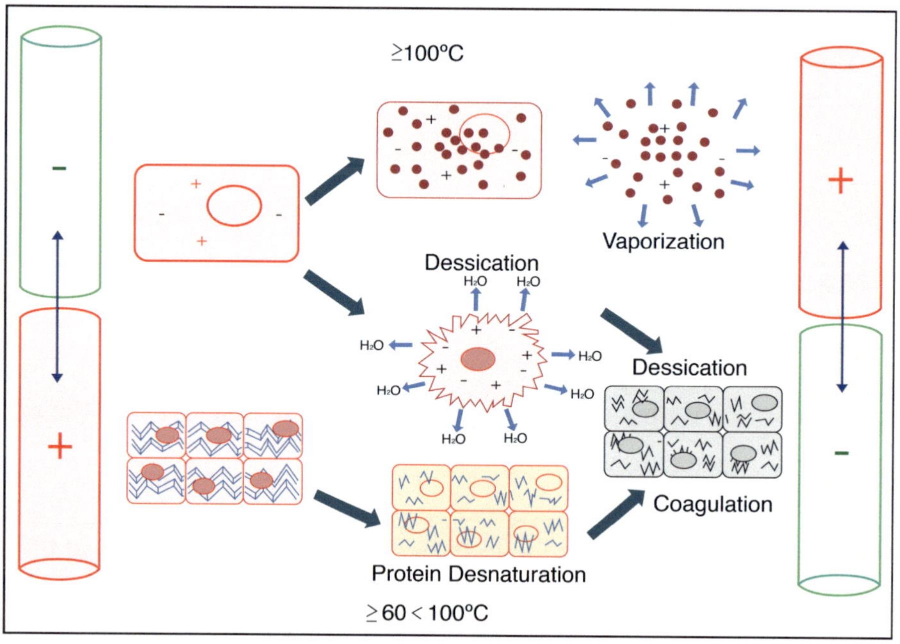

Fig. (6). Impact of elevation of tissue temperature at least 60°C but below 100°C. The first is tissue desiccation. The second is the rupture of hydrothermal bonds or crosslinks and reformation of these in a random fashion that includes bridging the gap between two opposing tissue surfaces.

An increase in tissue temperature represents a decrease in tissue impedance. Maximum decrease impedance is correlated with lesion depth while maximum heating is usually associated with lesion width.

The efficiency of tissue heating by RF can be achieved by i) improving heat production, which correlates with the intensity and duration of the RF energy deposited, and ii) decreasing heat loss mainly through convection into the blood pool [33].

The tissue effects observed are also related to the type of current applied, either conventional direct RF or pulsed RF [33]. Deep tissue destruction by the direct RF bipolar mode causes electrocoagulation. The technique uses high-frequency alternating current (300-750 kHz) for usually 30 to 60 seconds and up to 5 min, depending on the treatment. The size of the ablation site is dependent on several important factors: generator power, electrode contact area, tissue resistivity and location, and treatment duration [34]. This procedure represents a favorable therapy for liver malignancies, lung tumors, and kidney cancer, breast and bone tumors [35].

Application of significantly constant current by unipolar and bipolar modes produces superficial tissue destruction (electrodessication and electrofulguration), causing a greatest amount of lateral heat spread and destruction of the superficial tissue by dehydration and carbonization.

Pain relief [36, 37] and decrease of tumorous disorders of the brain and neck [35] are accomplished by pulse RF without heating the region and creating a histological lesion. The electrode-tip delivers a current of 50,000 Hz in 20-ms pulses, at a frequency of 2/s [38]. Heating a nerve at low temperatures (40- 45°C) may temporarily block conduction along the nerve with no physiologic lesion observed by the rapid recovery of function.

4. THERAPEUTIC APPLICATIONS

4.1. Transdermal Drug Delivery

The application of an alternating RF current between 100-500 kHz to the skin produces a structural disruption due to a vibration in motion of ions, causing a rapid destruction of cells close to the local application site. The formation of microchannels generated by the removal of the SC (by decomposition and vaporization) creates a pathway that may allow diffusion of lipophilic, hydrophilic and macromolecular actives. Due to the high velocity, it is assumed that electrochemical reactions do not take place and only heat conduction is responsible in the formation of microchannels. The micropores created (between 40 and 80 μm) are transitory, since the SC is shed naturally through the natural process of desquamation. The microchannels penetrate the superficial layers of the skin, causing minimal skin lesions or neural sensation.

The rate of drug delivery, reliant on the features of the microelectrode employed in the device, is controlled by the number and depth of microchannels created.

There are some studies that emphasize the use of RF as a promising technology for controlled transdermal delivery of molecules that penetrate the skin poorly.

The first studied that evidenced the transient aqueous microchannels across the skin was reported by Sintov *el al.* [2]. The penetration of two drugs, granisetron hydrochloride (pKa 9.4; MW 348.9 Da) and diclofenac sodium (pKa 4.0; MW 318.1 Da) was evaluated using a high-voltage current RF device.

Granisetron is a 5-hydroxytryptamine type 3 (5-HT_3) receptor antagonists that has demonstrated good performance to control and prevent chemotherapy-induced emesis [39]. Granisetron is strongly binding to the 5-HT(3) receptors and it is commonly associated with a long action (up to 24 h). This molecule is less susceptible to variation in patient response because it is not metabolized *via* enzymes of the cytochrome P450 (CYP) system (usually associated to polymorphism potentially affecting drug efficacy), but instead metabolized by members of the CYP3A subfamily [40].

Unfortunately, treatment efficacy with granisetron depends not only on the dose (1-2 mg, with systemic bioavailability of ~60% [41]), but also on the duration of treatment and the route of administration. Common routes are oral or intravenous (IV) administration, both impractical for chronic treatments. The oral route can lead to low drug absorption particularly in patients prone to vomiting, and the IV administration required trained staff using aseptic techniques for administration.

Sodium diclofenac, a phenylacetic acid derivative is a nonsteroidal anti-inflammatory (NSAID) analgesic agent used to treat mild to moderate pain resulting from minor surgery, trauma and dysmenorrhea, symptoms of rheumatoid arthritis, degenerative joint disease, and ankylosing spondylitis. Diclofenac exerts its action *via* inhibition of prostaglandin synthesis by inhibiting cyclooxygenase-1 (COX-1) and cyclooxygenase-2 (COX-2) [42].

The dose of diclofenac is usually 75 - 150 mg/day, generally given in 3 divided daily doses (25-50 mg), representing a disadvantage relative to less frequent administration with other drugs such as naproxen in rheumatoid arthritis, for instance [42].

The efficacy of diclofenac is also achieved when formulated as delayed-release tablets, however, it should be administered (25mg) four to five times daily in treatments such as ankylosing spondylitis. Other routes of administration are intramuscular, (IM) injection or rectal suppository, both usually uncomfortable for patients.

In the study, an array of needle like electrodes, connected to a microprocessor is placed at the skin application site (Fig. 7). An alternating RF current was applied to the electrodes in order to generate heat and create aqueous microchannels into the skin [2].

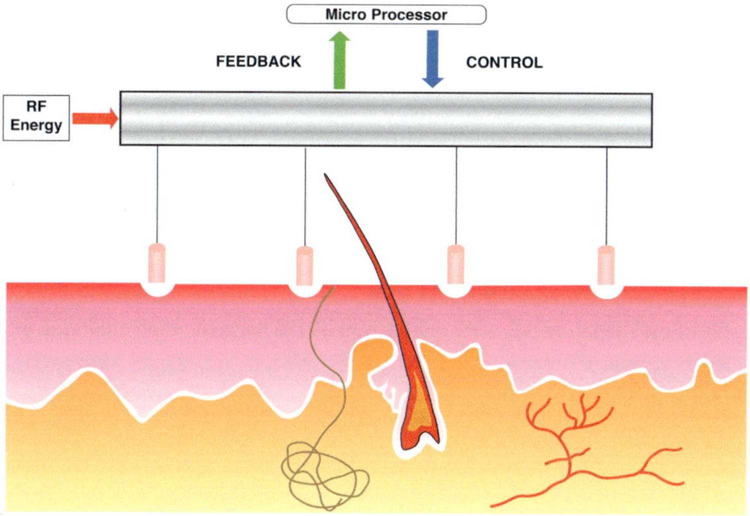

Fig. (7). Radiofrequency microchannels (Adapted by permission from Sintov *et al.* Radiofrequency-driven skin microchanneling as a new way for electrically assisted transdermal delivery of hydrophilic drugs, J Control Rel 89 (2): 311-320 Copyright 2003 Elsevier Science B.V.).

The permeation studies were performed *in vitro* using porcine skin model, and *in vivo* using rats. The RF device (ViaDerm Transpharma Ltd, Israel) uses a disposable array composed by stainless steel microelectrodes (100µm length, and 40 µm diameter; 200 microelectrodes/cm^2) mounted on a polycarbonate structure. The device is activated by pressure, once it is placed on the skin at the application area. Repeated applications (200 V- 250 V and 380 V) were performed at a frequency of 100 kHz for 1ms, 5ms and 15 ms, *in vivo* and *in vitro*, respectively.

The results showed significant steady state fluxes of both granisetron (41.6 μg/cm²/h) and diclofenac (23.0 μg/cm²/h) administered by patches after pretreatment with Viaderm. Diclofenac plasma levels in the pre-treated rats using an array at 250 V reached plateau levels of 1.47 ±0.33 μg/ml after 6h, as compared to levels of 0.16± 0.04 1 μg/ml obtained with the non-treated rats (Fig. **8**).

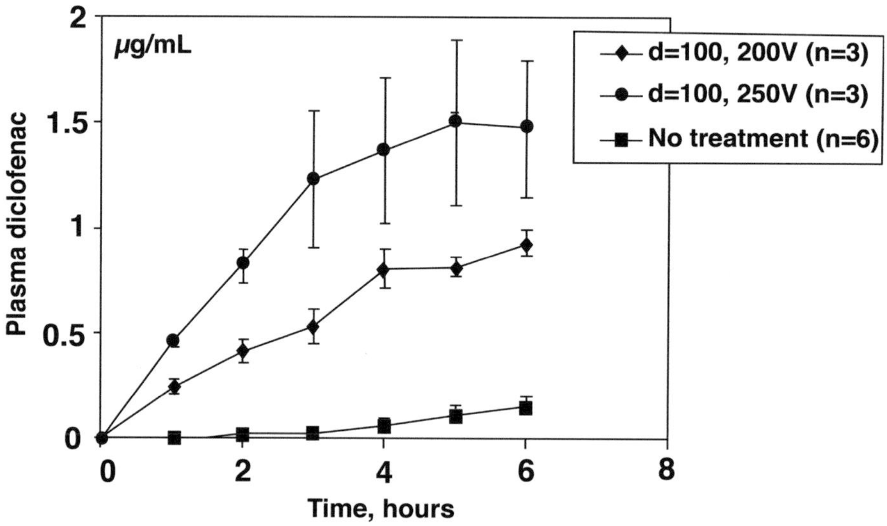

Fig. (8). Plasma levels of diclofenac in rats after application of 1% hydroalcoholic solution on 2.8 cm² surface area. (♦) skin pretreatment with RF currents of 200 V (100 kHz, 5 bursts); (•) skin pretreatment with RF currents of 200 V; (▪) passive diffusion. (Adapted by permission of AC Sintov *et al.* Radiofrequency-driven skin microchanneling as a new way for electrically assisted transdermal delivery of hydrophilic drugs, J Control Rel 89 (2): 311-320 Copyright 2003 Elsevier Science B.V).

Similarly, application of 1.4 cm granisetron patches (3% in cross-linked hydrogel) after pretreatment with radiofrequency (200 V, 100 kHz, 5 bursts) resulted in a plasma level of 239.3±43.7 ng/ml after 12 h, ~30-fold higher than the plasma levels achieved after 24h of passive diffusion (Fig. **9**). According to the permeability coefficients calculated, electrostatic attraction/repulsion ratios of both molecules may drive the migration along aqueous microchannels, being this effect more important for granisetron (cation) than diclofenac (anion). The relevance of the solubility properties of the actives (particularly for hydrosoluble granisetron) also plays an important role on their skin permeation. RF microchanneling did not produce any erythema or edema during the pretreatment process. The tissue around the microchannels created (30 μm diameter and 70 μm depth) did not present any pathological changes.

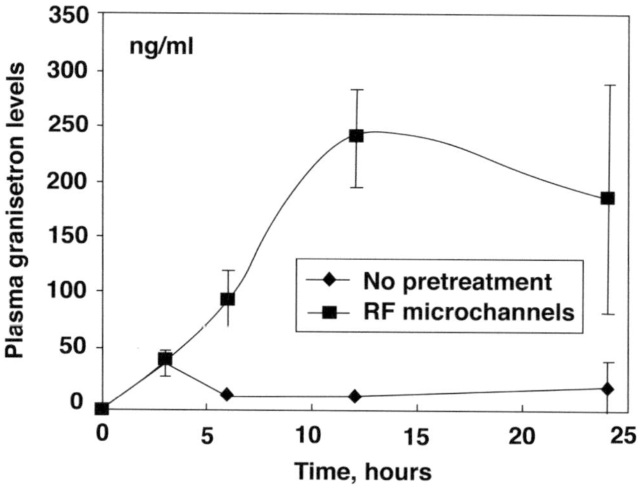

Fig. (9). Plasma levels (ng/ml) of granisetron in rats after application of 3% aqueous solution in Vigilon hydrogel patches. The passive diffusion through untreated skin is represented by the diamond-shaped symbols. (Adapted by permission of AC Sintov *et al.* Radiofrequency-driven skin microchanneling as a new way for electrically assisted transdermal delivery of hydrophilic drugs, J Control Rel 89 (2): 311-320 Copyright 2003 Elsevier Science B.V).

Iontophoresis, another physical method using microcurrent to enhance transdermal drug delivery has also been suggested to improve GST transport (GST 40 mM, (-Na+) [43]. A current density of 0.3mA/cm^2 was applied trough Ag/AgCl electrodes for 5h. Comparison with the present study shows that RF technique is less efficient to deliver GST resulting in a 4-fold lower flux (0.69 μg/cm^2/min (GST 32mM, (-Na+) compared to that obtained by iontophoresis (2.45 μg/cm^2/min) [43].

Growth hormone, also known as somatotropin or somatropin, is a 191-amino acid protein secreted by somatotropic cells of the anterior pituitary gland. It is indicated to treat GH deficiency, idiopathic short stature, chronic kidney disease, Turner syndrome, Prader-Willi syndrome, AIDS-related wasting, fat accumulation associated with lipodystrophy in adults, SHOX haploinsufficiency, children born small-for-gestational age and Noonan syndrome [44]. One of the major disadvantages of hGH is its short plasma half-life, 3.4 hours after subcutaneous (SC) injection and 0.36 hours after intravenous (IV) injection [45]. rhGH (recombinant hGH) dose consists of daily subcutaneous injections or three IM injections/week, which is uncomfortable and painful for patients. Moreover, this may be associated to low efficacy and increasing health care costs, with people (principally teenagers) missing two injections per week [46]. RF non-invasive technique, among long-lasting preparations to achieve a longer half-life, may represent an alternative delivery method to avoid such disadvantages.

Levin *et al.* evaluated the bioavailability and bioactivity of human growth hormone (hGH) (22 kDa) across RF by microchannels of 200/cm^2 created in the skin [47]. Printed-like patches of 1.4 cm^2 with different concentrations of protein were applied on rat or guinea pigs (GPs) skin after the creation of microchannels. A high bioavailability of 75% and 33% (relative to s.c. injection), respectively, was attributed to the formation of a localized concentration of hGH *in situ*. The diffusion mediated through the microchannels by a concentration gradient led to a significant delivery rate and peak blood level of the drug. The maximal efficient dose observed in both rats and GPs was 300 μg per 1.4 cm^2 patch area. Elevated levels of systemic insulin-like growth factor-1 (IGF-1) demonstrated the bioactivity of the protein. Some limitation factors were identified such as diffusion rate across the microchannels, restoration (healing) of channels, dissolution rate of hGH from the patches, metabolism of the protein by the skin and the animal model.

A Phase I clinical trial was conducted by TransPharma in 2007 to evaluate the safety, efficacy and tolerability of Viaderm to deliver hGH transdermally.

ViaDerm system comprises a handheld electronic device that used RF energy to create microscopic pores and a 5cm^2 dry hGH patch. The ViaDerm-hGH™ completed Phase I clinical trials in 2010 [19] obtaining promising results.

In order to position the efficacy of RF to improve hGH delivery with respect to other technologies, a study with microneedles is described below. Microneedles have been identified as the most developed system for the minimally-invasive application of hGH, despite their adverse effects (redness and swelling) [46].

Carboxymethylcellulose and trehalose 600 μm-microneedles, for instance, have demonstrated 71% absolute bioavailability of rhGH following administration of about 170 μg in male hairless rats, with minimal transient erythema [48].

A two-layered chondroitin dissolving microneedle containing solid dispersion of rhGH showed extents of absolute bioavailability of ~100% [49]. Self-dissolving micropiles of rhGH (dose of 200 μg/kg) formulated with dextran (used as a base) was studied in rats. A bioavailability of 87.5% of rhGH has been shown, compared to IV injection of rhGH (dose of 5 μg/kg) [50].

Kam *et al.* investigated the transdermal delivery of testosterone-cyclodextrin complex (model drug of ~2500 Da) *in vitro* and *in vivo* by the application of ViaDor™ (150 microchannels/cm^2), a RF device that generates an alternating electrical current at a frequency between 100 to 500 kHz [51].

The study was performed in two parts. i) An *in-vivo evaluation* performed on live hairless guinea pigs (GPs) using 2 mg dry patches of testosterone applied on the abdomen region. The animals were sacrificed at different timing points once the microchannles were created and skin samples, containing the application areas were collected. ii) An *in-vitro* delivery study was then conducted using the collected skin samples (4x4 cm) using Franz diffusion cells and a solution of testosterone-cyclodextrin at 2%.

As expected, testosterone permeability gradually decreased as the healing process progressed. A rapid decrease in the pseudo steady-state flux (39.6 μg/cm^2.h) at time 0, compared to fluxes after 36 h (1.08 μg/cm^2.h) were observed *in vitro*.

Testosterone pharmacokinetics profile obtained from the GPs pre-treated with ViaDor reached plasma levels of 31.8±12.1 ng/ml at 4 hrs. A significant decrease in testosterone concentration (9.3 ± 6.6 ng/ml) was observed when the patch was applied 8 h post-RF application (Fig. **10**). Application of a second patch replacing a first patch applied 8h immediately after RF treatment shows a similar behavior. However, this patch results in a 1.8 fold decreased in concentration (17.1 ± 14.8 ng/ml; replacement group).

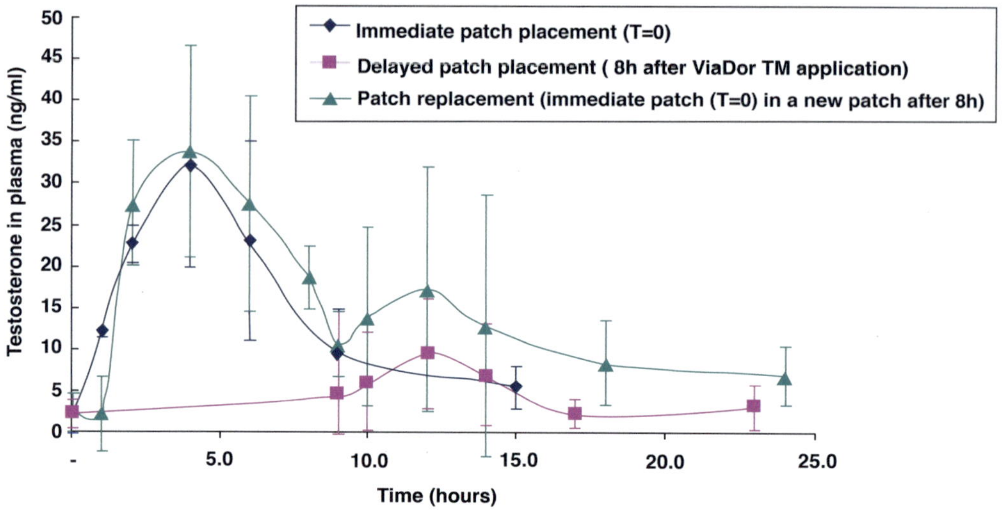

Fig. (10). Testosterone-cyclodextrin complex transdermal permeation in Guinea pigs following ViaDorTM treatment and patch. (Adapted by permission of Y. Kam *et al.* Radio Frequency-Microchannels for Transdermal Delivery: Characterization of Skin Recovery and Delivery Window, Pharmacol. Pharm. 2012, 3, 20-28, Copyright © 2012 Sci Res).

The histological findings confirmed that healing occurs immediately after the microchannels formation and the 24h period will gradually set the stage for the healing process of the epidermis.

Kim *et al.* [52] have shown *in vitro* and *in vivo* the influence of RF fluency and the molecular size of fluorescence isothiocyanate (FITC) dextrans on delivery rate and permeability of α-bisabolol (MW 222.37 Da), arbutin (MW 272.25 Da) and epidermal growth factor (EGF) (MW 6,045 Da). The RF-microporator employed consists of a reusable electronic controller to measure the impedance of skin that help to adjust the current applied during the ablation process, and a disposable array of 100 stainless steel electrodes (1 mm length x 250 µm diameter) spaced 1.5 mm apart. Micropores created were of 50 µm wide and 70-100 µm deep. For the *in vitro* tests, excised hairless mouse skin was subjected to 300 V; 500 kHz; 1 ms burst length, 5 bursts; power 100%. The skin permeability of FITC dextran (MWs: 4,000, 10,000, 20,000 or 40,000 Da) was measured as a function of RF fluence.

The efficacy of RF technology for topical delivery of α-Bisabolol and EGF (formulated in PBS or vehicle containing PEG 400) was conducted in animals randomly assigned to UV control, test and reference groups [52].

The topical delivery of α-Bisabolol was evaluated in 32 female F5 melanin hairless mice. UVB radiation was applied 3 times/week for 3 weeks with 300 mJ/cm^2 per exposure. α-bisabolol or vehicle solution was applied once daily for 4 weeks from the day after the last tanning session. RF microporation (100% fluence; 5 bursts) was applied 2 times/week (RF treatment group) before treatment with the solution. The degree of pigmentation was evaluated using a chromameter.

EGF topical delivery was tested in 60 female hairless mice. UVB radiation was applied to the back of the animal 3 times/week at 100 mJ/cm^2 per exposure [52]. EGF or vehicle was applied once daily from the day after 6-week UVB irradiation to the day of sacrifice (Day 84). RF microporation fluence was similar at that described for α-bisabolol. The degree of aging was assessed by TEWL (transepidermal water loss), skin thickness and wrinkle formation.

The results showed a ~ 22.0-fold increase in flux of FITC dextran with MW of 10,000 Da compared to the control with 100% fluence. Only the RF pre-treatment with fluence above 80% allowed the passage of FITC dextran with MW 40,000 Da. High fluence seemed to produce deeper microchannels through the SC and epidermis. However, the permeation improvement by RF fluence was not proportional to the MW. Although the larger molecular size molecules generally exhibited greater increase of flux compared to the smaller actives, the flux enhancement due to the creation of microchannels was reduced as the molecular weight increased above 20,000. This decrease in diffusivity through the microchannels was attributed due to their larger size.

In vitro flux data of Arbutin (MW 222 Da) and EGF (MW 6,045 Da) formulated in PBS across the skin showed an enhancement ratio of ~3 to ~7, respectively by passive diffusion and RF microporation application [52].

The flux of α-bisabolol through excised hairless mouse skin followed RF pre-treatment resulted in an enhancement factor of only 1.4. These data corroborates not only the effect of hydrophilic properties and molecular size on the skin permeation enhancement by microchannels, but also the impact of the vehicle. The viscosity of polyether compounds on the partitioning through the epidermis layer may also play an important role on the penetration enhancement of high molecular weight compounds.

In vivo studies showed a positive feedback with the combination of RF microporation and α-bisabolol delivery on UV-induced pigmentation at 0, 7, 14, 21, and 28 days. α-Bisabolol with or without RF microporation seemed to reduce pigmentation from 14 days after treatment [52]. RF microporation in combination with single vehicle also showed a depigmenting effect. The biopsy obtained after 28 days of topical application of the active demonstrated that the number of melanocytes was significantly decreased after RF microporation and α-bisabolol treatment.

RF microporation seemed to improve wrinkle formation by UVB irradiation. The parameters for the wrinkles were significantly reduced in the UV +RF microporation+EGF group compared to other UV-exposed groups. The effect of RF microporation with or without topical application of EGF on UV-irradiated skin showed well oriented collagen fibers with a density similar to the density of that of the normal skin. Considering the clinical results and synergistic effect with the active ingredients, further studies with larger population and different animal models must be performed. Different formulation vehicles may also be investigated as they have an impact on the efficacy of actives.

4.2. Cutaneous Gene Therapy

The skin is a valued target for gene therapy due to its accessibility and monitoring of the presence and expression of inserted genes. [53]. Promising approaches related to the correction of genetic disorders include those with a significant impact on skin [54], various forms of melanoma [55] and diabetic wound healing [56 - 58]. Gene therapy is becoming a relevant approach for acquired diseases (Fig. **11**), including various forms of cancers, principally for patients who do not respond to conventional therapies and infectious diseases.

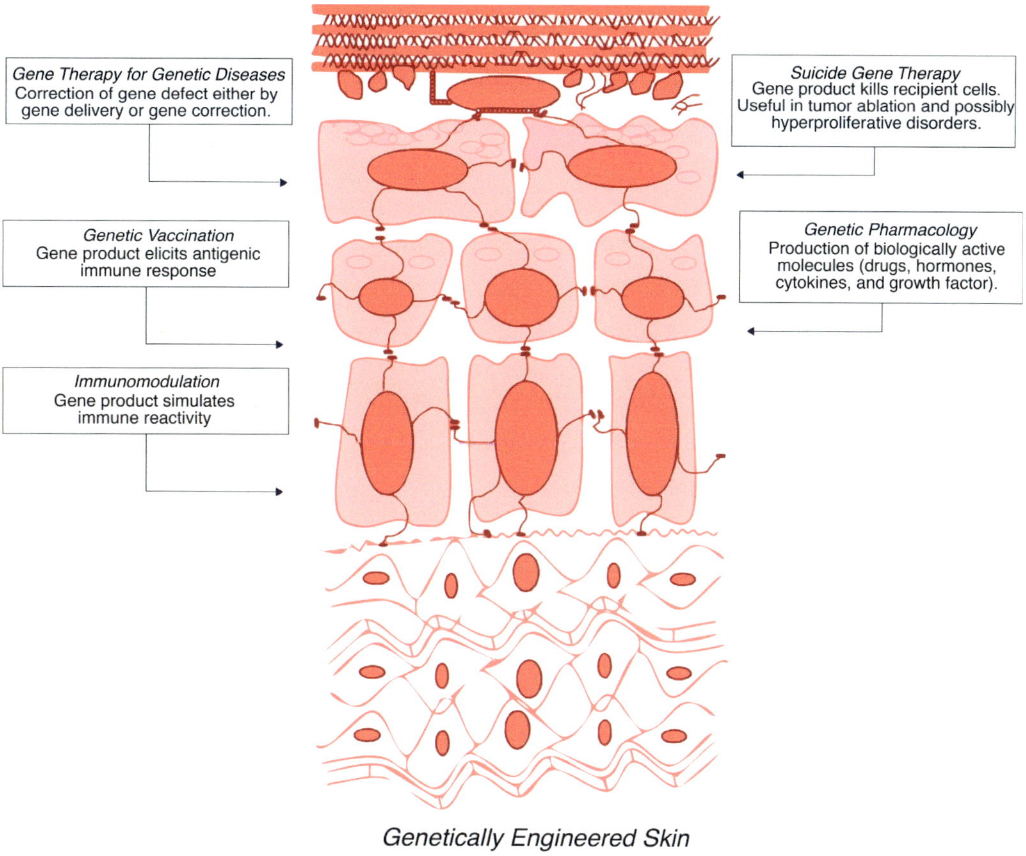

Fig. (11). Different approaches of gene therapy.

Genetic vaccination, for instance represents an interesting approach of cutaneous therapy due to its efficiency and low cost compared to other immunization techniques, such as the use of recombinant proteins [59 - 62]. The insertion of DNA into the skin leads to expression of the foreign antigen as a result of the capabilities of Langerhans cells to stimulate an immune reaction. Genetic pharmacology is another promising application of gene therapy. By the administration of DNA fragments (encoding therapeutically beneficial genes to the tissue), a defective gene is either to prevent from producing its protein or to increase the concentration of normal protein produced in the body.

The physicochemical properties of hydrophilic DNA molecule and SC represent a great challenge of delivering genes to the viable skin [3].

There are a number of physical methods used to successfully deliver gens to the skin. The gene gun approach is commonly used to “accelerate” small DNA-coated gold particles into target cells or tissues. Due to their small size, DNA-bound structures carried by the particles can enter the cell membrane, dissociate from them and expressed. A previous experiment with the gene gun has shown significant levels of epidermal grow factor receptor expression to stimulate epidermal growth *in vivo* [63].

Direct DNA intradermal injection of naked DNA has shown a high level of gene expression by increasing the ionic strength, being most evident in the subdermal smooth muscle cells and epidermal cells [64].

Microneedles coated with DNA have demonstrated to improve protection against influenza and to enhance immunogenicity to Hepatitis C [59, 60].

The use of ultrasound (US) combined with herpes simplex virus thymidine kinase gene-loaded microbubbles have been suggested as a new gene delivery technique to treat liver tumor [65].

Electroporation has also become an attractive technology for gene transfer [66]. This technique has shown a ~ 83-fold increase in transgene expression, relative to naked DNA injection in a porcine model. Transfected cells included adipocytes, fibroblasts, and mononuclear cells with dendritic processes [67].

There are some studies that investigate the use of RF for delivery of genetic material that may result in gene expression.

Birchall *et al.* confirmed the ability of ViaDerm™, previously described in section 5.4.1., to facilitate targeted and controlled delivery of a mammalian expression plasmid and subsequent gene expression within the viable epidermis [68]. Studies were conducted with full thickness breast skin that was exposed to RF application (5 bursts of 700 us, 290 or 330V at 100 kHz) using a disposable array of electrodes of 100 or 50um with a density of 100 electrodes/cm^2 in a total area of 1.4 cm^2.

Application of 50 μm electrode arrays facilitated reproducible permeation across the skin, allowing 5% diffusion of the applied 100 nm fluorescein nanoparticles, compared to the application of 100 μm electrode arrays that led to a variable permeation enhancement and disruption of the membrane (Fig. **12**).

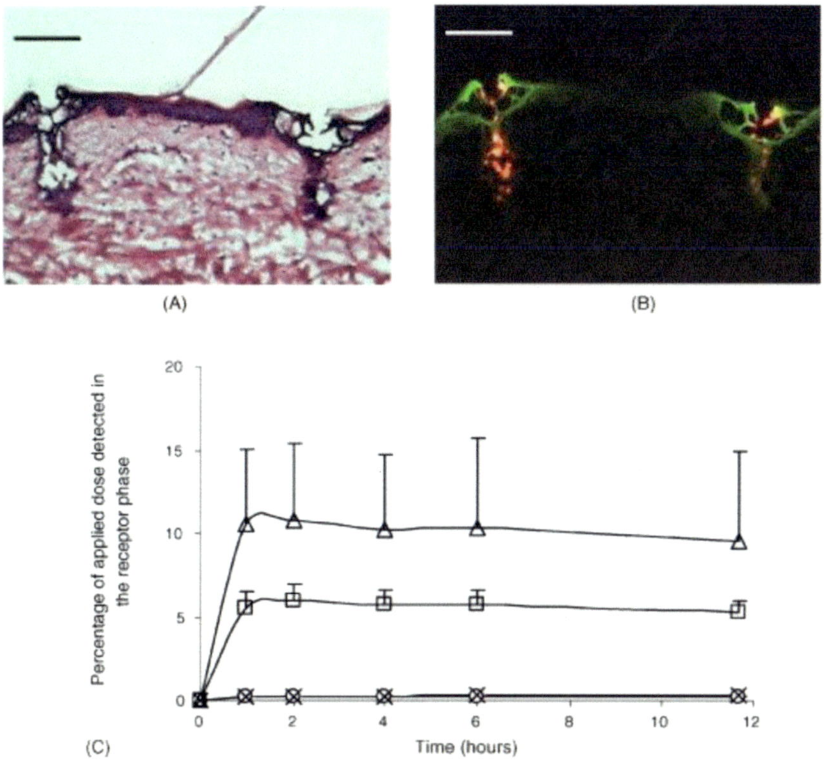

Fig. (12). Light (**A**) and fluorescent (**B**) photomicrographs of RF-microchannels containing fluorescent nanoparticles. Original magnification = 100×, bar = 100 μm; (**C**) diffusion of fluorescent nanoparticles through ViaDerm™ treated epidermal membranes. Data presented as percentage of topical nanoparticle dose detected in the receptor phase of Franz cells over a 12 h period.. (○) Untreated skin—PBS donor phase, (×) Untreated skin—topical nanoparticles, (□) 50 μm array ViaDerm™iaDermning fluorescent nanoparticles. (△) 100 μm array ViaDerm™ treated skin—topical nanoparticles (N = 3 ± S.D.). (Adapted by permission from Birchall *et al.* Cutaneous gene expression of plasmid DNA in excised human skin following delivery *via* microchannels created by radio frequency ablation. Int. J. Pharm., 2000; 18 (1); 177 - 188 Copyright Elsevier B.V. 2006).

Gene expression profiles of human organ culture were used to predict the efficacy of β-galactosidase reporter plasmid DNA applied alone to ViaDerm™ treated skin. The author reports the presence of intense blue staining related to substantial reporter gene expression (Fig. **13a** and **13b**) in the epidermis with no detection of expression in tissue treated with RF device and probed with the control (Fig. **13c**). The expression was predominantly adjacent to the RF microchannels (Fig. **13d** and **13e**). It was also observed that the extent and level of expression may be significantly higher by treating the skin prior and after application of the DNA solution.

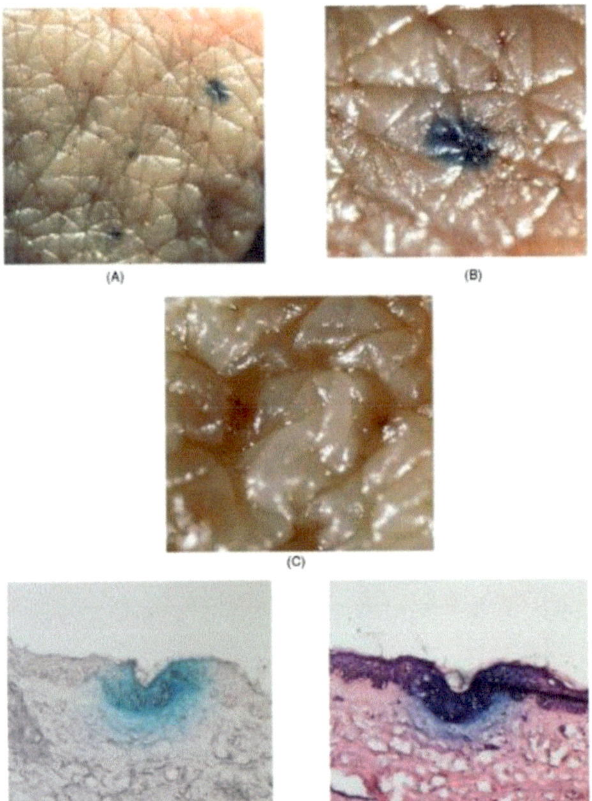

Fig. (13). Photomicrographs of ViaDerm™ treated human skin stained for β-galactosidase expression (50 μm arrays). (**A**) En face stereomicroscopy; (**B**) en face light microscopy, original magnification = 40×; (**C**) en face stereomicroscopy of ViaDerm™ treated human skin treated with the pEGFP-N1 plasmid; (**D**) unstained cryosection, original magnification = 100×; (**E**) H&E stained cryosection, original magnification = 100×, bar = 100 μm. (Adapted by permission from Birchall *et al.* Cutaneous gene expression of plasmid DNA in excised human skin following delivery *via* microchannels created by radio frequency ablation. Int. J. Pharm., 2000; 18 (1); 177 - 188 Copyright Elsevier B.V. 2006).

Radiofrequency-induced heat therapy (RFHT) has been suggested as a good alternative to treat cutaneous leishmaniosis (CL) [69]. CL is an infection caused by Leishmania parasites transmitted by the bite of phlebotomine sand flies, and manifests as localized hypo-pigmented skin lesions or redness that may become chronic, producing tissue destruction and disfigurement. The optimal therapy for CL comprises daily systemic injections or weekly intralesional inoculations of pentavalent antimonials for at least 3 weeks. These drug treatments may present important side effects and poor patient compliance due to routes of administration.

Some technologies such as cryotherapy and heat therapy have been used to treat CL [70, 71 - 76]. Cryotherapy, for instance is effective to treat dry and small lesions (<1 cm) without antimonials, however it requires several applications of liquid nitrogen on the affected tissues (7 - 21days) [70].

Good results have been obtained with RFHT when compared to administration of antimonial drugs in the treatment of CL [72, 73, 75, 76]. The therapy consists of controlled and localized delivery of RF under local anesthesia into injuries for usually 30-60 sec to generate heat and produce a secondary burn in the upper dermis, destroying damaged tissue while causing minimal damage to healthy underlying tissue.

Bumb *et al.* showed the long-term efficacy and safety of a single application of RFHT compared to intralesional sodium stibogluconate (SSG) injection in the treatment of CL by L. tropica [77]. 100 patients were randomized in a 1:1 ratio to receive either RFHT (one application 30-60s, depending on the thickness of the lesion) or SSG injection. The patients were follow-up every 2 weeks for 4 months to control healing process and then at 5, 6, 9, 12 and 18 months to monitor clinical therapy rate. The results did not show any statistical difference in terms of healing (between 6 and 104 weeks) following SSG injection compared to RFHT treatment. The clinical therapy rates after 6 months were 98% and 94%, for RFTH and SSG treatments, respectively. No recurrence of infection was recorded in patients up to 12-18 months after the beginning of treatment.

A 12-month follow-up study conducted by Aronson *et al.* showed that RFH therapy may be as effective as systemic sodium stibogluconate treatment, and much safer in inducing lesion healing in US soldiers who had acquired L. major infection in Iraq [75]. Moreover, RF treatment has been reported to be highly effective in the treatment of CL caused by L. tropica in immunocompromised patients refractory to sodium stibogluconate administration [74]. The patients showed no recurrence of illness 18 months after the treatment.

The potential mechanisms that may be responsible for RFH therapy-induced are not well defined yet. The main assumption involves direct destruction of parasites by heat followed by stimulation of the immune response due to release of parasite antigen from destroyed tissue, which leads to the rapid upregulation of a protective response.

Lobo *et al.* showed the effect of heat therapy on systemic effects assessed by modulation of systemic cytokine response, following RF application compared to Glucantime™ therapy in patients infected with L. braziliensis [76]. Cytokine expression was assessed by normal peripheral blood mononuclear cells after 0, 14 and 28 days after initiation of treatment. The results did not revealed any significant differences between the two therapies, showing a similar cytokine response compared to the induced by the antimonial treatment.

Further studies primarily on the efficacy of RFH in short and long-term therapies caused by other Leishmania types should be established in order to consider this technology as a new therapeutic alternative for leishmaniosis.

4.3. Non-Surgical Dermatologic Treatments

4.3.1. Acne and Scars

Acne vulgaris can affect individuals at any age and may have a deep impact in their quality of life. Moderate and severe acne vulgaris requires several months or even year's regimen of systemic or topical medications, with numerous visits to the clinic. Patients may possibly show adverse effects due to the frequent use of common medication or lack of response to alternative drugs. Therefore, there is a need to investigate new techniques to improve current therapies.

Some physical methods have been proposed to treat acne such as laser ablation, chemical peeling and surgery [78]. However, those are intended to decrease the sequel of scars rather than cure the active disease.

Non-ablative RF has been used to soften acne scars imperfections by the stimulation of new collagen production [79]. Some examples are listed below.

Ramesh *et al.* evaluated efficiency of a new matrix-tunable RF technology in 30 Indian patients with ice pick, box and rolling acne scars (2 to 20 mm) pre-treated with oral antibiotics, exfoliating agents (tretinoin), and eventually subcision for deeper box type scars [80]. Each scar was treated at 1 month intervals and evaluated by visual scale (digital photographs) expressed in terms of progression rate. Data were collected every 15 days for a period of 6 months. The results show clinical improvement, ranging from 50% to 70%, after 2 and 6 months, respectively. However, the response of patients varied with the type of scars: ice pick type of scars reported the maximum improvement (20% excellent, and 80% good results) compared to predominant box type scars, which showed moderate to poor improvement (55%). Rolling type scars reported variable data (20% excellent, 50% good and 20% poor results).

Gold *et al.* [81] evaluated the efficacy of a fractional bipolar RF treatment (3 applications/ month), using a hand-held applicator (Matrix RF, Syneron, Inc.) on slight to moderate acne scars in 13 females (~36 years old; skin type I-V). Improvement on acne scar severity and tolerance, evaluated by a physician during the 1-3 months follow-up visits was considerably reduced. Patient's satisfaction was significant (67-92%).

Cho *et al.* [82] demonstrated an improvement in the grade of mild to moderate acne scars and large facial pores in more than 70% of a population of 30 patients when using a fractional RF microneedle therapy. Skin surface roughness and dermal density was also enhanced, whereas TEWL and sebum measurement did not change.

Chandrashekar *et al.* [83] conducted a retrospective study in 31 patients of skin types III-V with moderate and severe facial acne scarring to test efficacy and safety of four serial microneedling fractional RF treatments during 6 months (with 6 weeks intervals between each session). Microneedles penetration depth was limited to either 3,5 mm in predominant ice pick scars and mixed scarring or 1.5 mm on forehead, temple areas and arcas with bony prominences. Energy settings of 35 W- 40 W at depths of 3.5 mm with successively lower energy levels (30 W-35 W, 25 W-30 W, respectively), at lower penetration depths were applied.

Goodman & Baron's acne scar grading system [84] showed 80.64% improvement by 2 grades, and 19.35% by 1 grade in 31 patients with Grade 3 and 4 scars. Rolling and box scars showed better response than icepick scars. The treatment confirmed transient side effects such as mild erythema, post-inflammatory hyperpigmentation and track marks of the device.

The epidermal permeability of steroids induced by ablative RF in combination with low frequency ultrasound (US) technology has been investigated as a method to treat hypertrophic scar treatment [85]. Four areas were treated with steroids, nose, knee, neck and mandibular. A fractional RF applicator (45 watts x 3 passes) with a tip of 110 stainless pins was applied on to the skin. Triamcinolone acetonide (1 ml; 20 mg/mL) was dropped on the perforated surface and finally, the US was applied (50 Hz; intensity= 80%) 30-60s per lesion. The combined treatment (RF + US) was carried out every 3-4 weeks until therapeutic progress. A dermatologic examination was conducted every 21 days during treatment and after 30, 90, 180 days and one year after the last session. The results show a significant improvement after 1 session in patients with scars on nose and mandibular zones. Scars on the neck and on the knee showed a marked improvement after 4 sessions. This method appears to enhance the efficiency of steroids by increasing their skin penetration while apparently reducing the possibilities of localized atrophy and irregular form of the treated lesion. However, further studies with longer follow-up and representative populations should be evaluated in order to corroborate such outcome.

Rongsaard and Rummaneethorn [86] showed the clinical and side effects of fractional bipolar RF compared to those of fractional erbium-doped (ED) 1,550 nm laser in 20 subjects with atrophic acne scars Fitzpatrick skin type III-V. The data do not demonstrated statistical difference between the two treatments. However, relevant improvement in skin texture was observed with the ED laser. Some side effects such as pain, transient facial erythema, and scab formation were noticed with both technologies. Pain scores were significantly higher with ED laser in relation to RF treatments.

Trelles *et al.* [87] studied the efficacy of a unipolar fractional ablative RF technology (iPixel™ RF, Alma Lasers, Caesarea, Israel) with acoustic pressure on acne scarring over 2 and 6 months in 19 patients who underwent 4 treatment sessions at 3-week intervals. The results showed after 2 months 57% of fading on total scarring on the face and 49% on the back and shoulders; 62% and 58% was observed after 6 months, respectively. No side effects to the ablation were observed.

The trials illustrated in this section have shown the best results for resolution of acne and scars showing an improvement in superficial appearance. The appreciation of such effects occurs most likely after different passes and several sessions and, include a relatively long post-treatment period. Side effects are not negligible; transient pain and erythema (usually resolve within few days) was also observed. Further research is to be conducted to determine targeted RF parameters to treat specific atrophic acne subtypes. Furthermore, the long-term responses of treatment (alone or in combination with topical drugs) should also be carefully investigated.

4.3.2. Hyperhidrosis

Hyperhidrosis is an important disorder in which an excessive sweating is produced by the eccrine sweat glands due to overactive cholinergic innervation. The most common alternatives used to treat this condition such as iontophoresis, topical aluminum chloride and botulinum toxin are mainly palliative [88]. Surgery represent a permanent cure however, this technique have the risk of significant adverse effects and complications. Ultrasound has been recently employed to treat hyperhidrosis [89], however, this initial work has not provided a well comprehension of the damage made to the glands and the affordability of the treatment with respect to other technologies, if it is legitimately used for this purpose [89]. Radiofrequency has been investigated as a non-invasive modality to treat this disease by compromising the electrochemical activity of the sweat glands.

Kim *et al.* [90] assessed the application of bipolar fractional microneedling radiofrequency (FMR at intervals of 4 weeks for primary axillary hyperhidrosis (PAH)) in 20 patients. The microneedles delivered 1 MHz from a surface of 0.5 to 3.5 mm below the surface of the skin. The protocol included 2 passes for 150 ms at 25 V; 70% of patients observed more than 50% improvement in sweating. The results showed a decrease in the number and size of both apocrine and eccrine glands 1 month after the final treatment (n=3). Transitory side effects such as tingling, swelling and redness were observed in the affected areas, but were apparently resolved within 1 week.

Fatemi Naeini *et al.* [91] have observed a significant improvement of the treated site after three sessions of fractionated microneedle radiofrequency (FRM) at 3-week intervals treatment in 25 patients with severe PAH. Hyperhidrosis disease severity scale (HDSS) showed after 21 weeks a 1.8 -fold decrease with respect to the controlled side. The follow-up evaluation revealed 79% of 1 or 2-score decrease in HDSS. A decrease number of the sweat glands in the affected side (histological evaluation) confirmed those findings.

Additional studies in this field considering higher population and longer observation periods are needed. Control of variables affecting sweat production, as well as suitable features such as amount of energy applied, depth of penetration and long-term response to treatment should be tested in order to evaluate the advantages of RF therapy to treat hyperhidrosis. In addition, targeted energy parameters to treat different types of the disorder should be also explored.

4.3.3. Skin Tightening

Skin laxity represents an unpleasant sign of aging that may occur anywhere on the body, most noticeable on the face but may also be predominant on the hands, abdomen, thighs, neck, *etc.* It is a general atrophy that results from the change in viscoelasticity properties of the skin due to age (breakdown of collagen and elastin binding fibers) and repeated mechanical forces. Surgery has been a standard treatment for many years, however there is an increased tendency to use non-invasive alternatives that results in shorter recovery time.

The most common treatments are dermal fillers to soften the shadowing around some parts of the face, making the jowls of cheek appear less prominent. A second option is skin tightening devices such as infrared (IR), laser (erbium laser or CO_2) and RF. The main mechanism of action of these treatments is the heating of the dermal and subdermal regions while reducing damage to the epidermis.

Limited studies evidenced biologically the use of RF energy to treat skin laxity. England *et al.* [92] has examined the tissue interaction of monopolar RF heating and cross-linked fillers in a young pig model over a period of 4 months. The outcome showed an increase in fibroplasia with hyaluronic acid, hydroxylapatite and polylactic acid. A significant increase in collagen deposition was observed for hydroxylapatite.

Shumaker *et al.* [93] reported, as a second part of the previous study, the effect of the five fillers injected in a juvenile farm pig. Fillers were analyzed histologically 5 days, 2 weeks, or 1 month after treatment. RF treatment caused significantly increases in the inflammatory and fibrotic responses but showed few histological changes when associated with the filler substances.

Several clinical studies usually based on qualitative measurements report improvements of skin texture and laxity.

Fitzpatrick and colleagues, for instance, run a blinded clinical trial in 86 patients who were treated with monopolar RF energy (Thermage; Solta Medical). Fitzpatrick wrinkle score showed improvements in 83.2% of treated periorbital areas. Photographic evaluation showed that 61.5% of eyebrows were lifted by at least 0.5 mm [94].

Alster and Tanzi *et al.* used monopolar RF (ThermaCool; Thermage Corp., Hayward, CA) to treat cheek, submental, and neck mid-to-moderate laxity in 50 patients (skin phototypes I-IV). Fluences from 97 to 144 J/cm^2 and 74 to 134 J/cm^2, on the cheeks and neck were evaluated respectively [95]. In general, significant improvement and patient satisfaction were reported.

More recently, Edwards *et al.* [96] evaluated the clinical efficacy of a monopolar RF device with a vibrating tip (Thermage CPT System; Solta Medical) on mild to moderate facial skin laxity in forehead, cheek, jawline, and upper neck in 64 patients. The energy levels applied were between 14 and 24 J/cm^2, with ~900 pulses delivered. 80% of the volunteers expressed minor correction of skin laxity and 55% noticed an improvement of skin texture. Skin laxity correction was apparently improved after 7 months out of treatment compared with those after 1-3 months. No prolonged pain was informed in any patient treated.

Chipps *et al.* [97] used 3D photography to assess the effectiveness and patient satisfaction of a novel application of monopolar RF on rhytids and laxity of the face and neck. 49 subjects received a total of 2 RF treatments (Pelleve; Ellman International Inc.) with one month interval. The treated area received at least 5 passes, reaching a temperature of 41-43°C. 85% of patients observed an improvement in their skin appearance and smoothness, and 62% in skin brightness. However, some factors may have affected the interpretation of results such as uncontrolled hydration of the patient at the time of evaluation, alignment of head and neck when taking the images and digitalization of photographs.

Vega *et al.* [98] tested the efficacy of the cited monopolar RF system (Pellevé S5 Wrinkle Treatment Generator; Ellman) to tighten the skin of the hands in 31 women with a median age of 56 years. 3 treatments were performed with an interval of 2 weeks. The outcome showed a visible improvement of the appearance of the treated hands in 89% of patients based on the visual Global Aesthetic Improvement Scale after 3 months.

Key *et al.* [99] presented at the American Society for Laser Medicine and Surgery Conference (April 4-6, 2014; Phoenix, AZ), a new approach of skin tightening by the use of skin thermal imaging with RF auto-feedback probe heating. 70 patients underwent treatment with or without lipoaspiration at subsurface temperatures of 50°C to 60°C. The results demonstrated an improvement on a 4-point skin laxity score in 70% of patients. Apparently, no significant adverse events were observed due to the monitoring of temperature.

4.3.4. Reduction of Adipose Tissue Volume

Localized subcutaneous fat deposits may negatively impact patients self-esteem and easily affect their quality of life. The medical contouring approaches used to improve such skin conditions include liposuction, abdominoplasty, and thigh lifts, among other procedures. However, those treatments have risk of adverse effects and need long recovery periods.

Non-contact radiofrequency has been suggested to transitory reduced fat deposits due to an increase in temperature [100]. Fat cells present a higher resistance to radio waves than surrounding tissues. The heat produced by RF application may modify the cell membrane, increasing in this way its permeability and thus, boosting their metabolic activity which will lead to an increase in vascular perfusion [101]. The connective tissue is also affected by RF energy as it boosts the production of heat shock proteins and collagen, which is reflected as improved skin tone and elasticity.

Franco *et al.* [102] evaluated the feasibility of controlling heating volume applied to subcutaneous adipose tissue by RF technology. Fluctuations in the distribution of the electric potential were characterized at the skin surface of human skin samples at 500 kHz, 1, 2, 3, and 4 MHz. An increase in frequency provoked a decrease in electric potential at the skin surface, from the centre to the edge of the RF applicator. The data showed that within a 3 cm subcutaneous fat layer, the absorbed power was 40% less at the bottom than that at the top of the layer for 500 Hz. Uniform heating was corroborated at the same frequency.

Franco *et al.* [103] assessed subsequently the feasibility of using such non-invasive RF device to induce harmful thermal damage to subcutaneous adipose tissue. Cultured adipocyte cells were subjected to hyperthermic conditions: 45, 50, 55, 60, and 65° C during 1, 2, and 3 min. *In vitro* cell viability decreased from 89% to 20% at increase temperatures of 45°C to 50°C, respectively, during 1 min exposure. *In vivo* studies showed an increase in temperature (50°C) of adipose tissue at 7-12 mm depth, while the temperature of superficial tissue was <30°C during RF contact. Histology evaluations did not show any abnormality in epidermal and dermal layers. However, subcutaneous vascular alterations were perceived within ~4 -19 mm depth from the skin surface.

Mlosek *et al.* [104] showed the efficacy the RF, monitored by high-frequency US to treat cellulites in 28 women. The thickness of epidermis, dermis and subcutaneous layers as well as the length of the subcutaneous tissue bands growing into the dermis were examined among other parameters. A tripolar device T1 (Beauty Light Science and Technology CO., Ltd, Beijing, China) was used, starting with an application of 110 J /cm^2 and then increased up to 10-20 J /cm^2. Patients underwent 8 procedures 7-8 day's interval period. The results obtained by ultrasound monitoring showed a significant decrease in subcutaneous tissue thickness when using radiofrequency (thickness before and after therapy was 17.152 mm and 14.924 mm, respectively). 25 women (89%) who were subjected to RF treatment experienced a decrease in cellulite after therapy. The reduction of cellulite by one degree in the scale was observed in 20 patients (71%), and by 2 degrees only in five patients (17%). No statistically significant changes were observed in the placebo group.

Milanese *et al.* [105] investigated the influence of whole-body vibration (WBV) alone and in combination with localized RF on fat deposits in the abdominal, buttock and thigh region in 44 young individuals during an 8-week trial, 2 sessions per week. Application of WBV+RF led to a significant reduced in skinfold thickness at several sites, more importantly at the thigh site.

Kim *et al.* [106] observed a reduction of fat deposits combining phosphatidylcholine (PPC) injections with RF to shorten the period of oedema and swelling. 1-year follow-up demonstrated that the reduction of fat deposit was well sustained.

McDaniel *et al.* [107] studied a monopolar RF device with cooling (Exilis Elite, BTL Industries, Framingham, MA) to evaluate the selective effect of heating fat, causing disintegration of adiposites and apoptosis in a porcine model. The study was done in three Vietnamese pigs and delivered to an area of 20x10 cm (duration of treatment 20 min, 30 s). Biopsy samples were taken before and after treatment. The temperature on the surface of the skin and in different layers of the skin tissue was measured by infrared and by internal probe monitored by ultrasound examination. Apoptosis was monitored by the TUNEL method. The results showed changes in the temperature in the subcutaneous layers. The apoptotic index increased from 7% before the first treatment to approximately 53% after treatment, showing a substantial apoptic process. After three months, the apoptotic index seemed to be decreased back to around 11%.

Adato *et al.* [108] propose the use VelaShape II device (Syneron Medical Ltd, Yokneam, Israel) that associates bipolar RF, ultrasound and infrared with tissue manipulation to reduce adipose tissue volume. One treatment per week for 6 weeks was applied to 35 patients in specific zones (abdomen/flank, buttock, or thigh areas). A follow-up period of 3 months after completion of the treatment protocol was carried on. A gradual decrease in patient circumferences and improvement in skin tightening was observed. 93% patients demonstrated variable changes (1-60%) in fat layer thickness.

Fajkošová *et al.* [109] investigated the efficiency of non-contact RF device Vanquish™ for body contouring as a non-invasive tool to reduce fat and circumferences of abdomen. Treatment consisted of 4 sessions performed once a week for 30 min in 40 subjects. The homogeneity of heat distribution and temperature of the skin surface were controlled. The results showed an average of 4.93 cm decrease in abdominal circumference in 75% of the population. Mild to moderate erythema was also observed.

Boisnic *et al.* [110] has recently published a clinical and biological assessment of a device associating suction-coupled RF heating and ultra-short pulse duration, high voltage electrical pulses for the long-term reduction of adipose tissue. Abdominal fat was treated once a week for 6 weeks in 21 subjects. Biopsies from the treated and untreated regions were obtained. Measurement of apoptosis rate, and dermal thickness, among others were determined. Reduction of abdominal circumference (~2.3%), subcutaneous adipose tissue thickness (~4%) and adipose tissue weight (~4.7%) were observed during 3-months follow-up. Adipocytes from histological samples showed a decreased in size with increased levels of apoptosis.

There is still lack of long-term efficacy reports and complete description of side effects using non-contact RF technology for reduction of subcutaneous adipose tissue. Extended studies more objectivized that describe targeted parameters for the treated zones, the mechanism of action and the safety of use of the technology, particularly long-term examinations in representative populations with significant subcutaneous fat deposits (*i.e.*, overweight or obese) must be accomplished in order to consider this technique as a therapeutic alternative.

4.3.5. Melasma

Non-contact RF has been employed in association with topical agents to treat skin pigmentation. There are few clinical trials that report an effect on such problematic. Cameli *et al.* [111], for instance investigated the efficacy and safety of monopolar RF and delivery of phytocomplex containing 1% kojic acid. In this study, 15 patients affected by melasma underwent 6 sessions of treatment at 1-week intervals. The outcome was evaluated at time 0, 1 and 6 months after treatment using digital and ultraviolet computerized image analysis of skin color. Hyperpigmentation was significantly reduced at 1 and 6 months compared with baseline. The average melanin score, and the average erythema values showed a significant reduction.

Yoshida *et al.* [112] evaluated an intense pulsed-radio frequency system (IPL-RF; Aurora, Syneron Medical, Yokneam) that utilizes electrical and optical energy in combination with topical application of vitamin D3 ointment (Oxarol, Chugai Pharmaceutical, Tokyo, Japan) to treat light brown spots, also called cafe au lait spots, on skin in people with Neurofibromatosis 1 (NF1). During the study, the skin temperature was kept at 5°C to prevent heat damage, the light range varied from 580-980 nm and the RF energy range was 15-20 J/cm^3. Patients follow a mean of 8.5 treatments over a period of 6-12 months at 2-4 weeks. The efficacy rate was mainly moderate in all patients particularly in response to treatment of small spots rather that cave-au-lait spots. Improvement was observed between the 3rd and 10th sessions of treatment. Apparently, application of Vitamine D3 and RF has a synergistic effect for lightening by impacting both the melanin production from melanocyte and the transportation of melanin to keratinocytes.

The described treatments may represent an option to treat melasma; however, further trials to elucidate the mechanism of action and safety with other active drugs should be performed in order to consider the combined therapy as an alternative to treat pigmented lesions.

4.4. Orthopedic Treatments

The use of RF in orthopedic has been grown in the last decade. The benefits of such procedures reside in the production of heat that targets collagen-based connective structures.

A non-contact monopolar-capacitive coupled RF (mcRF) has shown the ability to increase temperatures above 50°C in tendons and ligaments, leading to the activation of the wound healing response without damaging the surrounding structures [4].

Previous studies in cadaveric specimens demonstrated that collagen changes after application of mcRF are dose dependent. Anatomical structures from 2 upper and lower extremities were exposed to RF application. The temperatures recorded at the targeted structures every second showed an increase of above 50 °C during the treatment. A progressive pattern of collagen denaturation, assessed by histological analysis evidenced correlation with the temperatures measured [113].

The tissue interactions between 5 fillers injected in a pig model and the application of monopolar RF heating were evaluated by England *et al.* in two studies [114]. The synergy of RF and fillers (cross-linked human collagen (Cosmoplast), hyaluronic acid (Restylane), calcium hydroxylapatite (Radiesse), polylactic acid (Sculptra), and liquid injectable silicone (Silikon 1000)) was studied during 4 months. An increase in fibroplasia and collagen deposition of RF treatment mainly associated with Restylane, Radiesse, and Sculptra fillers was observed. No apparent risk of local burns and influence of RF application on filler persistence in the skin were observed. In a second study [115], skin samples treated with dermal fillers were subjected to RF application. Histology evaluation was conducted at 5 days, 2 weeks, or 1 month after treatment. The results demonstrated important histological changes and wound healing response with RF according to the type of filler material.

Application of mcRF to treat pain associated with lateral elbow tendinopathies has been studied in 39 patients with a variety of nonsurgical therapies (*e.g.* nonsteroidal anti-inflammatory drugs, corticosteroid injections, and braces) [5]. Patients were treated with mcRF by applying 10 additional pulses, of a total of 100 pulses, directly to the point of maximum sensitivity, without local anaesthesia. 81% patients present a good response after a follow-up of 423 days.

Cronkey and LaPorta have investigated the usage of 6 instruments for detection of changes associated to functional ankle instability [116]. 20 patients were treated with a single session with the application of mcRF. The Cumberland Ankle Instability Tool demonstrated good sensitivity, detecting changes that correlated with patient's responses. 78% of the patients treated presented successfully results, from which 87.5% confirmed significant improvement in functional ankle stability.

mcRF would offer a new non-invasive choice for tendinopathies and sprained ligaments as this does not interfere with surgical procedures. However, additional studies on RF parameters to target specific zones as well as safety studies targeting representative populations should be performed in order to further explore the potential of the technology in this field.

4.5. Chronic Pain Treatments

Transcutaneous-pulsed (non-invasive) RF has been employed to treat pain but its clinical efficacy remains still controversial.

Malilk and Benzon conducted in 2007 a bibliographic research related to the application of pulsed RF in the adjacent area of a neural structure, resulted in only two controlled randomized trials out of 44, and only one trial reported efficiency of such technology [117].

Chao *et al.* analyzed 154 dossiers of patients with lumbar or cervical radicular pain caused by herniated intervertebral disk or preceding failed surgery [118]. Patients were subjected to pulsed RF therapy in 2 to 4 spinal levels, separately. Follow-up period went from 1 week to 1 year post-treatment. The results showed a good response to pulsed radiofrequency and a short-term pain relief (up to 6 months).

Taverner *et al.* recently reported a retrospective assessment of transcutaneous-pulsed RF treatment therapy on shoulder pain over a 4-year period [119]. The case review showed a single treatment performed in 13 patients presenting painful shoulders between 2006 and 2010 in an outpatient location. Two-thirds of the treated patients reported pain relief for around 1 year.

Taverner and Loughnan reported in a second phase controlled study with 51 patients with shoulder pain sustained reductions in pain at night, with activity and functional improvement at 4 and 12 weeks with active transcutaneous-pulsed RF [120]. No complications were apparently observed.

Stall has examined the use of non-invasive pulsed RF energy on recurrent migraine pain associated with occipital neuralgia [121]. Non-invasive pulsed RF was applied for 30 min twice daily directly over the occiput and upper cervical spine. 3 of 4 patients reported a decrease in occurrence and severity of non-prostrating and prostrating migraines compared to initial symptoms. Combining non-invasive pulsed RF with occipital nerve blocks showed a marked improvement in all symptoms.

Additional randomized controlled clinical trials with long-term follow-up must be further considered. The effect of heating on biological processes should also be elucidated in order to understand the role of pulsed RF in the management of chronic pain syndromes.

5. DEVICES

5.1. Transdermal RF Drug Delivery Systems

Avrahami *et al.* [122] patented a transdermal apparatus that make RF current pass between two or more electrodes through the tissue in order to generate at least one micro-channel in the SC to improved transdermal transport of the component. This device can be used alone for skin pre-treatment followed by a patch or mask application. Microchannels are created by the breakdown in the SC generated by the lateral capacity currents produced between the electrodes after application of AC current at 1 kHz and 300 kHz. The device is capable of monitoring the electrical resistance of skin. The method claims to cause ablation at the SC during a fist period for 1ms in order to assist the transport of a substance through the treated area during a second period of 200 ms, following to the first time period.

Avrahami *et al.* [123] patented in 2003 an electronic card (skin patch) to promote the administration of active substances by RF application. The device comprises a substance storage compartment, a sensor that generates a signal responsive to a physiological parameter, one or more electrodes adapted to be placed at respective sites on the skin, and a substance release element adapted to receive the signal, and drive some of the electrodes to apply a current capable of ablating the SC. Such device includes a sensor adapted to measure a physiological parameter such as transepidermal water loss (TEWL), temperature, skin impedance, blood pressure. The control unit (adequate to configure a current frequency between 1 kHz and 300 kHz) includes a motherboard to regulate all parameters of the electrical energy delivered to the electrode, to control micro-channel formation. In addition, the device comprises a communications unit, adapted to receive the signal and to transmit information to a computer external to the device.

A miniature, self-contained device and methods to porate the skin and deliver or extract an active compound transdermally was patented by Avrahami *et al.* in 2003 [124]. The device includes a cover for supporting at least one spark-generating electrode in the skin, and a control unit, which causes electrical current to pass through the electrode and generate one or more sparks between the electrode and the SC to create micro-channels. The number of sparks is measured by adjusting the magnitude and timing of the voltage applied to the electrodes. *In vitro* data showed that this technique at a density of 100 pores/cm^2 enhanced the penetration of acetaminophen through pig ear skin, which resulted in a 10-fold increase compared to untreated skin. In equivalent assessments, a 2.5 increase in drug permeation compared to the untreated group was observed after application of a formulation containing 1% diclofenac and 10% ethyl alcohol, confirming that the physicochemical properties of active agents definitely influence pore density to attain significant permeation values.

A handled device containing a plurality of electrodes, adapted to roll over the skin while maintaining electrical contact was patented by Avrahami *et al.* in 2004 for transdermal drug delivery and analyte extraction [125]. The driving electrode may move over the receiving electrodes automatically. The power source is adapted to drive the dynamic electrode to apply a current at a magnitude sufficient to perforate the SC. The application unit includes a reservoir to contain the drug composition and a conduit to transfer the substance to the application site at a controlled flow rate. This technology was marketed by TransPharma Medical as RF-MicroChannel Technology™ and was applied first in the ViaDerm™ drug delivery system.

Levin *et al.* (2005) [126] patented a method for transdermal delivery of water insoluble drugs, preferably steroids, utilizing the ViaDerm™ system. The patent claims on a system capable of delivering efficiently a water insoluble drug, which is formulated in a water-soluble media, into the blood, while causing minimal irritation and sensitization to the skin.

G. Levin and D. Daniel [127] patented a method for delivering active anti-emetic agents transdermally using a hydrophilic medical patch using ViaDerm™ technology. Clinical trials showed high plasma levels of granisetron over a period of 24 hours in patients treated with ViaDerm+granisetron-patch. Patients subjected to oral therapy demonstrated high levels of granisetron for shorter periods of time with an unsteady drug concentration in plasma. ViaDerm and granisetron patches produced similar (slight) irritation.

Levin *et al.* described a delivery system for topical application of poorly water-soluble cosmetic agents useful in treating cellulite, hyper-pigmentation, skin aging, and acne in association with Viaderm™ [128]. Significant results *in vitro* were confirmed for salicylic acid (0.2%), caffeine (3% and 1.5%), hydroquinone (2%) from solutions of commercial products.

Levin *et al.* patented in 2007 a device for effective topical administration of antigens comprising Viaderm™ [129, 130]. The delivery system is useful for immunization against bacterial, viral, and fungal antigens and for treating tumors and allergies. Results reported that Viderm™ facilitated transdermal immunization with ovoalbumin and trivalent influenza, compared to subcutaneous and intramuscular vaccination routes, in male guinea pigs. Apparently the RF device may shorten the time for appearance of titers of IgG and IgA antibodies.

TransPharma Medical Ltd. and Eli Lilly announced in 2010 encouraging results from a 4-week Phase 1 trial of a pocket-sized device ViaDerm-hPTH (1-34) (human parathyroid hormone) for the treatment of osteoporosis.

A blind placebo-controlled on the safety, tolerability, pharmacokinetics (PK) and pharmacodynamics (PD) of hPTH(1-34) (Forteo, injected form) was performed in 60 postmenopausal Japanese women. hPTH(1-34) was administered 28 days in transdermal doses of 30, 50, and 80 µg *via* the ViaDerm system. The results of the trial demonstrated a well tolerance with ViaDerm-hPTH(1-34), with PK and PD dose responses corresponding to the escalating hPTH(1-34) doses of the ViaDerm patches.). Phase 1 and Phase 2a studies were conducted later in Central and South America and Europe with similar doses, showing a similar performance of the technology to that of the previous study. Transpharma Medical has been acquired by Syneron Medical (Israel) and developed the Viador® device (formerly described as ViaDerm™) for transdermal drug delivery.

5.2. Non-invasive RF Systems Used in Skin Procedures

Conventional RF systems used in non-surgical dermatologic procedures are differentiated by the configuration of electrodes and corresponding electromagnetic fields.

Fractional RF systems mention in this section refers to the use of needles as electrodes to deliver fractionated bipolar or multipolar energy among several active and return needles. An electrode array is patterned to divide the treatment field into multiple RF thermal zones with intervening areas of untreated tissue.

Some of the typical RF devices used in non-invasive dermatologic procedures are listed above.

THERMAGE®. Solta Medical (CA, USA) was the first FDA approved monopolar device operating at 6.78 MHz for non-invasive treatment of the periorbital rhytids in 2002 and for the full face in 2004 [131]. Thermage NXT, the next generation device associates monopolar delivery, capacitive coupling and integrated cooling in one system to treat eyes, face and body. Recently, a new Comfort Pulse Technology™ (CPT) handpiece that uses vibration to make the procedure even more comfortable has been launched.

ACCENT® (Alma Lasers, IL, USA) uses both unipolar RF (for volumetric heating of adipose tissue) and bipolar RF (for more superficial non-volumetric heating) and operates at 40.68 MHz [132]. The unipolar handpiece provides RF energy without the need of a return electrode. The energy penetrates to a depth of up to 20 mm, heating the skin without damage to the tissue surface. Unipolar handpiece uses higher energy (100-200 watts) since it heats a bigger tissue volume. The system includes also a bipolar handpiece to provide more superficial heating from 60-100 watts, depending on the treatment area. The unipolar handpice consist of an RF resonance mechanism including a thermo-electric coupling cooler with pushbutton activation. The temperature skin is monitored with a laser thermometer.

PELLEVE™ (Ellman International, Oceanside, NY) operates in monopolar mode at 4.0 MHz and bipolar mode at 1.7 MHz. Line frequency is 50-60 Hz [133]. The PelleFirm System has received FDA clearance for tissue heating and the temporary reduction in the appearance of cellulite.

REGEN XL (Pollagen Ltd, Jerusalem, Israel) is a tripolar RF technology which simultaneously treats deep and superficial skin layers without damaging the epidermis by using multiple poles, lower energies can be delivered into the skin from each pole, making the treatments much more pleasant as compared with the original monopolar RF systems [134]. Max. output power is 30 Watts with an output frequency of 1 MHz.

ALMA SWEATX (Alma Lasers, USA) is used for hyperhidrosis and osmidrosis treatments. The diaelectric heating achieved with an RF frequency is of 40.68 MHz. Unipolar technology operates via a single electrode, delivering focused RF energy to the gland depth [135].

EVOLASTIN device (Syneron Medical Ltd, Yokeam, Israel) includes tiny like-microneedles electrodes of 1-2 mm [136]. The treatment delivers measured energy directly into the skin using 32g needles. The heating transmitted between paired needles is fractional and localized. Patient requires anesthesia by infiltration of lidocaine into the treated zone.

FRACTORA (Invasix, Yokeam, Israel) uses a reusable handpiece into which a disposable tip with variable density and array of microneedles of usually 1 mm is inserted [137]. The non-ablative tip has a 60-pin array that may reach 150 µm - 300 µm depth; a 60-pin 600 µm depth tip that gets a moderate to high epidermal impact, and a 120-pin 3000 µm depth tip for a very deep dermal impact. A sensor to monitor the skin temperature is included in the surface probe to assure safe parameters.

INFINI (Lutronic Corporation, South Korea) is capable of delivering energy in increments of 2.5 W in 20 equally graded energy level settings (level 1-2.5 W to level 20-50 W) [138]. The duration of each energy pulse can be set from 10 ms to 1,000 ms. The system consists of a disposable tip with gold-plated needles. The entire length of the needle is insulated. The depth of the needles can be adjusted from a minimum of 0.5 mm to a maximum of 3.5 mm. Clinical trials claimed on the use of this device in the fields of rejuvenation, tightening loose skin, axillary hyperhidrosis, and acne scars. 2-3 treatments of 30 min are recommended, achieving perceptible effects around 4-6 months post-treatment.

INTRACEL (Jeysis, Seoul, South Korea) contains 49-microneedles electrodes in 1cm^2 with only 0.3mm exposed at the top where RF energy is emitted [139]. Needles are insulated, thus michochannels formed at the skin surface are not exposed to thermal damage during RF emission, decreasing the risk of pigmentation and spares. Treatments with such device claim to treat acne scars and facial pores. Microneedles dimensions may be 0.5, 0.8, 1.5, or 2.0 mm long, and maximum device's power is 700 W.

PIXELRF (Fractional micro-plasma RF technology, Alma lasers, Buffalo Grove, IL) creates plasmas at the skin surface [132]. Plasma is a partially ionized gas that contains charged carriers and it is generated by electrical discharges in gases. When the plasma contacts the skin, it produces superficial micro-thermal injury of the SC under certain conditions. Multiple RF plasma micro-discharges are created in a gap between an applicator and the surface of the tissue. An array of pins (roller) is disposed in the front side on the applicator. RF electrical discharges are generated between the majority of the pins and respective points on the skin *via* gas. It operates in a unipolar mode. The micro-perforations produce holes of 100-150μm in depth with diameter of 80-120 μm.

EMATRIX SYSTEM (Syneron-Candela, CA, USA) used fractionated bi-polar radio frequency via an array of multielectrode pins to produce dermal heating. Sublative energy applied up to 62 mJ/pin [141].

POLLOGEN LEGEND™ (Pollagen Ltd, Jerusalem, Israel) incorporates VoluDermTM HE, a micro-needle RF technology, TriLipo® using non-invasive

RF energy and Dynamic Muscle Activation [134].

V-TOUCH ™ (Viora, NJ, USA) system uses RF energies at 0.8MHz, 1.7MHz and 2.45MHz [140]. The second generation of fractional RF technology is available only with the Viora V-FR hand piece with vacuum and cooling features producing less painful, safer, and more controlled treatments, with the ability to target specific applications, according to the skin layer.

ePRIME (Syneron, CA, USA) uses an array of micro-needles to deliver bipolar RF energy (460 kHz) to the skin. Cartridge contains 8 pairs of needles. Treatment duration is 3-5 s, 0.2 s increments.

INFINI (Lutronic, USA) delivers bipolar RF energy (1 MHz) via insulated gold-coated microneedles creating controllable fractionated thermal coagulation points within a specific layer of the dermis. 2 tip sizes are available, 49 or 16 microneedles. Treatment duration is 10 ms - 1,000 ms.

EDYMED PRO (USA) integrates real time impedance measurements assuring precise RF (1MHz) energy delivery adapted to each patients skin impedance. The device includes body and face hand pieces with disposable tip of 112 matrix spots.

5.3. Non-invasive RF Technology Associated to Other Energy Modalities

Combination of radiofrequency with other energy modalities such as lasers and light sources, and mechanical procedures like message and vacuum have been also investigated to improve clinical treatments and overcome safety issues.

ALUMA™ (Lumenis Inc., CA, USA) combines bipolar RF energy with a vacuum handheld tool [118]. Frequency 486 kHz, power of 2-10 W, pulse duration of 1-5 s.

ELOS™ (Syneron-Candela, CA, USA) combines optical energies (laser or light) with bipolar RF energy. The application of dual heating via optical and RF energy increases target temperature while maintaining epidermal protection [141]. Pulse repetition rate is 1-3 Hz and cooling is conducted at 5°C. RF energy goes from 25 J/cm^3 to 100 J/cm^3; spectrum 400 nm up to 2000 nm. All parameters depend on the applicator. The combinations of both energies, laser and RF, improve safety and limitations on the procedures compared to intense pulse light (IPL) and lasers.

POLARIS WR (Syneron Medical, Ltd.) used to treat fine lines, depth winkles and photo aging using RF energy associates to a diode laser (900 nm). RF ranges from 10 -100 J/cm^2 and the optical fluences are set from 10 - 50 J/cm^2. Both energies are delivered through the same bipolar electrode tip [142].

AURORA SR (Syneron Medical, Ltd.) is used to treat benign vascular and pigmented lesions, photo aging, and the first device in its class approved by the FDA for hair removal. It has an optical source (IPL) ranging from 560 nm -1200 nm. The energy delivered ranged from 5 - 25 J/cm^2 and dermal penetration achieve up to 4 mm skin depth.

LEGATO (Alma lasers) [142] combines microplasma iPixel RF technology with intermittent positive and negative acoustic pressure. RF energy delivered is 40.68 MHz.

Some bipolar devices utilize vacuum technology which may enhance the depth of heating achieved. These include TiteFx (Invasix) and Vtouch (Viora). Velashape II (Syneron) combines bipolar RF with vacuum as well as infrared light [143]. Venus Freeze (Venus Concept) uses an array of bipolar electrodes along with a magnetic pulse.

6. COST, RISKS AND SAFETY IN THE USE OF NON-INVASIVE RF TREATMENTS

RF technique may facilitate sustained delivery of drugs, achieving therapeutic levels by reducing peak dose related side effects and assuring drug levels above the minimal medical effect. The reduction of doses frequency could potentially improve the quality of life of patients, and easy-of-use of some devices may prevent the need for particular healthcare specialists, possibly decreasing the cost of treatments. However, RF transdermal methods relay on a 2-step process, application of energy to create microchannel and application of formulation. In order to have an opportune and regular use, the process of skin disturbance and drug delivery should be combined in the same system. In addition, long-term safety studies should be carried out in order to assure repeated use of such devices without causing irreversible skin damage.

This application also required an in-depth exploration in terms of efficiency and affordability compared to current physical enhancement techniques, more adaptable to be developed for home-use in order to position this technology as a convenient alternative in the transdermal field.

RF systems used in skin procedures should be further investigated as an alternative to achieve a strong effect, and relatively painless with rapid recovery times. It is also important to address further studies regarding the appropriate candidates for using such technique as effectiveness and safety will be based on individual needs, and those will be dependent not only on skin conditions (skin tone and quality) but also on general health and genetic conditions.

Non-ablative RF treatments will be relatively safe for men and women who are in good health. However, common side effects are usually present such as redness, temporary swelling, skin sensitivity, *etc*. Important side effects have been also observed when increasing fluences, producing fat necrosis and atrophic scaring particularly with monopolar devices. Controlling the number of passes (preferably multiple), applying low energy and getting the feedback from patients on heat sensation is relevant. Patient' perception and expectations are also crucial.

The most noted adverse effects with combined RF devices are principally tissue arcing, which can lead to scar formation. This is observed when the applicator is not well positioned on the target zone, causing that RF energy is not delivered deep enough, and pain associated with light sources. The inclusion of tips to treat specific area of the body has improved the RF procedures render them faster and more comfortable for patients.

People prone to have skin illnesses must have a medical advice prior to such procedures. Pregnant woman should not receive such treatments and patients using acne medications should discuss treatment with their doctor.

It is also important to mention that clinicians most inform their patients that RF non-ablative treatments would relatively help them to achieve younger, slimmer looking and/or healthy skin, but the results may not be seen for the first several months and may probably diminish after few months.

Important parameters to be fully investigated, particularly in tissue tightening may include appropriate patient selection as this is a key indicator for the success of this technique. Some areas of skin laxity without significantly dealing with muscular attachment appear to well respond to RF energy. However, data on long-term clinical studies on duration of results and need of a treatment maintenance is still missing.

The cost of skin procedures varies depending on diverse factors, such a geographical location of practitioners' office, their level of expertise, the skin condition of the patients and also the patient's desire results. On average, some examples of full treatments with RF medical instruments are shown in Table **1**.

Table 1. RF medical devices and treatments.

RF Instrument	FDA Approved	Procedure	Average Price (USD)	No of Sessions
Evolastin (Syneron Medical Ltd, Yokeam, Israel)	yes	electrocoagulation and hemostasis and treatment of wrinkles	3000 - 5000	1
Thermage (Solta Medical, USA)	FDA approved K132431	Tightening and countering	2000 to 3000	
Pelleve 2 (Ellman, USA)	FDA approved K102698	Wrinkles and rhytidis	1000 to 2000	
Venus Freeze (USA, Israel)	FDA approved K111670	Non-Surgical Body Contouring Cellulite Wrinkle Skin Tightening (Collagen, fat and tissues are heated up to 41 degrees centigrade and maintained for 10-15 minutes)	1000/session	6 sessions for the face/neck and 8-10 for the body
Aluma® Skin Renewal System (Lumenis, USA)	CE Marked FDA approved K051214	Wrinkle treatment and skin tightening	300/session	
Eprime (Syneron/Candela)	Yes	Improved skin tone and volume reduction of wrinkles	ePRIME microneedle cartridges price 350	

(Table 1) contd.....

RF Instrument	FDA Approved	Procedure	Average Price (USD)	No of Sessions
Endymed Pro (Endymed Medical, Israel)	CE Marked FDA approved K101510 & K120513		200-220 / 1h treatment	6 sessions required

CONCLUSION

RF technology dedicated to transdermal delivery and gene therapy appeared to be advantageous, suggesting an alternative for administration of therapeutic soluble molecules over a wide molecular weight range, achieving sustained drug flux. They may also offer a good possibility for immunizations as they are painless and safer compared to intramuscular or subcutaneous methods.

Non-contact RF methods used in medical skin procedures show encouraging results. However, most of the clinical trials showing favorable responses remain non-comparable due to independent means of evaluation. Furthermore, unipolar RF devices are usually associated to modest effects, while bipolar RF devices show to be less efficient in depth of penetration. Moreover, very few studies are designed to understand the effects of the technology at a cellular level. In addition, randomized controlled trials are still needed in order to make the evidence more robust. RF devices are significantly being evolved with the use of lower energy levels, larger and faster tips and multiple passes, improving device's efficiency and controlling by practitioners, and minimizing patient discomfort. Fractional RF devices demonstrate to be more tolerable and effective to treat wrinkle and facial laxity. However, the most common transient side effects, erythema and edema are still a disadvantage for patients.

The efficacy of non-invasive radiofrequency to treat different orthopedics problematics and chronic pain is still under investigation. Further trials, considering mechanism of action and better conditions that resulted in comparative efficacy data should be performed to get the finest way to use RF for such applications.

The major advantage of non-invasive RF treatments over ablative and surgical treatments is still the lower rate of side effects and less downtime required after treatment.

Promising trends for the next generation of the RF devices, particularly those combining different technologies have emerged. The ongoing challenges include increased therapeutic potential, reproducibility, device engineering for making devices more portable and re-usable, and affordability.

CONFLICT OF INTEREST

The author confirms that author has no conflict of interest to declare for this publication.

ACKNOWLEDGEMENTS

Declared none.

REFERENCES

[1] Cosman ER, Nashold BS, Ovelman-Levitt J. Theoretical aspects of radiofrequency lesions in the dorsal root entry zone. Neurosurgery 1984; 15(6): 945-50.
[http://dx.doi.org/10.1227/00006123-198412000-00035] [PMID: 6514169]

[2] Sintov AC, Krymberk I, Daniel D, Hannan T, Sohn Z, Levin G. Radiofrequency-driven skin microchanneling as a new way for electrically assisted transdermal delivery of hydrophilic drugs. J Control Release 2003; 89(2): 311-20.
[http://dx.doi.org/10.1016/S0168-3659(03)00123-8] [PMID: 12711453]

[3] Birchall J, Coulman S, Anstey A, *et al.* Cutaneous gene expression of plasmid DNA in excised human skin following delivery *via* microchannels created by radio frequency ablation. Int J Pharm 2006; 312(1-2): 15-23.
[http://dx.doi.org/10.1016/j.ijpharm.2005.12.036] [PMID: 16469457]

[4] Whipple TL. From mini-invasive to non-invasive treatment using monopolar radiofrequency: the next orthopedic frontier. Orthop Clin North Am 2009; 40(4): 531-535, x.
[http://dx.doi.org/10.1016/j.ocl.2009.06.006] [PMID: 19773059]

[5] Weber T, Kabelka B. Noninvasive monopolar capacitive-coupled radiofrequency for the treatment of pain associated with lateral elbow tendinopathies: 1-year follow-up. PM R 2012; 4(3): 176-81.
[http://dx.doi.org/10.1016/j.pmrj.2011.11.003] [PMID: 22342819]

[6] Cevc G. Lipid vesicles and other colloids as drug carriers on the skin. Adv Drug Deliv Rev 2004; 56(5): 675-711.
[http://dx.doi.org/10.1016/j.addr.2003.10.028] [PMID: 15019752]

[7] Diblíková D, Kopečná M, Školová B, *et al.* Transdermal delivery and cutaneous targeting of antivirals using a penetration enhancer and lysolipid prodrugs. Pharm Res 2014; 31(4): 1071-81.

[http://dx.doi.org/10.1007/s11095-013-1228-8] [PMID: 24271238]

[8] Karande P, Mitragotri S. Enhancement of transdermal drug delivery *via* synergistic action of chemicals. Biochim Biophys Acta 2009; 1788: 2362-73.

[9] Karande P, Jain A, Mitragotri S. Insights into synergistic interactions in binary mixtures of chemical permeation enhancers for transdermal drug delivery. J Control Release 2006; 115(1): 85-93. [http://dx.doi.org/10.1016/j.jconrel.2006.07.001] [PMID: 16935378]

[10] Newton SJ. Chemical penetration enhancers. Int J Pharm Compd 2013; 17(5): 370-4. [PMID: 24459781]

[11] Gratieri T, Alberti I, Lapteva M, Kalia YN. Next generation intra- and transdermal therapeutic systems: using non- and minimally-invasive technologies to increase drug delivery into and across the skin. Eur J Pharm Sci 2013; 50(5): 609-22. [http://dx.doi.org/10.1016/j.ejps.2013.03.019] [PMID: 23567467]

[12] Cázares-Delgadillo J, Naik A, Ganem-Rondero A, Quintanar-Guerrero D, Kalia YN. Transdermal delivery of cytochrome C--A 12.4 kDa protein--across intact skin by constant-current iontophoresis. Pharm Res 2007; 24(7): 1360-8. [http://dx.doi.org/10.1007/s11095-007-9294-4] [PMID: 17457661]

[13] Dubey S, Kalia YN. Electrically-assisted delivery of an anionic protein across intact skin: cathodal iontophoresis of biologically active ribonuclease T1. J Control Release 2011; 152(3): 356-62. [http://dx.doi.org/10.1016/j.jconrel.2011.03.004] [PMID: 21397646]

[14] Blagus T, Markelc B, Cemazar M, *et al.* In vivo real-time monitoring system of electroporation mediated control of transdermal and topical drug delivery. J Control Release 2013; 172(3): 862-71. REMOVED HYPERLINK FIELD [http://dx.doi.org/10.1016/j.jconrel.2013.09.030] [PMID: 24113487]

[15] Pierre MB, Rossetti FC. Microneedle-based drug delivery systems for transdermal route. Curr Drug Targets 2014; 15(3): 281-91. [http://dx.doi.org/10.2174/13894501113146660232] [PMID: 24144208]

[16] Weiss R, Hessenberger M, Kitzmüller S, *et al.* Transcutaneous vaccination *via* laser microporation. J Control Release 2012; 162(2): 391-9. [http://dx.doi.org/10.1016/j.jconrel.2012.06.031] [PMID: 22750193]

[17] Cameli N, Abril E, Mariano M, Berardesca E. Combined use of monopolar radiofrequency and transdermal drug delivery in the treatment of melasma. Dermatol Surg 2014; 40(7): 748-55. [PMID: 25111347]

[18] Kim J, Jang JH, Lee JH, *et al.* Enhanced topical delivery of small hydrophilic or lipophilic active agents and epidermal growth factor by fractional radiofrequency microporation. Pharm Res 2012; 29(7): 2017-29. [http://dx.doi.org/10.1007/s11095-012-0729-1] [PMID: 22399389]

[19] Singh TR, Garland MJ, Cassidy CM, *et al.* Microporation techniques for enhanced delivery of therapeutic agents. Recent Pat Drug Deliv Formul 2010; 4(1): 1-17. [http://dx.doi.org/10.2174/187221110789957174] [PMID: 19807682]

[20] Lolis MS, Goldberg DJ. Radiofrequency in cosmetic dermatology: a review. Dermatol Surg 2012;

38(11): 1765-76.
[http://dx.doi.org/10.1111/j.1524-4725.2012.02547.x] [PMID: 22913399]

[21] Beasley KL, Weiss RA. Radiofrequency in cosmetic dermatology. Dermatol Clin 2014; 32(1): 79-90.
[http://dx.doi.org/10.1016/j.det.2013.09.010] [PMID: 24267424]

[22] Millar NL, Murrell CAC. Heat Shock Proteins in Tendinopathy: Novel Molecular Regulators. Mediators of Inflammation 2012; 12(ID 436203): 7.

[23] Whipple TL. From mini-invasive to non-invasive treatment using monopolar radiofrequency: the next orthopedic frontier. Orthop Clin North Am 2009; 40(4): 531-535, x.
[http://dx.doi.org/10.1016/j.ocl.2009.06.006] [PMID: 19773059]

[24] Takahashi N, Tasto JP, Ritter M, *et al.* Pain relief through an antinociceptive effect after radiofrequency application. Am J Sports Med 2007; 35(5): 805-10.
[http://dx.doi.org/10.1177/0363546506297085] [PMID: 17267771]

[25] Rhim H, Goldberg SN, Dodd GD III, *et al.* Essential techniques for successful radio-frequency thermal ablation of malignant hepatic tumors. Radiographics 2001; 21(Spec No): S17-35.
[http://dx.doi.org/10.1148/radiographics.21.suppl_1.g01oc11s17] [PMID: 11598245]

[26] Pilla AA. Mechanism and Therapeutic Applications of Time-Varying and Static magnetic Fields. Boca Raton: CRC Press 2007; pp. 353-84.

[27] Gazelle GS, Goldberg SN, Solbiati L, Livraghi T. Tumor ablation with radio-frequency energy. Radiology 2000; 217(3): 633-46.
[http://dx.doi.org/10.1148/radiology.217.3.r00dc26633] [PMID: 11110923]

[28] electrotherapy.org. Hertfordshire: electrotherapy on the web. Avaible from: www.electrotherapy.org , [cited: March 2015];

[29] Challis LJ. Mechanisms for interaction between RF fields and biological tissue. Bioelectromagnetics 2005; 7 (Suppl. 7): S98-S106.
[http://dx.doi.org/10.1002/bem.20119] [PMID: 15931683]

[30] Al-Mandeel MM, Watson T. The thermal and nonthermal effects of high and low doses of pulsed short wave therapy (PSWT). Physiother Res Int 2010; 15(4): 199-211.
[http://dx.doi.org/10.1002/pri.460] [PMID: 20186887]

[31] Rhim H, Goldberg SN, Dodd GD III, *et al.* Essential techniques for successful radio-frequency thermal ablation of malignant hepatic tumors. Radiographics 2001; 21(Spec No): S17-35.
[http://dx.doi.org/10.1148/radiographics.21.suppl_1.g01oc11s17] [PMID: 11598245]

[32] Munro MG. Fundamentals of electrosurgery, Part I: Principles of Radiofrequency Energy for Surgery, The SAGES Manual on the Fundamental Use of Surgical Energy. New York: Springer 2012; pp. 15-59.
[http://dx.doi.org/10.1007/978-1-4614-2074-3_2]

[33] Sachdeva S, Dogra A. Radiofrequency ablation in dermatology. Indian J Dermatol 2007; 52: 134-7.
[http://dx.doi.org/10.4103/0019-5154.35091]

[34] Healey TT, Dupuy DE. Radiofrequency ablation: a safe and effective treatment in nonoperative patients with early-stage lung cancer. Cancer J 2011; 17(1): 33-7.
[http://dx.doi.org/10.1097/PPO.0b013e318209176f] [PMID: 21263265]

[35] Habash R. Bioeffects and therapeutic applications of electromagnetic energy. Boca Raton: CRC Press 2007; pp. 277-90.
[http://dx.doi.org/10.1201/9781420062854]

[36] Mikeladze G, Espinal R, Finnegan R, Routon J, Martin D. Pulsed radiofrequency application in treatment of chronic zygapophyseal joint pain. Spine J 2003; 3(5): 360-2.
[http://dx.doi.org/10.1016/S1529-9430(03)00065-2] [PMID: 14588947]

[37] Sherman RA, Acosta NM, Robson L. Treatment of migraine with pulsing electromagnetic fields: a double-blind, placebo-controlled study. Headache 1999; 39(8): 567-75.
[http://dx.doi.org/10.1046/j.1526-4610.1999.3908567.x] [PMID: 11279973]

[38] Bogduk N. Pulsed radiofrequency. Pain Med 2006; 7(5): 396-407.
[http://dx.doi.org/10.1111/j.1526-4637.2006.00210.x] [PMID: 17014598]

[39] Olver IN. Update on anti-emetics for chemotherapy-induced emesis. Intern Med J 2005; 35(8): 478-81.
[http://dx.doi.org/10.1111/j.1445-5004.2005.00879.x] [PMID: 16176471]

[40] Tan M. Granisetron: new insights into its use for the treatment of chemotherapy-induced nausea and vomiting. Expert Opin Pharmacother 2003; 4(9): 1563-71.
[http://dx.doi.org/10.1517/14656566.4.9.1563] [PMID: 12943486]

[41] Sweetman S, Ed. Martindale: the complete drug reference. 33rd ed., London: Pharmaceutical Press, Electronic version 2003.

[42] Gan TJ. Diclofenac: an update on its mechanism of action and safety profile. Curr Med Res Opin 2010; 26(7): 1715-31.
[http://dx.doi.org/10.1185/03007995.2010.486301] [PMID: 20470236]

[43] Cázares-Delgadillo J, Ganem-Rondero A, Quintanar-Guerrero D, López-Castellano AC, Merino V, Kalia YN. Using transdermal iontophoresis to increase granisetron delivery across skin *in vitro* and *in vivo*: effect of experimental conditions and a comparison with other enhancement strategies. Eur J Pharm Sci 2010; 39(5): 387-93.
[http://dx.doi.org/10.1016/j.ejps.2010.01.008] [PMID: 20096354]

[44] Richmond E, Rogol AD. Current indications for growth hormone therapy for children and adolescents. Endocr Dev 2010; 18: 92-108.
[http://dx.doi.org/10.1159/000316130] [PMID: 20523020]

[45] Webster R, Xie R, Didier E, *et al.* PEGylation of somatropin (recombinant human growth hormone): impact on its clearance in humans. Xenobiotica 2008; 38(10): 1340-51.
[http://dx.doi.org/10.1080/00498250802413856] [PMID: 18802875]

[46] Cai Y, Xu M, Yuan M, *et al.* Developments in human growth hormone preparations: sustained-release, prolonged half-life, novel injection devices, and alternative delivery routes. Eur J Pharm Sci 2010; 39: 387-93.
[PMID: 20096354]

[47] Levin G, Gershonowitz A, Sacks H, *et al.* Transdermal delivery of human growth hormone through RF-microchannels. Pharm Res 2005; 22(4): 550-5.
[http://dx.doi.org/10.1007/s11095-005-2498-6] [PMID: 15846462]

[48] Lee JW, Choi SO, Felner EI, Prausnitz MR. Dissolving microneedle patch for transdermal delivery of human growth hormone. Small 2011; 7(4): 531-9.
[http://dx.doi.org/10.1002/smll.201001091] [PMID: 21360810]

[49] Fukushima K, Ise A, Morita H, *et al.* Two-layered dissolving microneedles for percutaneous delivery of peptide/protein drugs in rats. Pharm Res 2011; 28(1): 7-21.
[http://dx.doi.org/10.1007/s11095-010-0097-7] [PMID: 20300802]

[50] Ito Y, Ohashi Y, Shiroyama K, Sugioka N, Takada K. Self-dissolving micropiles for the percutaneous absorption of recombinant human growth hormone in rats. Biol Pharm Bull 2008; 31(8): 1631-3.
[http://dx.doi.org/10.1248/bpb.31.1631] [PMID: 18670103]

[51] Kam Y, Sacks H, Mevorat-Kaplan K, *et al.* Radio Frequency-microchannels for transdermal delivery: characterization of skin recovery and delivery window. Pharmacol Pharm 2012; 3: 20-8.
[http://dx.doi.org/10.4236/pp.2012.31004]

[52] Kim J, Jang J-H, Lee JH, *et al.* Enhanced topical delivery of small hydrophilic or lipophilic active agents and epidermal growth factor by fractional radiofrequency microporation. Pharm Res 2012; 29(7): 2017-29.
[http://dx.doi.org/10.1007/s11095-012-0729-1] [PMID: 22399389]

[53] Hengge UR, Walker PS, Vogel JC. Expression of naked DNA in human, pig, and mouse skin. J Clin Invest 1996; 97(12): 2911-6.
[http://dx.doi.org/10.1172/JCI118750] [PMID: 8675706]

[54] Coulombe PA, Lee CH. Defining keratin protein function in skin epithelia: epidermolysis bullosa simplex and its aftermath. J Invest Dermatol 2012; 132(3 Pt 2): 763-75.
[http://dx.doi.org/10.1038/jid.2011.450] [PMID: 22277943]

[55] Brown CK, Kirkwood JM. Targeted therapy for malignant melanoma. Curr Oncol Rep 2001; 3(4): 344-52.
[http://dx.doi.org/10.1007/s11912-001-0088-2] [PMID: 11389820]

[56] Lee P-Y, Chesnoy S, Huang L. Electroporatic delivery of TGF-beta1 gene works synergistically with electric therapy to enhance diabetic wound healing in db/db mice. J Invest Dermatol 2004; 123(4): 791-8.
[http://dx.doi.org/10.1111/j.0022-202X.2004.23309.x] [PMID: 15373787]

[57] Lee PY, Li Z, Huang L. Thermosensitive hydrogel as a Tgf-beta1 gene delivery vehicle enhances diabetic wound healing. Pharm Res 2003; 20(12): 1995-2000.
[http://dx.doi.org/10.1023/B:PHAM.0000008048.58777.da] [PMID: 14725365]

[58] Lee PY, Cobain E, Huard J, Huang L. Thermosensitive hydrogel PEG-PLGA-PEG enhances engraftment of muscle-derived stem cells and promotes healing in diabetic wound. Mol Ther 2007; 15(6): 1189-94.
[PMID: 17406344]

[59] Song JM, Kim YC, O E, Compans RW, Prausnitz MR, Kang SM. DNA vaccination in the skin using microneedles improves protection against influenza. Mol Ther 2012; 20(7): 1472-80.
[http://dx.doi.org/10.1038/mt.2012.69] [PMID: 22508490]

[60] Gill HS, Söderholm J, Prausnitz MR, Sällberg M. Cutaneous vaccination using microneedles coated

with hepatitis C DNA vaccine. Gene Ther 2010; 17(6): 811-4.
[http://dx.doi.org/10.1038/gt.2010.22] [PMID: 20200562]

[61] Hu J, Han R, Cladel NM, Pickel MD, Christensen ND. Intracutaneous DNA vaccination with the E8 gene of cottontail rabbit papillomavirus induces protective immunity against virus challenge in rabbits. J Virol 2002; 76(13): 6453-9.
[http://dx.doi.org/10.1128/JVI.76.13.6453-6459.2002] [PMID: 12050357]

[62] de Oliveira CI, Nascimento IP, Barral A, Soto M, Barral-Netto M. Challenges and perspectives in vaccination against leishmaniasis. Parasitol Int 2009; 58(4): 319-24.
[http://dx.doi.org/10.1016/j.parint.2009.07.013] [PMID: 19698801]

[63] Nanney LB, Paulsen S, Davidson MK, Cardwell NL, Whitsitt JS, Davidson JM. Boosting epidermal growth factor receptor expression by gene gun transfection stimulates epidermal growth *in vivo*. Wound Repair Regen 2000; 8(2): 117-27.
[http://dx.doi.org/10.1046/j.1524-475x.2000.00117.x] [PMID: 10810038]

[64] Chesnoy S, Huang L. Enhanced cutaneous gene delivery following intradermal injection of naked DNA in a high ionic strength solution. Mol Ther 2002; 5(1): 57-62.
[http://dx.doi.org/10.1006/mthe.2001.0511] [PMID: 11786046]

[65] Zhou SJ, Li SW, Wang JJ, *et al.* High-intensity focused ultrasound combined with herpes simplex virus thymidine kinase gene-loaded ultrasound-targeted microbubbles improved the survival of rabbits with VX□ liver tumor. J Gene Med 2012; 14(9-10): 570-9.
[http://dx.doi.org/10.1002/jgm.2668] [PMID: 22941868]

[66] Somiari S, Glasspool-Malone J, Drabick JJ, *et al.* Theory and *in vivo* application of electroporative gene delivery. Mol Ther 2000; 2(3): 178-87.
[http://dx.doi.org/10.1006/mthe.2000.0124] [PMID: 10985947]

[67] Drabick JJ, Glasspool-Malone J, King A, Malone RW. Cutaneous transfection and immune responses to intradermal nucleic acid vaccination are significantly enhanced by *in vivo* electropermeabilization. Mol Ther 2001; 3(2): 249-55.
[http://dx.doi.org/10.1006/mthe.2000.0257] [PMID: 11237682]

[68] Birchall J, Coulman S, Anstey A, *et al.* Cutaneous gene expression of plasmid DNA in excised human skin following delivery via microchannels created by radio frequency ablation. Int J Pharm 2006; 312(1-2): 15-23.
[http://dx.doi.org/10.1016/j.ijpharm.2005.12.036] [PMID: 16469457]

[69] Bumb RA, Satoskar AR. Radiofrequency-induced heat therapy as first-line treatment for cutaneous leishmaniasis. Expert Rev Anti Infect Ther 2011; 9(6): 623-5.
[http://dx.doi.org/10.1586/eri.11.50] [PMID: 21692665]

[70] Asilian A, Sadeghinia A, Faghihi G, Momeni A. Comparative study of the efficacy of combined cryotherapy and intralesional meglumine antimoniate (Glucantime) *vs.* cryotherapy and intralesional meglumine antimoniate (Glucantime) alone for the treatment of cutaneous leishmaniasis. Int J Dermatol 2004; 43(4): 281-3.
[http://dx.doi.org/10.1111/j.1365-4632.2004.02002.x] [PMID: 15090013]

[71] Layegh P, Pezeshkpoor F, Soruri AH, Naviafar P, Moghiman T. Efficacy of cryotherapy *versus* intralesional meglumine antimoniate (glucantime) for treatment of cutaneous leishmaniasis in children.

Am J Trop Med Hyg 2009; 80(2): 172-5.
[PMID: 19190206]

[72] Sadeghian G, Nilfroushzadeh MA, Iraji F. Efficacy of local heat therapy by radiofrequency in the treatment of cutaneous leishmaniasis, compared with intralesional injection of meglumine antimoniate. Clin Exp Dermatol 2007; 32(4): 371-4.
[http://dx.doi.org/10.1111/j.1365-2230.2007.02405.x] [PMID: 17376205]

[73] Reithinger R, Mohsen M, Wahid M, *et al.* Efficacy of thermotherapy to treat cutaneous leishmaniasis caused by Leishmania tropica in Kabul, Afghanistan: a randomized, controlled trial. Clin Infect Dis 2005; 40(8): 1148-55.
[http://dx.doi.org/10.1086/428736] [PMID: 15791515]

[74] Prasad N, Ghiya BC, Bumb RA, *et al.* Heat, Oriental sore, and HIV. Lancet 2011; 377(9765): 610.
[http://dx.doi.org/10.1016/S0140-6736(10)61495-X] [PMID: 21315946]

[75] Aronson NE, Wortmann GW, Byrne WR, *et al.* A randomized controlled trial of local heat therapy *versus* intravenous sodium stibogluconate for the treatment of cutaneous Leishmania major infection. PLoS Negl Trop Dis 2010; 4(3): e628.
[http://dx.doi.org/10.1371/journal.pntd.0000628] [PMID: 20231896]

[76] Lobo IM, Soares MB, Correia TM, *et al.* Heat therapy for cutaneous leishmaniasis elicits a systemic cytokine response similar to that of antimonial (Glucantime) therapy. Trans R Soc Trop Med Hyg 2006; 100(7): 642-9.
[http://dx.doi.org/10.1016/j.trstmh.2005.08.011] [PMID: 16274713]

[77] Bumb RA, Prasad N, Khandelwal K, *et al.* Long-term efficacy of single-dose radiofrequency-induced heat therapy *vs.* intralesional antimonials for cutaneous leishmaniasis in India. Br J Dermatol 2013; 168(5): 1114-9.
[http://dx.doi.org/10.1111/bjd.12205] [PMID: 23298394]

[78] Patel L, McGrouther D, Chakrabarty K. Evaluating evidence for atrophic scarring treatment modalities. JRSM Open 2014; 5(9): 2054270414540139.
[http://dx.doi.org/10.1177/2054270414540139] [PMID: 25352991]

[79] Simmons BJ, Griffith RD, Falto-Aizpurua LA, Nouri K. Use of radiofrequency in cosmetic dermatology: focus on nonablative treatment of acne scars. Clin Cosmet Investig Dermatol 2014; 7: 335-9.
[http://dx.doi.org/10.2147/CCID.S74411] [PMID: 25540589]

[80] Ramesh M, Gopal M, Kumar S, Talwar A. Novel Technology in the Treatment of Acne Scars: The Matrix-tunable Radiofrequency Technology. J Cutan Aesthet Surg 2010; 3(2): 97-101.
[PMID: 21031069]

[81] Gold MH, Biron JA. Treatment of acne scars by fractional bipolar radiofrequency energy. J Cosmet Laser Ther 2012; 14(4): 172-8.
[http://dx.doi.org/10.3109/14764172.2012.687824] [PMID: 22548644]

[82] Cho SI, Chung BY, Choi MG, *et al.* Evaluation of the clinical efficacy of fractional radiofrequency microneedle treatment in acne scars and large facial pores. Dermatol Surg 2012; 38(7 Pt 1): 1017-24.
[http://dx.doi.org/10.1111/j.1524-4725.2012.02402.x] [PMID: 22487513]

[83] Chandrashekar BS, Sriram R, Mysore R, Bhaskar S, Shetty A. Evaluation of microneedling fractional radiofrequency device for treatment of acne scars. J Cutan Aesthet Surg 2014; 7(2): 93-7. [http://dx.doi.org/10.4103/0974-2077.138328] [PMID: 25136209]

[84] Goodman GJ, Baron JA. Postacne scarring: a qualitative global scarring grading system. Dermatol Surg 2006; 32(12): 1458-66. [PMID: 17199653]

[85] Issa MC, Kassuga LE, Chevrand NS, Pires MT. Topical delivery of triamcinolone *via* skin pretreated with ablative radiofrequency: a new method in hypertrophic scar treatment. Int J Dermatol 2013; 52(3): 367-70. [http://dx.doi.org/10.1111/j.1365-4632.2012.05704.x] [PMID: 23414164]

[86] Rongsaard N, Rummaneethorn P. Comparison of a fractional bipolar radiofrequency device and a fractional erbium-doped glass 1,550-nm device for the treatment of atrophic acne scars: a randomized split-face clinical study. Dermatol Surg 2014; 40(1): 14-21. [http://dx.doi.org/10.1111/dsu.12372] [PMID: 24267397]

[87] Trelles MA, Martínez-Carpio PA. Attenuation of acne scars using high power fractional ablative unipolar radiofrequency and ultrasound for transepidermal delivery of bioactive compounds through microchannels. Lasers Surg Med 2014; 46(2): 152-9. [http://dx.doi.org/10.1002/lsm.22224] [PMID: 24474092]

[88] Walling HW, Swick BL. Treatment options for hyperhidrosis. Am J Clin Dermatol 2011; 12(5): 285-95. [http://dx.doi.org/10.2165/11587870-000000000-00000] [PMID: 21714579]

[89] Garcia J. Treatment of axillary hyperhidrosis/bromidrosis using VASER ultrasound. Aesthetic Plast Surg 2010; 34(1): 120. [http://dx.doi.org/10.1007/s00266-009-9457-2] [PMID: 20043152]

[90] Kim M, Shin JY, Lee J, Kim JY, Oh SH. Efficacy of fractional microneedle radiofrequency device in the treatment of primary axillary hyperhidrosis: a pilot study. Dermatology (Basel) 2013; 227(3): 243-9. [http://dx.doi.org/10.1159/000354602] [PMID: 24107595]

[91] Fatemi Naeini F, Abtahi-Naeini B, Pourazizi M, Nilforoushzadeh MA, Mirmohammadkhani M. Fractionated microneedle radiofrequency for treatment of primary axillary hyperhidrosis: A sham control study. Australas J Dermatol 2015; 56(4): 279-84. [http://dx.doi.org/10.1111/ajd.12260] [PMID: 25496000]

[92] England LJ, Tan MH, Shumaker PR, *et al.* Effects of monopolar radiofrequency treatment over soft-tissue fillers in an animal model. Lasers Surg Med 2005; 37(5): 356-65. [http://dx.doi.org/10.1002/lsm.20253] [PMID: 16240419]

[93] Shumaker PR, England LJ, Dover JS, *et al.* Effect of monopolar radiofrequency treatment over soft-tissue fillers in an animal model: part 2. Lasers Surg Med 2006; 38(3): 211-7. [http://dx.doi.org/10.1002/lsm.20292] [PMID: 16485274]

[94] Fitzpatrick R, Geronemus R, Goldberg D, Kaminer M, Kilmer S, Ruiz-Esparza J. Multicenter study of noninvasive radiofrequency for periorbital tissue tightening. Lasers Surg Med 2003; 33(4): 232-42.

[http://dx.doi.org/10.1002/lsm.10225] [PMID: 14571447]

[95] Alster TS, Tanzi E. Improvement of neck and cheek laxity with a nonablative radiofrequency device: a lifting experience. Dermatol Surg 2004; 30(4 Pt 1): 503-7.
[PMID: 15056138]

[96] Edwards AF, Massaki A, Fabi SG, *et al.* Clinical efficacy and safety evaluation of a new monopolar radiofrequency (mRF) device with comfort pulsed technology for the treatment of facial skin laxity: 10month experience with 64 patients. Dermatol Surg 2013; 39: 104-10.
[http://dx.doi.org/10.1111/dsu.12010] [PMID: 23153312]

[97] Chipps LK, Bentow J, Prather HB, *et al.* Novel nonablative radio-frequency rejuvenation device applied to the neck and jowls: clinical evaluation and 3-dimensional image analysis. J Drugs Dermatol 2013; 12(11): 1215-8.
[PMID: 24196328]

[98] Vega JM, Bucay VW, Mayoral FA. Prospective multicenter study for safety &efficacy unique RF device for hand wrinkles. J Drugs Dermatol 2013; 12: 24-6.
[PMID: 23377324]

[99] Key D. American Society for Laser Medicine and Surgery Conference. April 4-6, 2014; Going.

[100] Nassab R. The evidence behind noninvasive body contouring devices. Aesthet Surg J 2015; 35(3): 279-93.
[http://dx.doi.org/10.1093/asj/sju063] [PMID: 25691381]

[101] Hantash BM, Ubeid AA, Chang H, Kafi R, Renton B. Bipolar fractional radiofrequency treatment induces neoelastogenesis and neocollagenesis. Lasers Surg Med 2009; 41(1): 1-9.
[http://dx.doi.org/10.1002/lsm.20731] [PMID: 19143021]

[102] Franco W, Kothare A, Goldberg DJ. Controlled volumetric heating of subcutaneous adipose tissue using a novel radiofrequency technology. Lasers Surg Med 2009; 41(10): 745-50.
[http://dx.doi.org/10.1002/lsm.20876] [PMID: 20014265]

[103] Franco W, Kothare A, Ronan SJ, Grekin RC, McCalmont TH. Hyperthermic injury to adipocyte cells by selective heating of subcutaneous fat with a novel radiofrequency device: feasibility studies. Lasers Surg Med 2010; 42(5): 361-70.
[http://dx.doi.org/10.1002/lsm.20925] [PMID: 20583242]

[104] Mlosek RK, Woźniak W, Malinowska S, Lewandowski M, Nowicki A. The effectiveness of anticellulite treatment using tripolar radiofrequency monitored by classic and high-frequency ultrasound. J Eur Acad Dermatol Venereol 2012; 26(6): 696-703.
[http://dx.doi.org/10.1111/j.1468-3083.2011.04148.x] [PMID: 21692869]

[105] Milanese C, Piscitelli F, Simoni C, Pugliarello R, Zancanaro C. Effects of whole-body vibration with or without localized radiofrequency on anthropometry, body composition, and motor performance in young nonobese women. J Altern Complement Med 2012; 18(1): 69-75.
[http://dx.doi.org/10.1089/acm.2010.0324] [PMID: 22268971]

[106] Kim IS, Hyun MY, Park KY, Kim CW, Kim BJ, Kim MN. Phosphatidylcholine and bipolar radiofrequency for treatment of localized fat deposits. J Dermatolog Treat 2014; 25(4): 308-9.
[http://dx.doi.org/10.3109/09546634.2013.783198] [PMID: 23621400]

[107] McDaniel D, Fritz K, Machovcova A, Bernardy J. A focused monopolar radiofrequency causes apoptosis: a porcine model. J Drugs Dermatol 2014; 13(11): 1336-40.
[PMID: 25607699]

[108] Adatto MA, Adatto-Neilson RM, Morren G. Reduction in adipose tissue volume using a new high-power radiofrequency technology combined with infrared light and mechanical manipulation for body contouring. Lasers Med Sci 2014; 29(5): 1627-31.
[http://dx.doi.org/10.1007/s10103-014-1564-x] [PMID: 24687404]

[109] Fajkošová K, Machovcová A, Onder M, Fritz K. Selective radiofrequency therapy as a non-invasive approach for contactless body contouring and circumferential reduction. J Drugs Dermatol 2014; 13(3): 291-6.
[PMID: 24595574]

[110] Boisnic S, Divaris M, Nelson AA, Gharavi NM, Lask GP. A clinical and biological evaluation of a novel, noninvasive radiofrequency device for the long-term reduction of adipose tissue. Lasers Surg Med 2014; 46(2): 94-103.
[http://dx.doi.org/10.1002/lsm.22223] [PMID: 24535760]

[111] Cameli N, Abril E, Mariano M, Berardesca E. Combined use of monopolar radiofrequency and transdermal drug delivery in the treatment of melasma. Dermatol Surg 2014; 40(7): 748-55.
[PMID: 25111347]

[112] Yoshida Y, Sato N, Furumura M, Nakayama J. Treatment of pigmented lesions of neurofibromatosis 1 with intense pulsed-radio frequency in combination with topical application of vitamin D3 ointment. J Dermatol 2007; 34(4): 227-30.
[http://dx.doi.org/10.1111/j.1346-8138.2007.00258.x] [PMID: 17352718]

[113] Whipple T, Villegas D. Thermal and electric energy fields by noninvasive monopolar capacitive-coupled radiofrequency: temperatures achieved and histological outcomes in tendons and ligaments. PM R 2010; 2(7): 599-606.
[http://dx.doi.org/10.1016/j.pmrj.2010.02.012] [PMID: 20466613]

[114] England LJ, Tan MH, Shumaker PR, *et al.* Effects of monopolar radiofrequency treatment over soft-tissue fillers in an animal model. Lasers Surg Med 2005; 37(5): 356-65.
[http://dx.doi.org/10.1002/lsm.20253] [PMID: 16240419]

[115] Shumaker PR, England LJ, Dover JS, *et al.* Effect of monopolar radiofrequency treatment over soft-tissue fillers in an animal model: part 2. Lasers Surg Med 2006; 38(3): 211-7.
[http://dx.doi.org/10.1002/lsm.20292] [PMID: 16485274]

[116] Cronkey J, LaPorta G. Rating systems for evaluation of functional ankle instability: prospective evaluation in a cohort of patients treated with monopolar capacitive-coupled radiofrequency. Foot Ankle Spec 2012; 5(5): 293-9.
[http://dx.doi.org/10.1177/1938640012457941] [PMID: 23008239]

[117] Malik K, Benzon HT. Pulsed radiofrequency: a critical review of its efficacy. Anaesth Intensive Care 2007; 35(6): 863-73.
[PMID: 18084976]

[118] Chao SC, Lee HT, Kao TH, *et al.* Percutaneous pulsed radiofrequency in the treatment of cervical and

lumbar radicular pain. Surg Neurol 2008; 70(1): 59-65.
[http://dx.doi.org/10.1016/j.surneu.2007.05.046] [PMID: 18207554]

[119] Taverner MG, Loughnan TE, Soon CW. Transcutaneous application of pulsed radiofrequency treatment for shoulder pain. Pain Pract 2013; 13(4): 310-5.
[http://dx.doi.org/10.1111/j.1533-2500.2012.00582.x] [PMID: 22863196]

[120] Taverner M, Loughnan T. Transcutaneous pulsed radiofrequency treatment for patients with shoulder pain booked for surgery: a double-blind, randomized controlled trial. Pain Pract 2014; 14(2): 101-8.
[http://dx.doi.org/10.1111/papr.12059] [PMID: 23560519]

[121] Stall RS. Noninvasive pulsed radio frequency energy in the treatment of occipital neuralgia with chronic, debilitating headache: a report of four cases. Pain Med 2013; 14(5): 628-38.
[http://dx.doi.org/10.1111/pme.12078] [PMID: 23566238]

[122] Avrahami Z. Transdermal Drug Delivery and Analyte Extraction Field of the Invention WO Patent 2000027473 A1, 2000.

[123] Avrahami Z. Electronic card for transdermal drug delivery and analyte extraction US Patent 20030208152 A1, 2003.

[124] Avrahami Z. Sohn Ze ev. Monopolar and bipolar current application for transdermal drug delivery and analyte extraction US Patent 6611706 B2, 2003.

[125] Avrahami Z, Ze'ev S. Handheld apparatus and method for transdermal drug delivery and analyte extraction US Patent 20040230227 A1, 2004.

[126] Levin G, Stern M, Daniel D. Transdermal delivery system for water insoluble drugs US Patent 20050287217 A1, 2005.

[127] Levin G, Daniel D. Transdermal delivery system for anti-emetic medication US Patent 20050260252 A1, 2005.

[128] Levin G, Sacks H, Rudaev S. Transdermal delivery system for cosmetic agents US Patent 20070270732 A1, 2007.

[129] Levin G, Gershonowitz A, Gadasi H. Method and device for transdermal immunization US Patent 20070009542 A1, 2007.

[130] Levin G. Delivery system for transdermal immunization US Patent 20070292445 A1, 2007.

[131] solta.com. New York: Valeant Pharmaceuticals North America, LLC. Avaible from: http://www.solta.com/brands/thermage , [update: 2014; cited: March 2015];

[132] almalasers.com. Nürnberg: Alma Lasers Ltd. Avaible from: http://www.almalasers.com/ , [update: 2014; cited: March 2015];

[133] pelleve.com. New York: Cynosure, Inc. Avaible from: http://www.pelleve.com/ , [update: 2015; cited: March 2015];

[134] pollogen.com. Pollogen Ltd. Avaible from: http://www.pollogen.com/ , [update: 2014; cited: March 2015];

[135] Avaible from: http://www.almasweatx.com/ , [cited: March 2015];

[136] Goldberg DJ. Asthetic Dermatology. In: Lapidoth M, Halachmi S, Eds. Radiofrequency in

CosmeticDermatology.

[137] invasix.com. Irvine: Invasix. Avaible from: http://www.invasix.com/Fractora_7 , [cited: March 2015];

[138] international.lutronic.com. Burlington: Lutronic All. Avaible from: http://www.international.lutronic.com/infini , [update: 2016; cited: March 2015];

[139] intraceluk.com. Avaible from: http://www.intraceluk.com/ , [cited: March 2015];

[140] vioramed.com/int. New York: Viora. Avaible from: http://www.vioramed.com/ , [cited: March 2015];

[141] syneron-candela.com/int. Wayland: Syneron® Medical Ltd. Avaible from: http://syneron-candela.com/ , [update: 2016; cited: March 2015];

[142] Eckhouse FK. Adatto MA. Radiofrequency combinations. In: Lapidoth M, Halachmi S, Eds. Radiofrequency in Cosmetic Dermathology. Germany: Karger 2015; pp. 70-4.

[143] syneron-candela.com/int. Wayland: Syneron® Medical Ltd. Avaible from: http://syneron-candela.com/na/technology/velashape-technology , [update: 2016; cited: March 2015];

CHAPTER 6

Microneedles

Yunhua Gao*, **Yuqin Qiu** and **Suohui Zhang**

Key Laboratory of Photochemical Conversion and Optoelectronic Materials, Technical Institute of Physics and Chemistry, Chinese Academy of Sciences, Beijing, 100190, China

Abstract: Transdermal drug delivery is a well-accepted route of administration for therapeutical drugs. Skin is the largest area human body organ, however, the substantial barrier property of the skin stratum corneum limits practical value of transdermal route of drug administration. It has been proved that microneedle array devices can overcome the barrier characteristics of the stratum corneum and enhance the delivery of therapeutic medicines through skin. This chapter focuses on looking at the microneedle-mediated transdermal drug delivery for therapeutical applications. The definition of microneedles, enhancement mechanisms and devices in research or in the market are also depicted.

Keywords: Definition, Devices in research or in the market, Mechanisims of action, Microneedle, Therapeutical applications.

1. INTRODUCTION

Transdermal drug delivery (TDD) is convenient for the delivery of active pharmaceutical ingredients. The transdermal route offers some advantages compared with other noninvasive routes of drug delivery, such as the circumvention of first-pass hepatic metabolism, increased compliance and potential for controlled release. However, the clinical application of transdermal drug delivery has been limited because of the extremely low permeability of drugs through the stratum corneum [1].

* **Corresponding author Yunhua Gao:** Technical Institute of Physics and Chemistry, Chinese Academy of Sciences, Beijing, 100190, China; Tel/Fax: 0086-10-82543581; E-mail: yhgao@mail.ipc.ac.cn

José Juan Escobar-Chávez (Ed.)

Microneedle array devices with sub-millimeter needle-shaped structures was expected to overcome obstacles of the outermost skin layer, the stratum corneum. The concept of microneedles, piercing through the stratum corneum and increasing markedly drug skin permeability without stimulating sensory nerve endings and causing pain was first put forward by Gerstel MS and Place VA in 1976 [2]. And Henry *et al.*, demonstrated the proof of the concept experimentally in 1998 for transdermal drug delivery [3]. Since then, hundreds of preclinical studies have been reported. Microneedle technology has shown great effectiveness in promoting the penetration of macromolecules, hydrophilic substances, vesicles and nanoparticles. Recently, numerous types of microneedles have been clinically examined across a range of applications, including drug and vaccine delivery. The aim of this chapter is to give an overall picture of the main features of microneedles used for transdermal and topical drug delivery. The definition of microneedles, enhancement mechanisms, therapeutical applications and devices in research or in the market are depicted.

2. DEFINITION OF MICRONEEDLES

Microneedles are a kind of drug delivery device for the use in the percutaneous administration of a drug for local therapy or systemic therapy. Microneedles can be defined as solid or hollow according to its structure. The device generally comprises a multiplicity of micron sized needles which are attached to a base support. The typical height is range from 100 to 1000 μm (*e.g.* Fig. **1**). A variety of materials have been evaluated for the fabrication of microneedles, such as silicon, metal, ceramics and polymers [4, 5].

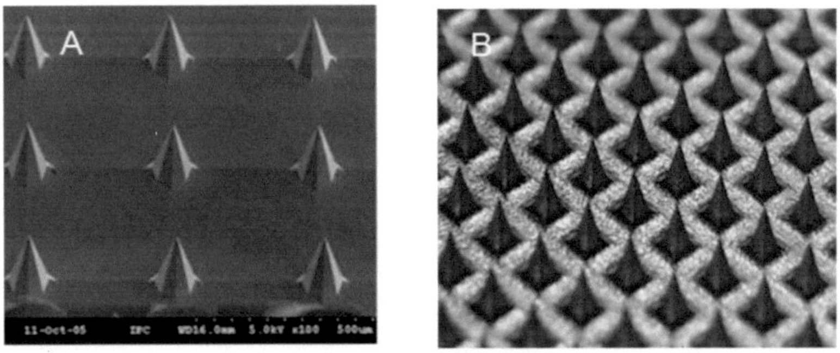

Fig. (1.1). A. Solid silicon microneedles, **B.** Solid metal microneedles (from author's lab).

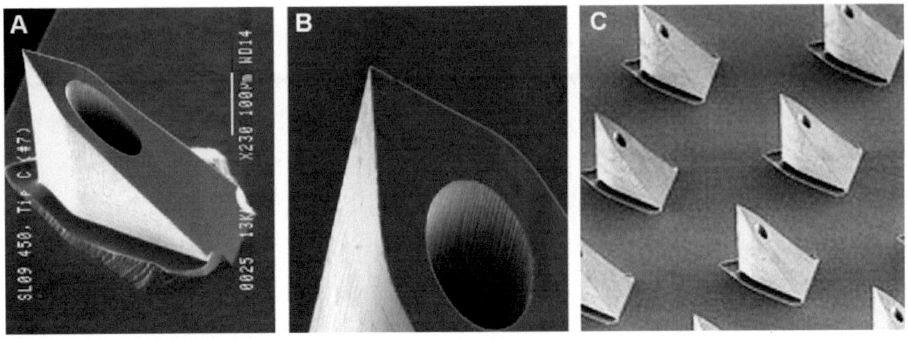

Fig. (1.2). Hollow silicon microneedles. (**A**) A single microneedle, (**B**) the microneedle tip, and (**C**) a microneedle array (Reprinted with permission from [6]. Elsevier (2009).

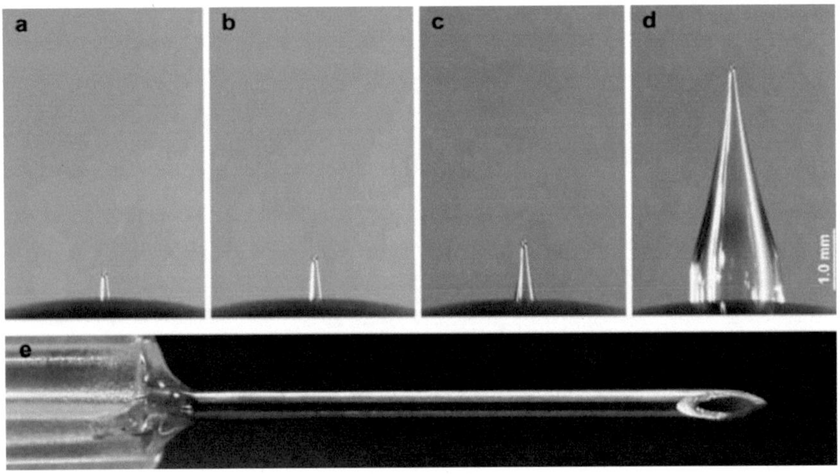

Fig. (1.3). Hollow microneedle used for intradermal infusion. Microneedles length (**a**) 0.5mm, (**b**) 0.75 mm, (**c**) 1 mm and (**d**) 4 mm, (**e**) Hypodermic needle (26-gauge). All images are obtained under bright field microscopy at the same magnification. (Reprinted with permission from [7]. Elsevier (2011)).

In addition, different terms have been reported in the literature base on the geometry or application of the needle, such as micropile [8], microstructure [9], microprojections [10, 11], micron sized lancets [12], microdevices [13], *etc* [14 - 18]. Despite of use of different terms, all these microneedles were for the same purpose, namely to pierce stratum corneum to form hydrophilic pathways by minimally invasive method without contacting the nerves of the skin to avoid bleeding or pain. Human volunteers have reported that a microneedle array having 5 × 10 arrays of 620 μm long stainless steel needles was not painful upon insertion [19]. Another study in 18 human volunteers reported that microneedle insertion was painless and caused only minimal irritation which lasted less than 2 h [20].

3. MECHANISIMS OF ACTION

The stratum corneum, about 15 microns thick when dry and about 40 microns thick when fully hydrated [21, 22], forms a barrier to prevent ingress of most topically applied drugs into the body. Successful passive transdermal drug delivery is accomplished by only a limited number of active molecules having certain physicochemical properties such as low molecular weight <500 Da, sufficient lipophilicity [23]. Without the manipulation of modern technology to achieve penetration enhancement, many important therapeutic peptides, proteins, vaccines, oligonucleotides or particles would be unavailable for percutaneous delivery.

The microneedles applied to the skin surface can piece mechanically the stratum corneum barrier and create hydrophilic microchannels. These microchannels created by microneedles readily permit transport of micromolecules such as vaccines and proteins or particles. The hydrophilic microchannels were investigated by Bankes *et al.* who reported that the permeability of naltrexone hydrochloride is higher than that of the corresponding base because the drug salt is easy to dissolve in the interstitial fluid filled spaces of the aqueous channels [24]. It has been reported that residual microchannel after microneedle removal are microns in size and the closure is after 72 h when kept under occlusion [25], but microchannels close shortly after microneedle application when microchannels are under no- occlusion or after patch removal [26]. However, we found the lifetime of residual microchannels in the rat skin by microneedle (680μm polymer microneedle) is about 12h under non-occlusion (Fig. **2**). Furthermore, Banks *et al.* has found that microchannel opening can keep seven days in the presence of diclofenac in the patch formulation [27]. In a single-blind study of 12 healthy volunteers to assess the effects of two microneedle arrays with 180 or 280 μ m high on microchannel closure, skin penetration was determined by external staining and TEWL measurement [28]. Indications of microchannel repair were obvious at 8–24 h post-insertion.

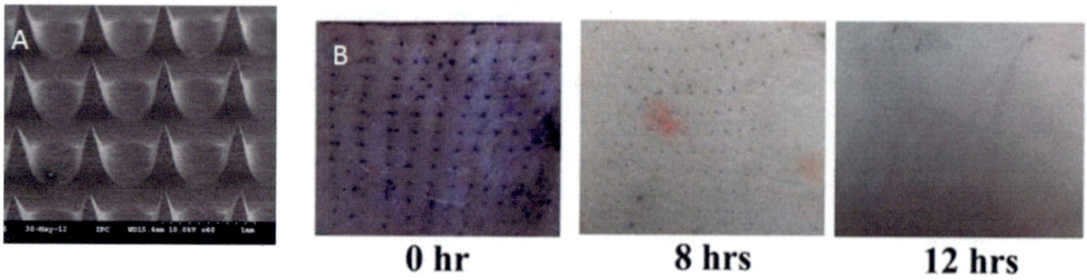

Fig. (2). A: Scanning electron micrograph of the microneedles of chondroitin sulfate (CS). Each microneedle measuring 680 μm in length, 380 μm by 380 μm in cross section at the base, and the radius of the tip is appropriately 10 μm. **B**: The recovery time of abdomen skins of rat treated by CS microneedles. CS microneedles were applied on several sites of abdomen skin rats, and one of these sites was stained by trypan blue at 0, 8 and 12 hrs after treatment. (from author's lab).

The depths of the microchannels in the skin by silicon microneedles (150μm) are about 80-90μm [6] and a depth of 110μm using maltose microneedles (500μm) were reported [29]. These differences may be from the needles' geometry, physical properties or the force of insertion. The studies on geometry and insertion mechanics of microneedle have been reviewed by Mark R. Prausnitz [30].

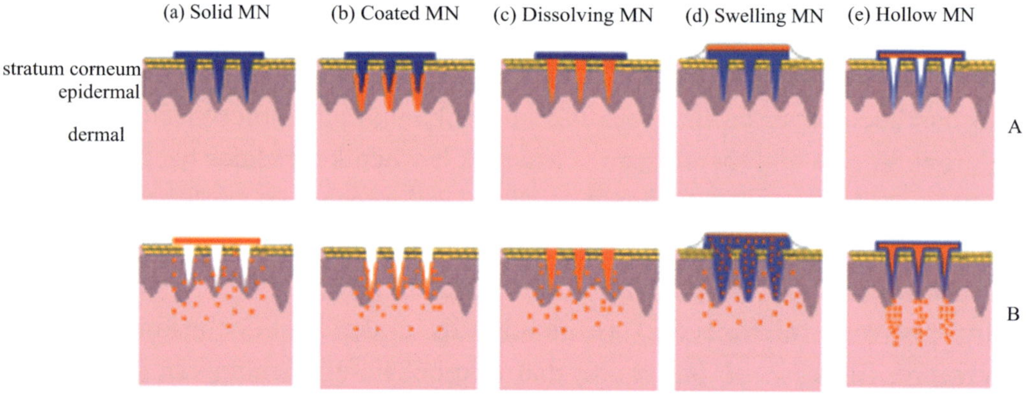

Fig. (3). Schematic of drug delivery with different designs of microneedles (MN). Microneedles are first applied to the skin (**A**) and then delivery drug (**B**). (**a**) Solid microneedles are used as a pretreatment. The microneedles are withdrawn followed by application of drug-containing patch (solid MN). (**b**) After insertion solid microneedles coated with dry drugs into the skin, the drug is deposited in the skin, the needles are then withdrawn (coated MN). (**c**) After insertion drug-loaded polymeric microneedles into the skin, microneedles are dissolved and the drug is released in the skin (dissolving MN). (**d**) After insertion polymeric microneedles into the skin, the drug is released through the hydrogel matrix upon microneedles swelling from a drug-loaded reservoir (Swelling MNs). (**e**) Hollow microneedles for injection of drug solution (hollow MN).

The mechanism of drug delivery depends on the microneedle design is shown in (Fig. **3**).

Table **1** summarizes benefits and limitations of these designs. Drugs may be delivered using microneedles by five different mechanisms: i) percutaneous diffusion of the drug through hydrophilic microchannels created in the skin by solid microneedles; ii) intradermal delivery by directly coating the drug onto solid microneedles; iii) intradermal delivery by incorporating the drug inside the water soluble or biodegradable polymer solid microneedles during fabrication (for microneedles that dissolve in the skin upon insertion); iv) intradermal diffusion of the drug through the swelling hydrogel conduits of polymer solid microneedles from a drug-loaded reservoir; or v) intradermal microinjection by delivering the liquid drug *via* hollow microneedles.

Table 1. Characteristics of different microneedles designs.

Microneedle Design	Characteristics and Benefits	Limitations
Solid Microneedles	► Made of metal, silicon, titanium, glass or polymer ► Low-cost manufacturing for polymer microneedles in FDA-approved medical material ► Improved mechnical strength and effective insertion ► Delivery depends upon drug diffusion (vertical or lateral) ► Diffusion through microchannels (microneedle withdrawm)	► Silicon or metal solid microneedle involved complicated fabrication ► Risk of breakage within the skin for silicon ► two-step application process ► Medical waste after use
Coated Microneedles	►Drug release is not dependent on the diffusion ►Without additional drug reservoir or microfluidics component ►Simple and easy to use drug patch for end user (similar to passive patch) Allows dose sparing	►Coating formulation and technique is the key to success ►Limited drug loading capacity (suitable only for highly potent molecules and vaccines) ►Essential to ensure coated drug was delivered (drug layer is easy to fall off when insertion) Limited needle sharpness ►Medical waste after use

(Table 1) contd.....

Microneedle Design	Characteristics and Benefits	Limitations
Dissolving Microneedles	► Drug loaded in microneedles ddissolves within minutes ► Controlled drug release possible ► No sharp medical waste after use. ► A variety of materials of biodegradable and biocompatible are suitable for manufacturing (sugars, polymer and others) ► Simple and economical micromoulding fabrication technique	►Limited drug loading capacity for hydrophobic drugs ►Not suitable for encapsulation of sensitive ►Careful selection of material required to ensure faster dissolution
Swelling Microneedles	►Made of crosslinked polymers which contain no drug themselves ►Suitable fabricating in a wide range of patch sizes and MN geometries ►Greater payload delivery than coated and dissolving microneedle ►Controlled drug release by the crosslink density of the hydrogel system	►Medical waste after use Ref [53].
Hollow Microneedles	►Microneedle with a central conduit for delivery of fluid formulations ►Rapid onset of drug action possible ►A more flexible doses	►Complicated and expensive fabrication technique ►Reduced mechanical strength as compared to solid microneedles especially when made with sillicon ►Blockage of the needle during insertion by skin tissue ►Need to regulate flow rate required (microfluidics component) ►Medical waste after use Ref [54 - 57].

The first design is solid microneedle-assisted delivery of drug. Solid microneedles can be pressed onto the skin to create microscopic channels. Drug or vaccine applied onto pretreated skin diffuses through these microchannels for local or systemic delivery. By piercing the skin, transdermal permeability of drug has been increased as many orders of magnitude [3] and shown to deliver compounds including hydrophilic drugs [31], lipophilic drugs [32], insulin [33 - 35], proteins (*e.g.*, hepatitis B surface antigen) [36], genetic material (*e.g.*, oligonucleotides, plasmid DNA) [37 - 40], nanoparticles [39, 40] and microparticles (*e.g.*, 2.0 µm sized FluoSpheres) [29] *in vitro* and *in vivo*. Solid microneedles also can be used by scraping the skin, and vaccines have been delivered to animal models and given satisfactory results [18, 41].

The second design is coated microneedles for intradermal drug delivery. Solid water-insoluble microneedles are first coated with a potent drug or vaccine and then these coated microneedles are pierced into the skin layers [42]. The coated microneedles are allowed to stay in the skin in a short time (about 1min) during the drug is dissolved in the skin layers and then withdrawn. Since microneedle arrays do not penetrate the skin to their full length, coatings should be applied to the tip or upper part of the microneedles. Coatings are usually applied by dipping microneedles in a drug formulation at the desired concentration, viscosity and surface tension to provide reproducible drug loading. Widera *et al.* coated titanium microneedles (width 100 µm and 35 µm thickness) with a model antigen ovalbumin (OVA) by applying the coating only to the tip of the microneedles. Higher loading dose was obtained by multiple coatings by repeatedly immersing the microneedles into the coating solution with a drying time of 5 sec between coatings [43]. Other investigators have further optimized coating process to uniformly coat both hydrophilic and hydrophobic molecules onto microneedles. Coatings of desmopressin, parathyroid hormone (PTH), bovine serum albumin, plasmid DNA, Influenza vaccine, and 1 – 20 µm microparticles, amongst others on microneedles have been demonstrated [44 - 46].

The third design is dissolvable microneedles for intradermal drug delivery. Drug is homogenously distributed in microneedle matrix material. Post-insertion, the microneedle tips are dissolved in the skin layers and releases drugs, which then drugs diffuse easily into the skin. The matrix materials for fabricating dissolvable microneedle have to be inert, safe biodegradable or water- soluble, sufficiently hard in dried form, and compatible with drug components. Most of materials tested are various polymers or sugars [4]. Dissolving microneedles have been demonstrated for delivery of many model compounds *in vitro* and *in vivo* [47 - 52].

The fourth design is swelling microneedles for intradermal drug delivery. The substrate materials of microneedle arrays were crosslinked polymers. The swelling microneedles themselves contain no drug. They rapidly absorb skin interstitial fluid during inserting skin to form continuous, hydrogel pathways. The drugs delivery is from attached - drug patch to the dermal microcirculation along the hydrogel conduits of microneedles. Donnelly *et al.* described that the swelling microneedles can be fabricated in a flexible patch sizes and geometries, easily sterilized. Such microneedles resist microchannels closure until they are totally removed from the skin. Release of active ingredients is no longer restricted by loading capacity for microneedles themselves. And percutaneous drug controlled release is now from the crosslink density of the hydrogel system instead of the stratum corneum. The swelling microneedles has been demonstrated for delivery both small molecules, such as metronidazole and theophylline, and biological macromolecules, such as insulin and BSA [53].

The fifth design is hollow microneedles for intradermal drug delivery. The hollow microneedles have a conduit within the needle and drug solution can be delivered *via* hollow microneedles using a driving force such as pressure (similar to syringe and needle). Most hollow systems additionally integrate with a drug or vaccine reservoir and fluid delivery system, such as a syringe, pump or other pressure-generating means, to accomplish delivery rather than relying on passive fluidic transport through the microneedles themselves. For the mechanisms involved in transdermal delivery of drug *via* hollow microneedles, studies have shown that, unless mechanisms exist in the delivery system to pressurize the drug solution reservoir, transfer of drug from the reservoir into the skin is controlled by Fick's laws of diffusion. In some cases, flux may exhibit non ideal behavior at higher drug concentrations, and high viscosity can decrease delivery rates. Partial retraction or vibration of the microneedle array after application may enhance the efficiency of delivery of the therapeutic agent [54 - 56].

4. THERAPEUTIC APPLICATIONS

One of the well-studied applications of microneedles is its use for percutaneous release of the drug. Table **2** summarizes the information of different microneedles that were used to deliver various drug molecules during *in vivo* preclinical and clinical studies (exclusive of vaccination studies). Some of these studies have been discussed in the following sub-sections.

Table 2. Results of some *in vivo* microneedles for drug delivery studies.

Drug	Microneedle (MN) Type	Needle Specifications	Model	References
5-aminolaevulinic acid (ALA) or methyl-5 -aminolaevulinate (MAL)	Solid stainless steel microneedle	2 mm long MN with 100 μm wide	3 patients with keratotic AKs and Bowen's disease	[58]
	Solid silicon microneedle arrays	270 μm long, 6 × 7 arrays with a diameter of 240 μm at the base and an interspacing of 750 μm	Nude mice	[59]
Albumin(radiolabelled)	Hollow silicon MN with a flexible poly-dimethylsiloxane reservoir	200μm long, 2×4 needles are spaced 1 mm apart	Mice	[60]
Antisense Oligonucleotides	Solid metal MN	430μm long, stainless steel MN array patch (2cm^2) with 240MN/cm^2	Hairless guinea pigs	[37]
Ascorbate-2-glycoside	Dissolving maltose MN	500μm long MN, 28 needles with a pitch of 350 μm	10 healthy adult volunteers for testing basic tolerance	[61]
Ascorbic acid	Dissolving microneedles with hyaluronic acid as matrix	220 + 20 μm long, 153 MN (17 x 9 array) patch with 2 x 1 cm^2	24 Korean women for 12 weeks for wrinkle improvement and safety	[62]
Basic fibroblast growth factor	Solid microneedle 33G	Nine 33-G microneedles	11 Korean women	[63]
Daniplestim	Dissolving maltose MN	500 μm long pyramidal MN in 6 layers(27 MN/layer)	Hairless rat	[64]
Desmopressin	Drug coated titanium MN array patch (Macroflux® patch)	200 μm long arrow head MN in an array of 321 MN/cm^2 in a 2cm^2 patch;Array was integrated into an hand held applicator device	Hairless Guinea Pig	[44, 65]
	Dissolving MN containing drug and chrondroitin sulfate or dextran as base polymer	500 μm long MN in an array of 100MN/cm^2	Male Wistar Hannover rats	[66]

(Table 2) contd.....

Drug	Microneedle (MN) Type	Needle Specifications	Model	References
Diclofenac	Solid stainless steel microneedle	800 μm long and 200 μm in width at the base in an arrays of 50 MNs	Healthy human volunteers with no history of dermatologic disease	[67]
Equine anti-tetanus toxin	3M's hollow Microstructured Transdermal System (hMTS)	500–900 μm long in an array of 18 MN/1.27 cm^2	Female domestic swine approximately 6–18 weeks old	[68]
Erythropoietin	Drug coated titanium MN array patch	Macroflux® patch, Array was integrated into an hand held applicator device	Hairless Guinea Pig	[69]
	Dissolving MN prepared using chrondroitin sulfate and dextrin or albumin as polymers	3.24 mm long (single MN) and 0.5mm basal diameter	Male ddY mice	[48]
Etanercept	Hollow steel MN (34 gauge)	1mm long	Female Yorkshire swine	[70]
Hexyl nicotinate (Vasodilators)	Hollow microneedle arrays		Human volunteers	[71]
Human growth hormone	Dissolving MN containing drug and chrondroitin sulfate or dextran as base polymer	500 μm long MN in an array of 100MN/cm^2	Male Wistar Hannover rats	[66]
	3M`s hollow Microstructured Transdermal System	500–900 μm long in an array of 18 MN/1.27 cm^2	Hairless Guinea Pig and domestic swine	[68]
	Drug coated titanium MN array patch (Macroflux® patch)	200 or 400 μm long MN	Hairless Guinea Pig	[72]
Human inmmumoglobulin G (IgG)	Dissolving maltose MN and Demaroller (solid metal MN)	Pylamidal maltose MN (81 needles in three layers) and 192 conical stainless steel MN (~700 μm long) stacked in 8 rows (Dermaroller)	Hairless rat	[73]
Ibuprofen sodium	Dissolving MN with copolymer poly(methylvinylether/maleic acid)	600 μm long and 300 μm in width at the base in an arrays of 361(19x19)MNs/0.49 cm^2	Human L-132 lung cells and rat	[52]

(Table 2) contd.....

Drug	Microneedle (MN) Type	Needle Specifications	Model	References
Insulin (Regular recombinant human insulin and insulin lispro)	Roller having solid stainless steel MN	250, 500, or 1000 μm long MN arranged in 24 circular array of 8 needles/row (total 192 needles) on a cylindrical drum	Male Sprague-Dawley rats	[74]
	Dissolving MN prepared using dextrin as base	3.24 mm long, one needle	Male ddY mice	[75]
	Solid metal MN	1000 μm long with 105 needle	Diabetic hairless rats	[33]
	Dissolving MN with poly(methylvinylether maleic anhydride	600 μm long and 300 μm in width at the base in an arrays of 11 x 11 MNs	Diabetic rats	[47]
	Hollow steel MN (34 gauge)	1mm long	Female Yorkshire swine	[70]
	Hollow silicon MN	400 μm long on 4 mm x 4 mm chips with 21 MNs	Sprague Dawley rats	[76]
	34 G hollow stainless steel	1.5 mm long	22 human subjects with type 1 diabetes	[77]
	Solid stainless microneedle arrays and Iontophoresis(0.2 mA/cm^2)	800 μm long MN in an array of 296 MN over 2cm^2	Sprague-Dawley rats	[78]
	Single hollow microneedle		Children and adolescents with type 1 diabetes	[79]
Insulin-like growth factor-1 (1 μg/mL), vascular endothelial	Solid microneedle 33G	Nine 33-G microneedles	11 Korean women	[64]
L-Carnitine	Solid silicon MN	150 μm long with 484 MNs/cm^2	Sprague-Dawley rats	[31]
Lidocaine(4%)	Metal acupuncture needle	<500μm in length	Human subjects	[80]
Low Molecular Weight Heparin (LMWH)	Dissolving MN constructed from chondroitin, dextran or dextrin	1.52 mm long single MN	Male Wistar rats	[81]
Methotrexate(Anticancer agents)	Dissolving maltose microneedles and Iontophoresis	500 μm long with 28 MNs	Male hairless rats	[82]
Methy nicotinate	Hollow MN array	200 μm long MN	Human subjects	[83]

(Table 2) contd.....

Drug	Microneedle (MN) Type	Needle Specifications	Model	References
Naloxone and Naloxone hydrochloride	3M`s hollow Microstructured Transdermal System	500-900 µm long (18MNs). Each MN had a 10-40 µm cannula for fluid delivery. Array was integrated into an hand held applicator device	Hairless Guinea Pig and domestic swine	[68]
Naltrexone. HCl	Solid stainless steel microneedle	800 µm long and 200 µm in width at the base in an arrays of 50 MNs	healthy human volunteers with no history of dermatologic disease	[67]
Naltrexone	Solid MNs		healthy human volunteers	[19]
6-β-Naltrexol hydrochloride	Solid stainless steel MN	750µm long MN in an array of 5 MN	Hairless guinea pig	[84]
Nicardipine Hydrochloride	Dissolving maltose MN	508 µm long with 27 MNs	Hairless rat	[85]
Ovalbimin	Coated microprojections	Silicon microprojections having lengths of 30,60 and 90um (3364 MN in 4mm x4mm area) integrated into a patch (5mm x5 mm area)	C57BL/6 female mice	[86]
Parathyoid Hormone (I-34, for osteoporosis treatment)	Drug coated titanium MN array patch (ZP-PTH--(Macroflux® patch)delivery technology	190 µm long arraow head MN in an array of 1300MN/2cm^2, arranged in hexagonal design	Phase 1 and Phase 2 clinical studies in human subjects	[45]
Pilocarpine	Coated metal MN	500-750 µm long MN coated with drug using dip coating process	New Zealand white rabbits	[87]
Retinoic acid	Dissolving polymer MN patch with sodium hyaluronate	300 (MH300) or 800 µm (MH800) long	HR-1 hairless mice; human for safety study	[88]

(Table 2) contd.....

Drug	Microneedle (MN) Type	Needle Specifications	Model	References
Retinyl retinoate	Dissolving microneedles with hyaluronic acid as matrix	220 + 20 μm long, 153 MN (17 x 9 array) patch with 2 x 1 cm^2	24 Korean women for 12 weeks for wrinkle improvement and safety	[62]
Somatropin	Hollow steel MN	1mm long (34 gauge)	Female Yorkshire swine	[70]

4.1. Drug Delivery

4.1.1. Insulin & Insulin Analogs

As one of the most widely used injectable drugs, insulin has received by far the most attention among the various biotherapeutics studied for microneedle-based drug delivery, including work with different microneedle design types and progressing through preclinical studies into human trials.

Compared with subcutaneous delivery of insulin, microneedle-based insulin delivery may increase patient comfort and compliance in self- administration. Moreover, studies conducted suggest pharmacokinetics (PK) and pharmaco-dynamic (PD) benefits for microneedle delivery compared with standard subcutaneous injection methods. Solid microneedles and dissolving microneedles loading insulin have been studied extensively in mice, diabetic rats and dogs [33, 48, 74, 75, 78, 89 - 91]. These approaches were shown to enable effective insulin delivery to reduce blood glucose levels. Hollow microneedles have been more widely used for insulin delivery and have progressed into human studies. The first report using microneedle for human insulin delivery was a clinical research trial in ten healthy adult males that evaluated delivery of insulin lispro dose *via* a rapid bolus injection with stainless steel hollow microneedles of three lengths (1.25, 1.50 or 1.75mm × 31 Ga) [92]. In this study and in subsequent similar studies, the results show that microneedle-based insulin intradermal delivery not only induced faster insulin absorption but also enabled more rapid onset and offset of metabolic effect on blood glucose levels than subcutaneous injection, which may have better control over postprandial blood glucose levels [93 - 95]. Expedited PK has been explained by rapid lymphatic uptake and distribution of protein drugs from the skin [70]. In addition, clinical trial showed that subjects found microneedles to be less painful, with only transient redness and edema reported as side effects [94,95].

The most recently study reported on microneedle insulin delivery in 22 subjects with type 1 diabetes examined the PK and PD effects of insulin lispro administered before two daily standardized breakfast and lunch, which is comparison of the microneedle-based intradermal (ID) with traditional subcutaneous (SC) injection [77]. Intravenous basal regular insulin was given throughout, and premeal blood glucose (BG) was adjusted to 115 mg/dl. This study indicates that intradermal lispro is absorbed significantly faster than SC and with greater consistency between doses and between subjects. Glycemic control expressed as percentage of time-in-range over 6 h post-prandially was not significantly improved, but this lack of difference may reflect the unusually tight control of postmeal glycemia with SC lispro dosing after individual dose optimization or potential basal over insulinization. In conclusion, ID insulin delivery is superior to SC infusion in speed of systemic availability and PK consistency and may improve postprandial glucose control.

Various human studies run with microneedle-delivered insulin have been consistent as a whole outcome and demonstrate that the rapid-onset PK effects afforded by microneedle administration can be achieved despite minor variations in insulin concentration, dose and type. Microneedle-delivered insulin as an alternative parenteral approach for ID insulin delivery has promising potential for application, and immunological considerations warrant further exploration in clinical use. Recently, we reported that percutaneous delivery insulin with solid microneedle assisted in rats, compared with subcutaneous delivery, significantly higher Levels of human anti-insulin antibody (AIA) were observed [96]. The increased immunogenicity of insulin delivery by microneedle might be due to the large number of immune cells in skin epidermal.

4.1.2. Parathyroid Hormone (PTH)

Zosano Pharma is developing a rapid transdermal delivery patch that includes a drug-coated array of titanium microneedles applied with a hand-held applicator.

ZP-PTH patch for the treatment of serious osteoporosis is being developed as an alternative to daily injections. The product delivers teriparatide (human parathyroid hormone, PTH (1-34)), a compound that stimulates formation of new bone and reduces the risk of fractures. The ZP-PTH patch system consists of a 2 cm^2 titanium microneedle array with 1300 microneedles/2 cm^2. Microneedles have an arrow-head shape with a length of 190 microns. The tips of the microneedles are coated with PTH (1-34). The coated microneedles are directly inserted into the superficial skin where the drug coating dissolves, producing high localized drug concentrations to drive systemic absorption. In a Phase I PK study, delivery of teriparatide with the ZP-PTH patch resulted in a rapid absorption to the plasma in healthy volunteers; time to maximum concentration was three-times shorter and apparent half-life twice shorter than conventional SC injection. In a Phase II, PK/PD study in 165 post-menopausal women with osteoporosis, teriparatide area under the plasma concentration-time curve (AUC) proportionally increased with dose (20, 30 and 40 μg) administered using the ZP-PTH patch. Inter-subject and intra-subject AUC variability was similar for all patch doses and comparable to SC injection. All patch doses produced a significant increase in spine bone mineral density. In addition, Phase 2 study showed that the ZP-PTH patch was well-tolerated and to be safe and effective in post-menopausal women with osteoporosis. The patch showed a consistent dose response effect for AUC and maximum concentration, and gains in bone mineral density at both the lumbar spine but also at the hip site. The PK profile of PTH delivery by the patch was constant at the 1-month and 6-month (last dose) time points. There was no effect of age, ethnicity or weight compared to injection. These results demonstrate that the transdermal microneedle system can deliver constant, therapeutically useful PTH PK profile. Based on the findings, the transdermal microneedle system is advancing to Phase III clinical study [10, 45, 97, 98].

4.1.3. Lidocaine & Other Local Anesthetics

Administration of lidocaine and other local anesthetics has been studied with both hollow and solid microneedles. In one study, lidocaine was coated on non-dissolving polymer microneedles (500 μm long) and administered to pigs [99].

Lidocaine dissolves promptly off the microneedles and into skin such that the 1-min wear time achieves or exceeds lidocaine tissue levels needed to cause analgesia. The lidocaine levels in the skin were interpreted as sufficient to cause prolonged local anesthesia. This study showed that the lidocaine coated microneedles produced comparable duration of analgesia but provided substantial improvements over conventional creams in regard to the rate of onset. Lidocaine was also injected into the skin of human subjects using single, hollow 500-µm microneedles and compared to conventional intradermal injection with 26-Ga hypodermic needles [99, 100]. Administration pain was recorded using Visual Analogue Scale (VAS) and the area and depth of numbness were determined at 0, 7.5 and 15 min after injection. This study demonstrates the local anesthesia caused by lidocaine delivery by either method was the same, the subjects reported distinct less pain associated with delivery using microneedles and expressed strong preference for that method over intradermal injection with a hypodermic needle.

A microinjection of methyl nicotine with hollow microneedles has also been shown in human subjects [71, 83]. Hollow 200-µm microneedles were used and compared against topical application. A Laser Doppler Perfusion Monitor was used to record maximum blood flow and the time to maximum blood flow at the treatment sites. Microneedle-injected sites showed an obvious faster time to maximum blood flow than topical application. Volunteers reported feeling pressure but no pain from the microneedles during the injections. This study showed microneedles aid in bypassing the stratum corneum and enhance drug delivery through it. We reported another clinical trial that solid silicon microneedle arrays (150 µm long) were tested in a randomized, double-blind study to determine if microneedles could facilitate topical anesthesia by 1% dyclonine cream in 25 healthy volunteers [101]. Dyclonine was applied after microneedle array and sham treatments on opposite forearms, after which subjects rated pain from a standardized pain stimulus at 5-min intervals over the following hour. Administration pain was recorded using a standard 100-mm VAS. The results showed that use of the microneedle array markedly shortened the time to achieve clinically significant reduction in pain and also led to a greater depth of local anesthesia.

4.1.4. Naltrexone & 6-β-Naltrexol

Naltrexone (NTX) is a potent opioid receptor antagonist used primarily in the management of opiate and alcohol dependence. NTX is a small, hydrophilic molecule. Administered orally undergoes significant first- pass metabolism with a highly variable systemic bioavailability. Passive transdermal delivery of naltrexone is limited by its hydrophilic nature, making naltrexone a good potential candidate for microneedle administration. In one study, solid microneedle with 50 MNs (620μm long) was used for pretreatment skin. NTX was delivered from a transdermal patch to healthy human subjects with and without pretreatment of the skin with MNs [19]. This study was conducted to determine whether NTX plasma levels were undetectable over the 72-h period following delivery from a standard transdermal patch without pretreatment. Pretreatment of skin with MNs, by contrast, achieved steady-state plasma concentrations within 2 h of patch application and were maintained for at least 48 h. This study demonstrates the feasibility of using microneedles to enhance transdermal delivery of a hydrophilic drug.

6-β-Naltrexol (NTXOL), the major active metabolite of naltrexone (NTX), a clinically useful molecule for alcohol abuse treatment, was evaluated with solid microneedle (MN) pretreat skin permeation enhancement of NTXOL's hydrochloride salt in hairless guinea pigs [84]. NTXOL·HCl and NTXOL base as conventional transdermal candidates are not suitable due to their physicochemical properties. In this study design, following microneedle array treatment, the gel patch system was applied for 72 h. The pharmacokinetic results shows increases of NTXOL·HCl in MN-enhanced plasma levels are most consistent up to 48 h and begin to vary up to 72 h, followed by immediate decreases in levels post patch removal. And even in the presence of MN's, NTXOL base enhancement was low. This study confirmed that the hairless guinea pig is an appropriate and efficient model for simultaneous evaluation of MN systems, transdermal pharmacokinetics, micropore lifetime, and skin irritation.

Microneedles applied to the skin create micropores, allowing transdermal drug delivery of skin-impermeable compounds. The above human study with this technique testified delivery of naltrexone (an opioid antagonist) for two to three days, and not all subjects maintained therapeutic levels beyond 48 h. These results suggest that the micropores were beginning to re-seal and the skin was restoring its barrier properties. A similar delivery timeframe was observed when NTXOL was administered to hairless guinea pigs with the same approach.

Topical application of diclofenac, a nonspecific cyclooxygenase (COX) inhibitor, could prolong micropore lifetime in hairless guinea pigs, allowing for seven days NTX delivery [27]. The delivery effectiveness of NTX for seven days following one microneedle treatment in humans was comfirmed, with co-application of diclofenac [67]. Human subjects were treated with microneedles, diclofenac (or placebo), and naltrexone. Impedance measurements were used as a surrogate marker to measure micropore formation, and plasma NTX concentrations were measured for seven days post-microneedle application. The study demonstrates that topical application of diclofenac to MN-treated skin can maintain micropore viability, allowing NTX delivery for seven days. These data demonstrate the immense potential of MN technologies for drug delivery over longer periods of time than what has been shown previously.

4.1.5. Retinoic Acid, Retinyl Retinoate & Ascorbic Acid

All-trans retinoic acid (ATRA), a natural retinoid, is the important biologically active form of retinoids. ATRA-loaded dissolving polymer MN patch as a simple, alternative therapeutic option to traditional surgical treatments for Seborrheic keratosis (SK) was tested in hairless mice and human subjects [88]. The MN patch induced epidermal hyperplasia and marked expression of heparin-binding epidermal growth factor-like growth factor mRNA and protein corresponding to ATRA activity in the skin of HR-1 hairless mice. The acceleration of stratum corneum turnover (SCT) was also observed by the dansyl chloride method. The skin irritation study in mice and safety study in humans were performed. The study data show that MN patches can offer an effective and safe means of ATRA delivery into the skin, and the ATRA-loaded MN patch appears to be an effective pharmaceutical product providing a novel therapeutic option for seborrheic keratosis.

Recently, ascorbic acid and retinyl retinoate loaded dissolving microneedle patches were evaluated for wrinkle improvement and safety of MNs in human [89]. Clinical studies were carried out on 24 Korean women for 12 weeks. Patients in group A were treated with retinyl retinoate- loaded dissolving microneedle patches, and patients in group B were treated with ascorbic acidloaded patches twice daily. Wrinkle improvement was assessed by skin Visiometer SV 600. Both the retinyl retinoate and ascorbic acid-loaded dissolving microneedle patches demonstrated statistically significant differences in all Visiometer R-values. In particular, highly significant differences were shown at skin roughness and arithmetic average roughness. Also, there were no side effects such as allergies or irritant contact dermatitis.

4.2. Physiotherapy

Microneedles have also been used for percutaneous Collagen Induction Therapy (CIT). CIT is a new therapy for skin cell regeneration. Microneedling is believed to break or disrupt old collagen strands in scars and promote damaged collagen removal and cause collagen growth immediately under the epidermis. The majority of microneedle technology is for non-surgicaland nonablative treatment of skin conditions such as ageing (wrinkles, lax skin), scarring (acne, surgical), photodamage, hyperpigmentation (age/brown spots) and hair loss (alopecia). The process accelerates and stimulates skin's natural repair without causing permanent epidermal damage. Derma rollers are available on the market for treatment of skin problems. Clinical Resolution Laboratory markets MTS Dermaroller, a cosmetic aid possessing needles that penetrate the skin up to a depth of 0.2–0.3 mm. Microneedling or dermaroller treatment was widely evaluated and confirmed that the expression levels of type I collagen and total collagen content is increased. No patient showed any visible signs of the procedure or hyperpigmentation [102 - 104].

Although dermarollers are easy to use, yet there are some disadvantages such as inability to treat small areas as the roller damages adjacent skin too. In addition, the pressure used for rolling insults the epidermis. All these difficulties led to introduction of automated microneedling devices to the market such as micro pen or micro derma stamp, similar to the microneedles patch. It is a pen-like instrument with handle, disposable needles. It has different modes of speed and controlled depth. Automated microneedling devices are easy to use as the user has to just put the device in stamping action on skin and the perpendicular movement of needle leads to penetration at required depth [105, 106].

4.3. Miscellaneous Application

For medical applications, solid microneedles have been developed for drug delivery into blood vessel walls [107]. Such microneedles were shown to transect the arterial wall in both normal and atherosclerotic vessels in rabbit *ex vivo*. Microneedles are a promising tool for delivering drugs or genes to the vessel wall to prevent restenosis. Microneedles have also been used for drug delivery to the eye. Microneedle, due to its extremely small size, could pierce across ocular tissues such as conjunctiva, sclera and or cornea for drug delivery to back or front of the eye. Jiang *et al.* reported pilocarpine delivered into to the corneal using coated microneedles [87]. The use of microneedles seems to be promising for ocular drug delivery; however safety issues such as needle breakage, accidental injury, application method for transdermal delivery will have to be settled. Hollow microneedles have also been used for painless blood samples and biological fluids [108, 109]. Blood samples are generally collected from capillaries by pricking the skin or from veins using evacuated collection tube. Microneedles can be used to obtain precise body fluids as well as blood samples from the capillaries in the dermis layer. This method has a greatest advantage which making the procedurc painless. Hence painless blood sampling using microneedles can be a very good alternative to hypodermic needles.

Mukerjee *et al.* first evaluated the influence of geometry and design of hollow microneedles on through the skin and capillary movement of interstitial fluid [109]. The silicon microneedles are machined to a shank height of 250–350 μm with 300 μm center-to-center spacing. The ability to extract interstitial fluid from human skin is successfully achieved and verified by the *in situ* measurement of glucose concentration. Researchers from North Carolina State University have developed extremely small hollow microneedles that can be used to deliver quantum dots into skin. This study opens the door to new techniques for diagnosing and treating a variety of medical conditions, including skin cancer [110].

4.4. Vaccination

4.4.1. Mechanism of Action

The skin is densely populated by resident antigen presenting cells (APCs), so has strong immunological function. Langerhans cells (LCs) and dermal dendritic cells (dDCs) are the main immunological skin cells [111]. Additionally, skin keratinocytes and other cells in epidermis and dermis can stimulate and control immune responses, by producing cytokines and chemokines. Comparing to subcutaneous fat and muscle tissue, the dermis and the epidermis have more quantities of DCs. Consequently, hypodermic injection, the main route of antigen delivery, will bypass the skin's immune cells leading to less efficient vaccination. Antigen trafficking studies have shown that vaccination *via* the skin results in more efficient antigen migration into lymph nodes than conventional intramuscular delivery. So the skin, the epidermis and dermis, is an ideal attractive target for vaccination.

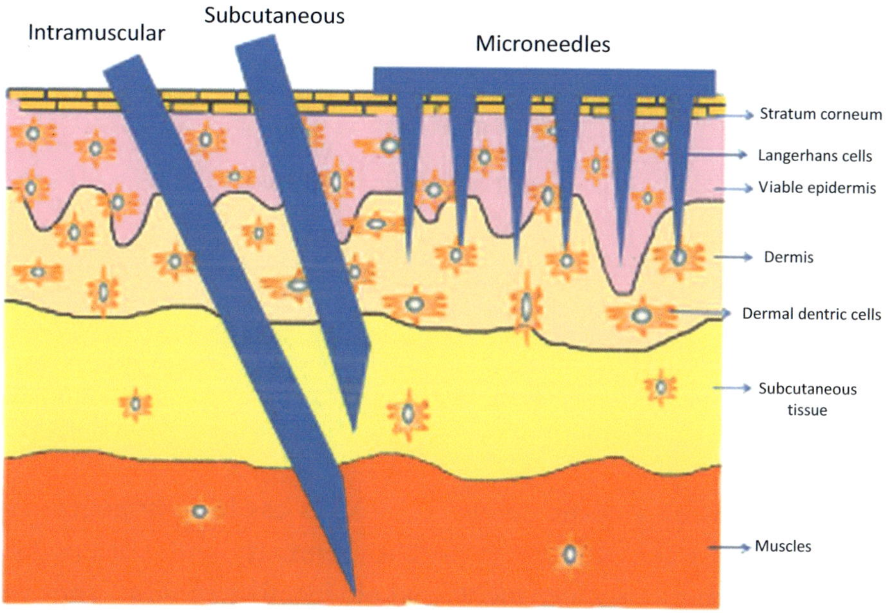

Fig. (4). Comparison between microneedle-based intradermal delivery and hypodermic needle-based conventional intramuscular and subcutaneous.

However, the present situation of transdermal delivery techniques still has difficulties. Intradermal injection is a manually difficult technique that requires the hand of professionally trained healthcarc personnel. MNs address this limitation and can make skin vaccination a practical clinical reality. MNs have been shown to penetrate the skin, across the stratum corneum barrier and create micron-scale pathways into the skin. These micropores created by MNs readily permit transport vaccines and realize the targeting of immunological cells in the epidermis and dermis (Fig. **4**). Motivated by these opportunities, vaccine delivery by different design of MNs has been the most widely studied.

4.4.2. Vaccine Platforms

MN-based vaccination has been extensively studied using a large number of model antigens and clinically relevant vaccines (Table **3**).

Table 3. Model antigens and clinically relevant vaccines studied in MN-based vaccinations.

Inactivated Viruses and Subunit Vaccines	Virus-like Particles	Live Attenuated Viruses	Bacterial Antigens	DNA
Influenza [46, 112 - 126] Rotavirus [127] HIV [128] Chikungunya virus [129] Rabies virus [130] Hepatitis B [36]	Influenza [131 - 137] HPV [138]	Adenovirus [139 - 141] MVA [141, 142] Measles [143] Japanese encephalitis [41]	BCG [144] Tetanus [123] Diphtheria [123, 145 - 148] Botulism [149] Malaria [123] *Yersinia pestis* [149, 150] Staphylococcus aureus [149] Anthrax [18, 149, 151]	Hepatitis B [15, 152] Hepatitis C [153] Influenza [117, 154, 155] HIV [140] Smallpox [156] Herpes simplex virus [157, 158]

Abbreviations: HPV, human papillomavirus; MVA, modified vaccinia virus Ankara; BCG, bacillus Calmette–Guérin; HIV, human immunodeficiency virus.

4.4.3. Influenza Vaccine

To date, the most studied vaccine delivered by MNs has been influenza vaccine. MN vaccination in the skin confers protective immunity with various forms of influenza vaccines. These vaccines include whole inactivated virus, split vaccine, subunit vaccine, virus like particles (VLPs), and DNA vaccines.

The delivery of whole inactivated influenza virus (WIV) using solid vaccine-coated MNs was evaluated in mice [126]. Vaccine-specific antibody responses and protection were induced in mice immunized in the skin at a comparable level as the standard intramuscular (IM) vaccination. However, requirements for high doses of influenza vaccines were postulated to be due to stability problems associated with dry coating of lipid-enveloped WIV vaccines onto solid MNs. Therefore, approaches for stabilization of vaccines during coating were investigated [159, 160]. These studies indicate that trehalose plays a critical role as a stabilizing agent in the protection of immunogenicity of influenza vaccines during preparation of coated MNs. Vaccination in the skin of mice using stabilized MN patch, therefore, elicits improved protective immunity with reduced vaccine doses [159, 160].

Despite the fact that WIV was more immunogenic compared to other forms, its use was discontinued in most countries and replaced with less reactogenic split or subunit influenza vaccines. In a study using metal MNs coated with licensed influenza subunit vaccines the magnitude and longevity of immune responses has been investigated [113]. The results demonstrate that stronger immune responses were induced after MN delivery of influenza subunit vaccine compared with IM delivery. Further findings demonstrate that skin immunization using metal MNs coated with an influenza subunit vaccine induces longer-lived immunity capable of conferring full protection and survival against lethal challenge with homologous virus. BD Soluvia™ is a prefillable delivery system that is integrated with a 1.5 mm long hollow needle, which enables intradermal delivery of a drug or vaccine. It was demonstrated in several clinical studies that the trivalent split inactivated influenza vaccines can be delivered intradermally using this device, and that a dose-sparing effect was achieved [161 - 163].

Similar to results with whole inactivated virus, use of trehalose in the MN coating with influenza HA VLPs preserved hermagglutination activity. MN immunization of mice in the skin with a single dose of stabilized influenza VLPs induced 100% protection against lethal infection, whereas unstabilized MN VLP vaccine induced only partial protection. Vaccination in the skin with stabilized MN VLP vaccine conferred superior protection to IM injection, potential dose sparing effects and rapid recall immune responses against influenza virus [164].

Influenza H5 HA endoding plasmid DNA vaccines were more immunogenic when delivered to the skin using MNs than by IM immunization with the same DNA vaccine. The inclusion of carboxymethylcellulose in the MN coating formulation was found to negatively affect antigen production by DNA vaccines [155]. On the other hand, coating of MNs with naked DNA vaccines in the absence of other excipients was feasible and found to be effective. Delivery of MN-coated DNA vaccines to the skin conferred dose sparing effects and induced improved protection compared to IM immunization [117].

4.4.4. Other Vaccines

4.4.4.1. Live Attenuated Viruses

Live attenuated virus vaccines are weakened forms of whole, mormally pathogenic viruses in which they are unable to replicate enough to cause illness, but still provoke an immune response that can protect against future infection. A study regarding the administration of a live attenuated Janpanese encephalitis vaccine in nonhuman primates provided higher neutralizing antibody titers and increased viremia duration by MN penetration than subcutaneous injection [41].

4.4.4.2. Inactivated Viruses and Subunit Vaccines

In case of inactivated viruses, a study of a clinically licensed rabies vaccine delivered by a 1 to 3 mm BD Soluvia MN syringe proved the safety and reliability of MN injection. The results showed that 1/4 dosage of the rabies vaccine was sufficient to produce higher sero-conversion rates than intramuscular injection [41]. In case of subunit vaccines, MN system was used to pretreat the skin for increase the permeability, and the hydrogel patch formulation was used as the carrier of hepatitis B surface antigen and cholera toxin B as an adjuvant. *In vivo* immunization studies carried out in mice showed that MN group can result in a longer duration of stable IgG titers compared with the IM group. Furthermore, CTB adjuvanted MN group could induce higher IgG titers compared with the group without CTB [36].

4.4.4.3. Virus-like Particles

A study involving the delivery of Gardasil, a commercially approved prophylactic human cervical cancer vaccine composed of the L1 VLP capsid of human papilloma virus, *via* Nanopatch (a densely-packed microprojection array), was reported to induce higher virus neutralizing antibody titers in mice than by IM immunization [138].

4.4.4.4. Bacterial Vaccines

Bacterial vaccines are constituted as a solution containing the intrinsic antigenic epitope portion of the bacterial polysaccharides or toxoids. The list of bacterial vaccines that have been formulated and administered by MNs is shown in (Table **3**). In case of anthrax, a noteworthy dose-sparing effect and a higher immune response than IM were reported in a rabbit model immunized by microcannula-shaped MNs delivering recombinant protective antigen (rPA) from Bacillus anthracis [151]. In another study, rats immunized by solid-state biodegradable MNs consisting of polyvinyl alcohol, trehalose, maltitol, hydroxypropyl-β-cyclodextrin and rPA showed comparable antibody responses similar to traditional delivery methods [9]. Protein-based diphtheria toxin (DT) was used as a model antigen in order to compare the activity of several adjuvants, such as LPS, Quil A, CpG abd cholera toxin (CT), when jointly administered in mice after MN pretreatment. Furthermore, DT combined with CT applied on MN -pretreated mouse skin induced a similar immune response to subcutaneous injection that delivered DT with alum [148]. In addition, another study loaded DT into N-trimethyl chitosan nanoparticles and delivered the vaccine, along with CT, into mice by MN treatment in order to improve the immunogenicity [146].

4.4.4.5. DNA Vaccines

A study examined the effects of MN based DNA vaccination of plasmids that encode a low dose of the vaginal herpes simplex virus (HSV) protein gD2. The results proved that the immune response compared favourably with that of conventional intramuscular DNA vaccination at a high dose, and provided to prevent lethal challenge with vaginal HSV-2 in a mouse model [158]. In another study, positively charged poly (lactic-co- glycolic) acid nanoparticles were coated with DNA plasmid solution expressing anthrax protective antigen, and the vaccine solution was used to immunize mice by dripping the solution onto skin that was pretreated with MN rollers [165]. As a result, transcutaneous DNA vaccination induced comparable responses to intramuscular administration, but a specific mucosal immunity and more balanced type 1 and 2 helper T cell responses. In another study, MNs composed of dissolvable polyelectrolyte multilayers encapsulating DNA vaccines for a model human immunodeficiency virus antigen has been developed, which promoted local transfection and prolonged persistence of antigens in the skin [166].

4.4.4.6. Clinical Trials

Since 2009, Sanofi Pasteur has obtained regulatory approval to market the first microinjection influenza vaccine Intanza1/IDFlu1/Fluzone1 in more than 40 countries including the USA, Canada, Australia and several European Union nations [167]. This vaccine uses BD™ Microinjection System that utilizing a MN for the delivery of the seasonal influenza vaccine. Nanopass Technologies LTD ("NanoPass") produces MicronJet™, a hollow MN device made of silicon (registered with the US FDA, the EU and other countries) for vaccine delivery. From 2013, NanoPass has been collaborating with the US center of Disease control and prevention (CDC) in conducting a large phase III trial of polio vaccine in infants in South East Asia [http://www.nanopass.com/content-c.asp?cid=22]. NanoPass has also supported a pandemic flu phase I study in 280 healthy adult volunteers using the MicronJet™ [168]. The Georgia Institute of Technology and Micron Biomedical have been awarded $2.5 million in grants from the Bill & Melinda Gates Foundation to advance the development of dissolvable microneedle patches for polio immunization. A phase 1 clinical trial will evaluate the possibility of using microneedle patches to deliver polio vaccines safely and effectively (http://www.news.gatech.edu/2015/02/23/polio-vaccination-microneedle-patches-receives-funding-patch-development-clinical-trial)].

4.4.4.7. Perspectives

MN-based systems for vaccine delivery have no doubt great potential. Most studies appear to show dose-sparing relative to conventional routes of administration. Delivery of vaccines to the skin is possible and would be easy to implement using a patch form of MNs as a self-administrative device, which might provide improved or comparable protection to intramuscular vaccination. Research into MN devices has more than 20 years. Most of the researches of MN-vaccine are still in the concept stage, and only a few was into clinical stages [162]. A number of factors must be considered before MN -based vaccination will become well-accepted in clinical practice, to the benefit of patients. Such as scalability of MNs fabrication, gap between animal study and human use, stability issues, dose problem, safety aspects, and so on. Research on MN devices for vaccine delivery was until recently more about solving the design and fabrication issues, while now focus is swiftly changing to the use and application of MNs for delivery of clinically relevant vaccines. It is therefore to be expected that vaccination will soon start becoming a needle-free practice.

5. COMBINATION OF MICRONEEDLE WITH ELECTRICALLY DRIVEN TECHNOLOGIES

5.1. Microneedle and Iontophoresis

Iontophoresis (ITP) enhances transdermal drug delivery by electrorepulsion and electroosmosis. Thus, iontophoresis can be used to drive ionized and unionized drugs across the skin. However, the range of drug molecules that can be delivered is limited by iontophoresis. And the application of a current density of over 0.5mA/cm^2 may cause the risk of irritation or other local skin reactions. Considering the issues mentioned above, the combination strategy of MN technology with iontophoresis has proposed and demonstrated [159 - 169]. The combination approach is anticipated to be beneficial because MN application will create aqueous pathways of low electrical resistance in the skin [170], and iontophoresis will be as the driving force to push the drug molecule across these pathways. Thus, the combination Technologies may lead to a synergistic enhancement in transdermal delivery and broaden the range of drugs suitable for transdermal delivery. Furthermore, the combination will allow the delivery using lower current density thus reducing the occurrence of adverse effects due to high electric dose.

To date the research of combination of ITP and MNs has focused on the use of MNs pretreatment and iontophoresis [169 - 176]. Few reports are about the combination of dissolving microneedles and iontophoresis [177, 178]. R. J. BABU group studied that the effect of lipophilicity of low molecular weight (MW) drug on the MN-mediated iontophoretic delivery *in vitro* [174]. Two hydrophilic molecules (atenolol: MW 266.00, pKa 9.37–9.63, Log P 0.23–0.57 and sotalol: MW 272.36, pKa 8.30-9.80, Log P−0.41–0.85) and two lipophilic molecules (propranolol: MW 259.35, pKa 9.26–9.50, Log P2.58–3.65 and acebutolol: MW 336.43, pKa 9.20–9.40, Log P1.43–1.87) were chosen as model drugs. Iontophoresis alone or MN alone increased the transdermal flux of the four drugs as compared with passive delivery. Microneedle- mediated iontophoretic flux during the current application period was higher than ITP alone or MN alone. The enhancement ratios for hydrophilic molecules, atenolol and sotalol, were 71- and 78-fold higher for ITP + MNs as compared with passive delivery. However, for lipophilic molecule, propranolol and acebutolol, there were 10-fold and 41-fold increase as compared with passive delivery. The results showed that the lipophilicity of the molecule plays a important role on the electrically assisted transdermal delivery of drugs across the aqueous pathways of microporated skin. Using the combination of ITP + MNs, hydrophilic drugs were delivered at a much higher rate as compared with lipophilic molecules.

Recently, M.Gujjar and A.K. Banga reported the results of a hydrophilicity and charged nature molecule glycopyrrolate that has a quaternary ammonium structure, a molecular weight of 380 Da and a log P of −1.18 [176]. Four methods of delivery were compared: passive, MNs, ITP, MNs-mediated ITP. The results showed that ITP significantly raised the delivery of glycopyrrolate compared to passive and microneedle mediated delivery. However, combination of MNs-mediated ITP did not result in any synergistic effect. Sugibayashi group reported the results of evaluation as two model compounds.

D_2O and fluorescein isothiocyanate (FITC)-dextrans (FDs average molecular weight of 3.8, 10.1, 39.0, 71.2 and 200.0 kDa, respectively) *in vitro* [169]. The results showed that the electroosmosis during iontophoresis through MN - pretreated skin was almost the same as through intact skin. The combination approach can further enhance the transdermal delivery of FDs high molecular compounds compared with MN pretreatment alone or iontophoresis alone, whereas no synergistic effect was found on the flux of D_2O. Another study with combination of drug-loaded dissolving MNs and ITP was reported [178]. Small hydrophilic compounds (theophylline, methylene blue, and fluorescein sodium), peptide (bovine insulin) and protein (fluorescein isothiocyanate—labelled bovine serum albumin (FTIC-BSA)) macromolecules were chosen as model drugs. The results showed that the combination of MN and ITP did not resulted in greater transdermal delivery of small molecular weight solute over either technique used alone, the delivery of peptide/protein was significantly enhanced.

These studies show that the synergistic effect of iontophoresis and microneedles appears to depend on the physicochemical properties of the drug such as molecular weight, structure, pKa, PI, LogP, pH and ionization. Even though the combination concept has been demonstrated to be effective in academic research, the commercial success of the product would be dependent upon several factors such as availability of technology, cost, stability of the electrodes, stability of the drug under applied current, accuracy of drug delivery issues.

5.2. Microneedle and Sonophoresis

Recently sonophoresis (SN) has also been shown to effectively deliver various water soluble therapeutic molecules. SN is a promising approach that involves the use of low frequency ultrasound waves for delivery of molecules to deep skin layers. The underlying mechanisms of SN are acoustic cavitation effects, the formation and collapse of gaseous cavities in the SC barrier [171] and thermal effects [172].

Sonophoresis as well as iontophoresis has been shown to result in synergistic effect on delivery of drug molecules, when used together with microneedle. Chen *et al.* evaluated the synergistic effect of low frequency ultrasound (20 kHz frequency, 0.5 W/cm^2 intensity and 20% duty Cycles) combined with 100 μm long hollow silicon microneedles in the delivery of calcein and bovine serum albumin across porcine skin. The results showed that the combination of SN and MNs greatly increased transdermal drug delivery rates compared to either technique alone [173]. HAN *et al.* also reported the the permeability of BSA when combining sonophoresis with 1.2mm or 1.5mm long solid microneedles [174]. The results indicated that the permeability of BSA is significantly increased when using the 15-W (20 kHz) ultrasound combined with the microneedles pre-treatment.

The combination of ultrasound and MNs provides an effective method for the delivery of hydrophilic macromolecule and shows a promising future. The portable ultrasound instrument is a common medical device in hospitals and likely to be obtained at a reasonable cost.

5.3. Microneedle and Electroporation

Electroporation uses controlled, millisecond electrical pulses to create temporary pores in the cell membrane. This action leasds to the formation of pores that allow macromolecule, such as DNA, proteins or antibodies, to enter the cell. Electroporation has also been investigated in combination with microneedles to enhance delivery of drugs through skin [175 - 178]. Dauqimont used hollow conductive microneedle both for DNA and proteins injection and for skin electroporation [175]. Yan *et al.* evaluated the synergistic effect of microneedle electrode array, called in-skin electroporation (IN-SKIN EP), to deliver fluorescein isothiocyanate dextran (FD, 4.3 kDa) as a model macromolecule, into the deeper skin tissues in hairless rat skin model [176]. The *in vitro* results indicated that IN-SKIN EP had a much higher skin permeability for FD-4 than MN alone or ON-SKIN EP (conventional EP treatment). Choi *et al.* reported the experiments of microneedle electrode array applying to red blood cells and human prostate cancer cells and demonstrated successful uptake of calcein (a green fluorescent marker compound that cannot cross intact cell membranes) and BSA by these cells [177, 178]. The uptake efficiency of small molecule calcein was higher than that of macromolecule BSA at a given condition. Further, DNA transfection of cells used the microneedle electroporation device was assessed. The results showed that the electrical active microneedle device could enable DNA delivery in skin.

In conclusion, the combination of micorneedles with electrically driven technologies will further help broaden the scope of drug delivery and has a promising future.

6. DEVICES IN RESEARCH OR IN THE MARKET

Microneedles technology was developed for administration of proteins, peptides, immunobiological, drugs and cosmetics as well as for bio-fluidic analysis. Commercial product development is also underway. Typical devices are shown in (Fig. **5**).

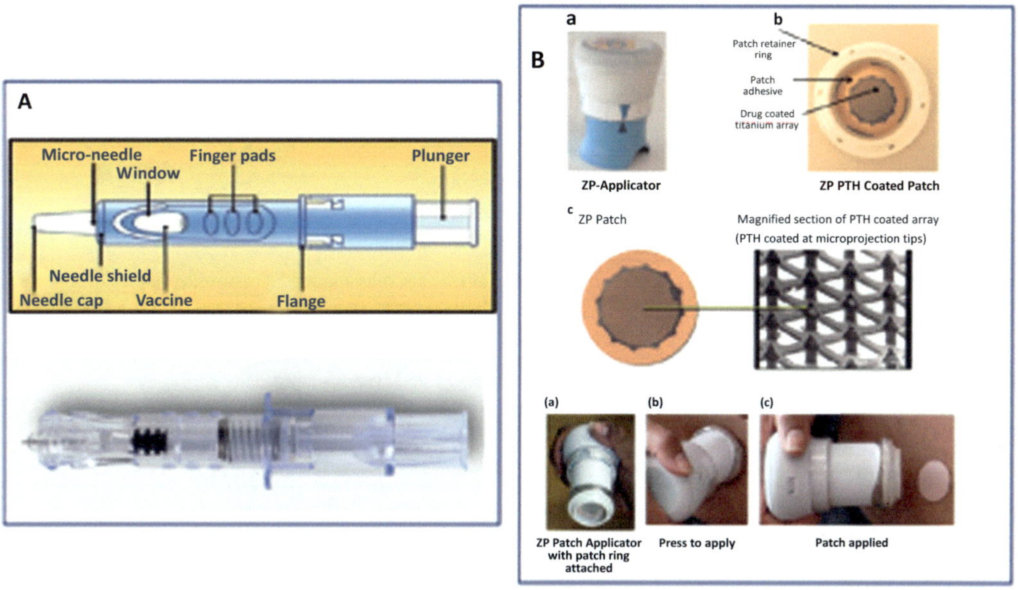

Fig. (5). A: The BD Soluvia™ microneedle delivery system (Reprinted with permission from [179] (Elsevier 2011)). **B:** Transdermal microprojection patch (ZP-patch) delivery system: **a.** applicator; **b.** drug-coated patch; **c.** microprojection array and coating at tips. (Reprinted with permission from [45, 180]. (Springer 2010 and John Wiley and Sons, 2009).

BD's Soluvia™ for intradermal vaccine delivery is already on market. Soluvia® is a single hollow microneedle that has a length of only 1.5 mm, ten times smaller than standard needles for the traditional intramuscular route. It is marketed worldwide prefilled with influenza vaccine for intradermal vaccination as Sanofi Pasteur IDflu®, Intanza® and Fluzone Intradermal®. Zosano Pharma has accomplished Phase 2 clinical trial with ZP-PTH, a coated microneedles, for parathyroid hormone (PTH) delivery. Corium has finished a Phase 1 safety and pharmacokinetic study of MicroCor PTH (1-34), a MicroCor dissolvable microneedles formulation of PTH, in healthy women. This results of the study showed that MicroCor PTH (1-34) was safe and well tolerated, with an excellent PK profile. Table **4** summarizes examples of marketed products based on microneedle technology, together with their possible use.

Table 4. Commercial status of microneedle-based transdermal products.

Brand Name	Manufactured By	Applications
AdminPen	AdminMed, USA	Liquid pharmaceutical formulation or cosmetics can be conveniently injected in to the skin. [http://adminmedical.com/adminpen]
BD Soluvia™	Becton Dickinson, USA	It is a prefillable microinjection system that is integrated with a tiny BD™ microneedle. It allows a drug or vaccine to be accurately delivered intradermally. [http://www.bd.com/pharmaceuticals/ products/microinjection.asp]
Cosmetics-SPE	Nanomed.Inc., China	It is solid silicon microneedles as a skin pretreatment followed by application of the active agents topically. [http://nanomed-devices.com/en/technology.html#2]
DebioJect	Debiotech, Switzerland	Useful for intradermal and hypodermic drug delivery and for interstitial fluid diagnostics. [http://www.debiotech.com/newsite/page/index.php? page=product_01&id=1&id_prod
Eclipse Micropen	Eclipse Aesthetics, LLC. USA	It is solid microneedles and a dermal micro-needling device used by skincare professionals worldwide. [http://www.eclipsemicropen.com/about/micropen-testimonials/]
Intanza/IDflu	Sanofi Pasteur,	first intradermal influenza vaccine marketed in Europe, Australia and Canada. [http://en.sanofi.com/Images/13920_20090226_amm_ intanza_idflu_en.pdf]
MicroCor	Corium International Inc., USA	It is dissolvable microneedles and can be used to deliver small as well as large molecules like proteins, peptides and vaccines. [http://www.coriumgroup.com/Products_MicroCor.html]
MicroHyala	CosMED Pharmaceutical Co.,Ltd., Japan	It is dissolvable microneedles containing hyaluronic acid that is released in the skin to treat wrinkles. [http://cosmed-pharm.co.jpenglish/microneedle.htm]
MicronJet	NanoPass Inc., Israel	It can be used with any standard syringe for painless delivery of vaccines and therapeutics. [http://nanopass.com/]

(Table 4) contd.....

Brand Name	Manufactured By	Applications
Microstructured transdermal system technology (MTS)	3M Corp., USA	The technology can be used to administer drugs including proteins in solid or liquid dosage form. [http://solutions.3m.com/wps/portal/3M/en_WW/3M-DDSD/Drug-Delivery-Systems/Technologies/Microneedle/]
Micro-Trans	Valeritas Inc., USA	It can deliver the drug into dermis without limitations of drug properties of physical and chemical or the patient's skin characteristics. [https://www.valeritas.com/technologies/micro-trans]
MTS-Rollers	Clinical Resolution Laboratory Inc., USA	It is solid microneedles and is used for transdermal delivery of cosmetics in deeper skin layers. [http://www.clinicalresolution.com/main/medicalsolutions.html]
NanoCare	NanoPass Inc., Israel	NanoCare applications for cosmetic enhancement. [http://nanopass.com/content-c.asp?cid=21]
TheraJect MAT™ (DrugMAT and VaxMat)	TheraJect Inc., USA	It is an array of rapidly dissolving micro-needles in a patch. Delivery to the epidermis is minimally invasive, without pain or blood. [http://www.theraject.com/about_us/more_aboutus.html]
ZP Patch	Zosano Pharma Inc., USA	Metallic microneedles (coated drugs) for the delivery of peptides and vaccines. [http://www.macroflux.com/]
ZP-PTH	Zosano Pharma Inc., USA	A product was developed for the treatment of severe osteoporosis [http://www.zosanopharma.com/index.php/20091106127/Research/Research-General/ZP-PTH.html]

CONCLUSIONS

Microneedles offer many advantages and opportunities to deliver drugs and vaccines more effectively. However, only a few are successfully marketed or in clinical so far. To further advance the microneedle technology, it is essential that the pharma companies involve in the research and development. The approach will hopefully lead to the commercialization of microneedles as a medical device for efficient delivery of therapeutic molecules. The development process of Intanza/IDflu and ZP-PTH proved this point. This will not only save resources but facilitate the product development process. In addition, appropriate selection of drug candidates with unmet therapeutic needs will be a key to the successful commercialization. Furthermore, to draft specific regulatory guidelines for development of microneedles is very necessary.

CONFLICT OF INTEREST

The authors confirm that they have no conflict of interest to declare for this publication.

ACKNOWLEDGEMENTS

This work was partially supported by the national key research and development plan of china (2016YFC1000900).

REFERENCES

[1] Smith EW, Maibach HI, Eds. Percutaneous penetration enhancers. Boca raton, FL: CRC Press 1995.

[2] Gerstel MS, Place VA. Drug delivery device. US Patent No. 3, 964, 482, 1976.

[3] Henry S, McAllister DV, Allen MG, Prausnitz MR. Microfabricated microneedles: a novel approach to transdermal drug delivery. J Pharm Sci 1998; 87(8): 922-5. [http://dx.doi.org/10.1021/js980042+] [PMID: 9687334]

[4] Kim YC, Park JH, Prausnitz MR. Microneedles for drug and vaccine delivery. Adv Drug Deliv Rev 2012; 64(14): 1547-68. [http://dx.doi.org/10.1016/j.addr.2012.04.005] [PMID: 22575858]

[5] van der Maaden K, Jiskoot W, Bouwstra J. Microneedle technologies for (trans)dermal drug and vaccine delivery. J Control Release 2012; 161(2): 645-55. [http://dx.doi.org/10.1016/j.jconrel.2012.01.042] [PMID: 22342643]

[6] Van Damme P, Oosterhuis-Kafeja F, Van der Wielen M, Almagor Y, Sharon O, Levin Y. Safety and efficacy of a novel microneedle device for dose sparing intradermal influenza vaccination in healthy adults. Vaccine 2009; 27(3): 454-9. [http://dx.doi.org/10.1016/j.vaccine.2008.10.077] [PMID: 19022318]

[7] Gupta J, Park SS, Bondy B, Felner EI, Prausnitz MR. Infusion pressure and pain during microneedle injection into skin of human subjects. Biomaterials 2011; 32(28): 6823-31. [http://dx.doi.org/10.1016/j.biomaterials.2011.05.061] [PMID: 21684001]

[8] Ito Y, Hasegawa R, Fukushima K, Sugioka N, Takada K. Self-dissolving micropile array chip as percutaneous delivery system of protein drug. Biol Pharm Bull 2010; 33(4): 683-90. [http://dx.doi.org/10.1248/bpb.33.683] [PMID: 20410606]

[9] Wendorf JR, Ghartey-Tagoe EB, Williams SC, Enioutina E, Singh P, Cleary GW. Transdermal delivery of macromolecules using solid-state biodegradable microstructures. Pharm Res 2011; 28(1): 22-30. [http://dx.doi.org/10.1007/s11095-010-0174-y] [PMID: 20535531]

[10] Ameri M, Daddona PE, Maa YF. Demonstrated solid-state stability of parathyroid hormone PTH(1-34) coated on a novel transdermal microprojection delivery system. Pharm Res 2009; 26(11): 2454-63. [http://dx.doi.org/10.1007/s11095-009-9960-9] [PMID: 20183917]

[11] Crichton ML, Ansaldo A, Chen X, Prow TW, Fernando GJ, Kendall MA. The effect of strain rate on the precision of penetration of short densely-packed microprojection array patches coated with vaccine. Biomaterials 2010; 31(16): 4562-72.
[http://dx.doi.org/10.1016/j.biomaterials.2010.02.022] [PMID: 20226519]

[12] Boehm RD, Miller PR, Daniels J, Stafslien S, Narayan RJ. Inkjet printing for pharmaceutical applications. Materials Today (Oxford, United Kingdom) 2014; 17: 247-52.
[http://dx.doi.org/10.1016/j.mattod.2014.04.027]

[13] Ochoa M, Mousoulis C, Ziaie B. Polymeric microdevices for transdermal and subcutaneous drug delivery. Adv Drug Deliv Rev 2012; 64(14): 1603-16.
[http://dx.doi.org/10.1016/j.addr.2012.09.035] [PMID: 23000744]

[14] van der Maaden K, Trietsch SJ, Kraan H, *et al.* Novel hollow microneedle technology for depth-controlled microinjection-mediated dermal vaccination: a study with polio vaccine in rats. Pharm Res 2014; 31(7): 1846-54.
[PMID: 24469907]

[15] Mikszta JA, Alarcon JB, Brittingham JM, Sutter DE, Pettis RJ, Harvey NG. Improved genetic immunization *via* micromechanical disruption of skin-barrier function and targeted epidermal delivery. Nat Med 2002; 8(4): 415-9.
[http://dx.doi.org/10.1038/nm0402-415] [PMID: 11927950]

[16] Fernando GJ, Chen X, Primiero CA, *et al.* Nanopatch targeted delivery of both antigen and adjuvant to skin synergistically drives enhanced antibody responses. J Control Release 2012; 159(2): 215-21.
[http://dx.doi.org/10.1016/j.jconrel.2012.01.030] [PMID: 22306334]

[17] Park K. Improving the reach of vaccines to low-resource regions with a needle-free vaccine delivery device and long-term thermostabilization. J Control Release 2011; 152(3): 329.
[http://dx.doi.org/10.1016/j.jconrel.2011.05.015] [PMID: 21600940]

[18] Mikszta JA, Sullivan VJ, Dean C, *et al.* Protective immunization against inhalational anthrax: a comparison of minimally invasive delivery platforms. J Infect Dis 2005; 191(2): 278-88.
[http://dx.doi.org/10.1086/426865] [PMID: 15609239]

[19] Wermeling DP, Banks SL, Hudson DA, *et al.* Microneedles permit transdermal delivery of a skin-impermeant medication to humans. Proc Natl Acad Sci USA 2008; 105(6): 2058-63.
[http://dx.doi.org/10.1073/pnas.0710355105] [PMID: 18250310]

[20] Bal SM, Caussin J, Pavel S, Bouwstra JA. *In vivo* assessment of safety of microneedle arrays in human skin. Eur J Pharm Sci 2008; 35(3): 193-202.
[http://dx.doi.org/10.1016/j.ejps.2008.06.016] [PMID: 18657610]

[21] Scheuplein RJ. Mechanism of percutaneous absorption. II. Transient diffusion and the relative importance of various routes of skin penetration. J Invest Dermatol 1967; 48(1): 79-88.
[http://dx.doi.org/10.1038/jid.1967.11] [PMID: 6018244]

[22] Anderson RL, Cassidy JM. Variation in physical dimensions and chemical composition of human stratum corneum. J Invest Dermatol 1973; 61(1): 30-2.
[http://dx.doi.org/10.1111/1523-1747.ep12674117] [PMID: 4718753]

[23] Arora A, Prausnitz MR, Mitragotri S. Micro-scale devices for transdermal drug delivery. Int J Pharm

2008; 364(2): 227-36.
[http://dx.doi.org/10.1016/j.ijpharm.2008.08.032] [PMID: 18805472]

[24] Banks SL, Pinninti RR, Gill HS, Crooks PA, Prausnitz MR, Stinchcomb AL. Flux across [corrected] microneedle-treated skin is increased by increasing charge of naltrexone and naltrexol in vitro. Pharm Res 2008; 25(7): 1677-85.
[http://dx.doi.org/10.1007/s11095-008-9578-3] [PMID: 18449628]

[25] Kalluri H, Banga AK. Formation and closure of microchannels in skin following microporation. Pharm Res 2011; 28(1): 82-94.
[http://dx.doi.org/10.1007/s11095-010-0122-x] [PMID: 20354766]

[26] Banga AK. Microporation applications for enhancing drug delivery. Expert Opin Drug Deliv 2009; 6(4): 343-54.
[http://dx.doi.org/10.1517/17425240902841935] [PMID: 19348604]

[27] Banks SL, Paudel KS, Brogden NK, Loftin CD, Stinchcomb AL. Diclofenac enables prolonged delivery of naltrexone through microneedle-treated skin. Pharm Res 2011; 28(5): 1211-9.
[http://dx.doi.org/10.1007/s11095-011-0372-2] [PMID: 21301935]

[28] Haq MI, Smith E, John DN, *et al.* Clinical administration of microneedles: skin puncture, pain and sensation. Biomed Microdevices 2009; 11(1): 35-47.
[http://dx.doi.org/10.1007/s10544-008-9208-1] [PMID: 18663579]

[29] Gupta J, Gill HS, Andrews SN, Prausnitz MR. Kinetics of skin resealing after insertion of microneedles in human subjects. J Control Release 2011; 154(2): 148-55.
[http://dx.doi.org/10.1016/j.jconrel.2011.05.021] [PMID: 21640148]

[30] Prausnitz MR. Microneedles for transdermal drug delivery. Adv Drug Deliv Rev 2004; 56(5): 581-7.
[http://dx.doi.org/10.1016/j.addr.2003.10.023] [PMID: 15019747]

[31] Zhang S, Qin G, Wu Y, *et al.* Enhanced bioavailability of L-carnitine after painless intradermal delivery *vs.* oral administration in rats. Pharm Res 2011; 28(1): 117-23.
[http://dx.doi.org/10.1007/s11095-010-0109-7] [PMID: 20387100]

[32] Qiu Y, Gao Y, Hu K, Li F. Enhancement of skin permeation of docetaxel: a novel approach combining microneedle and elastic liposomes. J Control Release 2008; 129(2): 144-50.
[http://dx.doi.org/10.1016/j.jconrel.2008.04.019] [PMID: 18538885]

[33] Martanto W, Davis SP, Holiday NR, Wang J, Gill HS, Prausnitz MR. Transdermal delivery of insulin using microneedles *in vivo.* Pharm Res 2004; 21(6): 947-52.
[http://dx.doi.org/10.1023/B:PHAM.0000029282.44140.2e] [PMID: 15212158]

[34] Wu Y, Gao Y, Qin G, *et al.* Sustained release of insulin through skin by intradermal microdelivery system. Biomed Microdevices 2010; 12(4): 665-71.
[http://dx.doi.org/10.1007/s10544-010-9419-0] [PMID: 20306299]

[35] Qiu Y, Qin G, Zhang S, Wu Y, Xu B, Gao Y. Novel lyophilized hydrogel patches for convenient and effective administration of microneedle-mediated insulin delivery. Int J Pharm 2012; 437(1-2): 51-6.
[http://dx.doi.org/10.1016/j.ijpharm.2012.07.035] [PMID: 22842625]

[36] Guo L, Qiu Y, Chen J, Zhang S, Xu B, Gao Y. Effective transcutaneous immunization against hepatitis B virus by a combined approach of hydrogel patch formulation and microneedle arrays.

Biomed Microdevices 2013; 15(6): 1077-85.
[http://dx.doi.org/10.1007/s10544-013-9799-z] [PMID: 23893014]

[37] Lin W, Cormier M, Samiee A, *et al.* Transdermal delivery of antisense oligonucleotides with microprojection patch (Macroflux) technology. Pharm Res 2001; 18(12): 1789-93.
[http://dx.doi.org/10.1023/A:1013395102049] [PMID: 11785702]

[38] Birchall J, Coulman S, Pearton M, *et al.* Cutaneous DNA delivery and gene expression in *ex vivo* human skin explants *via* wet-etch micro-fabricated micro-needles. J Drug Target 2005; 13(7): 415-21.
[http://dx.doi.org/10.1080/10611860500383705] [PMID: 16308210]

[39] Chabri F, Bouris K, Jones T, *et al.* Microfabricated silicon microneedles for nonviral cutaneous gene delivery. Br J Dermatol 2004; 150(5): 869-77.
[http://dx.doi.org/10.1111/j.1365-2133.2004.05921.x] [PMID: 15149498]

[40] Coulman SA, Barrow D, Anstey A, *et al.* Minimally invasive cutaneous delivery of macromolecules and plasmid DNA via microneedles. Curr Drug Deliv 2006; 3(1): 65-75.
[http://dx.doi.org/10.2174/156720106775197510] [PMID: 16472095]

[41] Dean CH, Alarcon JB, Waterston AM, *et al.* Cutaneous delivery of a live, attenuated chimeric flavivirus vaccine against Japanese encephalitis (ChimeriVax)-JE) in non-human primates. Hum Vaccin 2005; 1(3): 106-11.
[http://dx.doi.org/10.4161/hv.1.3.1797] [PMID: 17012854]

[42] Gill HS, Prausnitz MR. Coated microneedles for transdermal delivery. J Control Release 2007; 117(2): 227-37.
[http://dx.doi.org/10.1016/j.jconrel.2006.10.017] [PMID: 17169459]

[43] Widera G, Johnson J, Kim L, *et al.* Effect of delivery parameters on immunization to ovalbumin following intracutaneous administration by a coated microneedle array patch system. Vaccine 2006; 24(10): 1653-64.
[http://dx.doi.org/10.1016/j.vaccine.2005.09.049] [PMID: 16246466]

[44] Cormier M, Johnson B, Ameri M, *et al.* Transdermal delivery of desmopressin using a coated microneedle array patch system. J Control Release 2004; 97(3): 503-11.
[http://dx.doi.org/10.1016/S0168-3659(04)00171-3] [PMID: 15212882]

[45] Daddona PE, Matriano JA, Mandema J, Maa YF. Parathyroid hormone (1-34)-coated microneedle patch system: clinical pharmacokinetics and pharmacodynamics for treatment of osteoporosis. Pharm Res 2011; 28(1): 159-65.
[http://dx.doi.org/10.1007/s11095-010-0192-9] [PMID: 20567999]

[46] Kim YC, Quan FS, Compans RW, Kang SM, Prausnitz MR. Formulation and coating of microneedles with inactivated influenza virus to improve vaccine stability and immunogenicity. J Control Release 2010; 142(2): 187-95.
[http://dx.doi.org/10.1016/j.jconrel.2009.10.013] [PMID: 19840825]

[47] Migalska K, Morrow DI, Garland MJ, Thakur R, Woolfson AD, Donnelly RF. Laser-engineered dissolving microneedle arrays for transdermal macromolecular drug delivery. Pharm Res 2011; 28(8): 1919-30.
[http://dx.doi.org/10.1007/s11095-011-0419-4] [PMID: 21437789]

[48] Ito Y, Yoshimitsu J, Shiroyama K, Sugioka N, Takada K. Self-dissolving microneedles for the percutaneous absorption of EPO in mice. J Drug Target 2006; 14(5): 255-61.
[http://dx.doi.org/10.1080/10611860600785080] [PMID: 16882545]

[49] Ikejiri A, Ito Y, Naito S, Takada K. Two-and Three-Layered Dissolving Microneedles for Transcutaneous Delivery of Model Vaccine Antigen in Rats. J Biomater Nanobiotechnol 2012; 3: 325-34.
[http://dx.doi.org/10.4236/jbnb.2012.33030]

[50] Hiraishi Y, Nakagawa T, Quan YS, *et al.* Performance and characteristics evaluation of a sodium hyaluronate-based microneedle patch for a transcutaneous drug delivery system. Int J Pharm 2013; 441(1-2): 570-9.
[http://dx.doi.org/10.1016/j.ijpharm.2012.10.042] [PMID: 23137695]

[51] Zaric M, Lyubomska O, Touzelet O, *et al.* Skin dendritic cell targeting via microneedle arrays laden with antigen-encapsulated poly-D,L-lactide-co-glycolide nanoparticles induces efficient antitumor and antiviral immune responses. ACS Nano 2013; 7(3): 2042-55.
[http://dx.doi.org/10.1021/nn304235j] [PMID: 23373658]

[52] McCrudden MT, Alkilani AZ, McCrudden CM, *et al.* Design and physicochemical characterisation of novel dissolving polymeric microneedle arrays for transdermal delivery of high dose, low molecular weight drugs. J Control Release 2014; 180: 71-80.
[http://dx.doi.org/10.1016/j.jconrel.2014.02.007] [PMID: 24556420]

[53] Donnelly RF, Singh TR, Garland MJ, *et al.* Hydrogel-forming microneedle arrays for enhanced transdermal drug delivery. Adv Funct Mater 2012; 22(23): 4879-90.
[http://dx.doi.org/10.1002/adfm.201200864] [PMID: 23606824]

[54] Wonglertnirant N, Todo H, Opanasopit P, Ngawhirunpat T, Sugibayashi K. Macromolecular delivery into skin using a hollow microneedle. Biol Pharm Bull 2010; 33(12): 1988-93.
[http://dx.doi.org/10.1248/bpb.33.1988] [PMID: 21139238]

[55] Milewski M, Yerramreddy TR, Ghosh P, Crooks PA, Stinchcomb AL. *In vitro* permeation of a pegylated naltrexone prodrug across microneedle-treated skin. J Control Release 2010; 146(1): 37-44.
[http://dx.doi.org/10.1016/j.jconrel.2010.05.034] [PMID: 20678989]

[56] Wang PM, Cornwell M, Hill J, Prausnitz MR. Precise microinjection into skin using hollow microneedles. J Invest Dermatol 2006; 126(5): 1080-7.
[http://dx.doi.org/10.1038/sj.jid.5700150] [PMID: 16484988]

[57] Martanto W, Moore JS, Kashlan O, *et al.* Microinfusion using hollow microneedles. Pharm Res 2006; 23(1): 104-13.
[http://dx.doi.org/10.1007/s11095-005-8498-8] [PMID: 16308670]

[58] Kolde G, Rowe E, Meffert H. Effective photodynamic therapy of actinic keratoses and Bowen's disease using microneedle perforation. Br J Dermatol 2013; 168(2): 450-2.
[http://dx.doi.org/10.1111/j.1365-2133.2012.11153.x] [PMID: 22804095]

[59] Donnelly RF, Morrow DI, McCarron PA, *et al.* Microneedle-mediated intradermal delivery of 5-aminolevulinic acid: potential for enhanced topical photodynamic therapy. J Control Release 2008; 129(3): 154-62.

[http://dx.doi.org/10.1016/j.jconrel.2008.05.002] [PMID: 18556084]

[60] Häfeli UO, Mokhtari A, Liepmann D, Stoeber B. *In vivo* evaluation of a microneedle-based miniature syringe for intradermal drug delivery. Biomed Microdevices 2009; 11(5): 943-50. [http://dx.doi.org/10.1007/s10544-009-9311-y] [PMID: 19347587]

[61] Miyano T, Tobinaga Y, Kanno T, *et al.* Sugar micro needles as transdermic drug delivery system. Biomed Microdevices 2005; 7(3): 185-8. [http://dx.doi.org/10.1007/s10544-005-3024-7] [PMID: 16133805]

[62] Kim M, Yang H, Kim H, Jung H, Jung H. Novel cosmetic patches for wrinkle improvement: retinyl retinoate- and ascorbic acid-loaded dissolving microneedles. Int J Cosmet Sci 2014; 36(3): 207-12. [http://dx.doi.org/10.1111/ics.12115] [PMID: 24910870]

[63] Lee YB, Eun YS, Lee JH, *et al.* Effects of topical application of growth factors followed by microneedle therapy in women with female pattern hair loss: a pilot study. J Dermatol 2013; 40(1): 81-3. [http://dx.doi.org/10.1111/j.1346-8138.2012.01680.x] [PMID: 23039201]

[64] Katikaneni S, Li G, Badkar A, Banga AK. Transdermal delivery of a approximately 13 kDa protein--an *in vivo* comparison of physical enhancement methods. J Drug Target 2010; 18(2): 141-7. [http://dx.doi.org/10.3109/10611860903287164] [PMID: 19772395]

[65] Sathyan G, Sun Y-N, Weyers R, Daddona P, Staehr P, Gupta S. Macroflux® desmopressin transdermal delivery system: Pharmacokinetics and pharmacodynamic evaluation in healthy volunteers. AAPS J 2004; 6(S1): 665.

[66] Fukushima K, Ise A, Morita H, *et al.* Two-layered dissolving microneedles for percutaneous delivery of peptide/protein drugs in rats. Pharm Res 2011; 28(1): 7-21. [http://dx.doi.org/10.1007/s11095-010-0097-7] [PMID: 20300802]

[67] Brogden NK, Banks SL, Crofford LJ, Stinchcomb AL. Diclofenac enables unprecedented week-long microneedle-enhanced delivery of a skin impermeable medication in humans. Pharm Res 2013; 30(8): 1947-55. [http://dx.doi.org/10.1007/s11095-013-1036-1] [PMID: 23761054]

[68] Burton SA, Ng CY, Simmers R, *et al.* Rapid intradermal delivery of liquid formulations using a hollow microstructured array. Pharm Res 2011; 28(1): 31-40. [http://dx.doi.org/10.1007/s11095-010-0177-8] [PMID: 20582455]

[69] Ameri M, Peters E, Wang X, Daddona P, Maa Y-F. Erythropoietin (EPO) coated microprojection transdermal system: Pre-clinical formulation, stability and delivery. AAPS J 2009; 11(S2): T2245.

[70] Harvey AJ, Kaestner SA, Sutter DE, Harvey NG, Mikszta JA, Pettis RJ. Microneedle-based intradermal delivery enables rapid lymphatic uptake and distribution of protein drugs. Pharm Res 2011; 28(1): 107-16. [http://dx.doi.org/10.1007/s11095-010-0123-9] [PMID: 20354765]

[71] Sivamani RK, Stoeber B, Liepmann D, Maibach HI. Microneedle penetration and injection past the stratum corneum in humans. J Dermatolog Treat 2009; 20(3): 156-9. [http://dx.doi.org/10.1080/09546630802512679] [PMID: 19016065]

[72] Daddona P. Macroflux® transdermal technology development for the delivery of therapeutic peptides

and proteins. Drug Deliv Technol 2002; 2: 54-7.

[73] Li G, Badkar A, Kalluri H, Banga AK. Microchannels created by sugar and metal microneedles: characterization by microscopy, macromolecular flux and other techniques. J Pharm Sci 2010; 99(4): 1931-41.
[http://dx.doi.org/10.1002/jps.21981] [PMID: 19894263]

[74] Zhou CP, Liu YL, Wang HL, Zhang PX, Zhang JL. Transdermal delivery of insulin using microneedle rollers *in vivo.* Int J Pharm 2010; 392(1-2): 127-33.
[http://dx.doi.org/10.1016/j.ijpharm.2010.03.041] [PMID: 20347024]

[75] Ito Y, Hagiwara E, Saeki A, Sugioka N, Takada K. Feasibility of microneedles for percutaneous absorption of insulin. Eur J Pharm Sci 2006; 29(1): 82-8.
[http://dx.doi.org/10.1016/j.ejps.2006.05.011] [PMID: 16828268]

[76] Nordquist L, Roxhed N, Griss P, Stemme G. Novel microneedle patches for active insulin delivery are efficient in maintaining glycaemic control: an initial comparison with subcutaneous administration. Pharm Res 2007; 24(7): 1381-8.
[http://dx.doi.org/10.1007/s11095-007-9256-x] [PMID: 17387600]

[77] McVey E, Hirsch L, Sutter DE, *et al.* Pharmacokinetics and postprandial glycemic excursions following insulin lispro delivered by intradermal microneedle or subcutaneous infusion. J Diabetes Sci Technol 2012; 6(4): 743-54.
[http://dx.doi.org/10.1177/193229681200600403] [PMID: 22920798]

[78] Chen H, Zhu H, Zheng J, *et al.* Iontophoresis-driven penetration of nanovesicles through microneedle-induced skin microchannels for enhancing transdermal delivery of insulin. J Control Release 2009; 139(1): 63-72.
[http://dx.doi.org/10.1016/j.jconrel.2009.05.031] [PMID: 19481577]

[79] Norman JJ, Brown MR, Raviele NA, Prausnitz MR, Felner EI. Faster pharmacokinetics and increased patient acceptance of intradermal insulin delivery using a single hollow microneedle in children and adolescents with type 1 diabetes. Pediatr Diabetes 2013; 14(6): 459-65.
[http://dx.doi.org/10.1111/pedi.12031] [PMID: 23517449]

[80] Wilson JR, Kehl LJ, Beiraghi S. Enhanced topical anesthesia of 4% lidocaine with microneedle pretreatment and iontophoresis. Northwest Dent 2008; 87(3): 40-1.
[PMID: 18663870]

[81] Ito Y, Murakami A, Maeda T, Sugioka N, Takada K. Evaluation of self-dissolving needles containing low molecular weight heparin (LMWH) in rats. Int J Pharm 2008; 349(1-2): 124-9.
[http://dx.doi.org/10.1016/j.ijpharm.2007.07.036] [PMID: 17826015]

[82] Vemulapalli V, Yang Y, Friden PM, Banga AK. Synergistic effect of iontophoresis and soluble microneedles for transdermal delivery of methotrexate. J Pharm Pharmacol 2008; 60(1): 27-33.
[http://dx.doi.org/10.1211/jpp.60.1.0004] [PMID: 18088502]

[83] Sivamani RK, Stoeber B, Wu GC, Zhai H, Liepmann D, Maibach H. Clinical microneedle injection of methyl nicotinate: stratum corneum penetration. Skin Res Technol 2005; 11(2): 152-6.
[http://dx.doi.org/10.1111/j.1600-0846.2005.00107.x] [PMID: 15807814]

[84] Banks SL, Pinninti RR, Gill HS, *et al.* Transdermal delivery of naltrexol and skin permeability lifetime

after microneedle treatment in hairless guinea pigs. J Pharm Sci 2010; 99(7): 3072-80. [http://dx.doi.org/10.1002/jps.22083] [PMID: 20166200]

[85] Kolli CS, Banga AK. Characterization of solid maltose microneedles and their use for transdermal delivery. Pharm Res 2008; 25(1): 104-13. [http://dx.doi.org/10.1007/s11095-007-9350-0] [PMID: 17597381]

[86] Chen X, Prow TW, Crichton ML, *et al.* Dry-coated microprojection array patches for targeted delivery of immunotherapeutics to the skin. J Control Release 2009; 139(3): 212-20. [http://dx.doi.org/10.1016/j.jconrel.2009.06.029] [PMID: 19577597]

[87] Jiang J, Gill HS, Ghate D, *et al.* Coated microneedles for drug delivery to the eye. Invest Ophthalmol Vis Sci 2007; 48(9): 4038-43. [http://dx.doi.org/10.1167/iovs.07-0066] [PMID: 17724185]

[88] Hiraishi Y, Hirobe S, Iioka H, *et al.* Development of a novel therapeutic approach using a retinoic acid-loaded microneedle patch for seborrheic keratosis treatment and safety study in humans. J Control Release 2013; 171(2): 93-103. [http://dx.doi.org/10.1016/j.jconrel.2013.06.008] [PMID: 23791975]

[89] Ito Y, Ohashi Y, Saeki A, Sugioka N, Takada K. Antihyperglycemic effect of insulin from self-dissolving micropiles in dogs. Chem Pharm Bull (Tokyo) 2008; 56(3): 243-6. [http://dx.doi.org/10.1248/cpb.56.243] [PMID: 18310929]

[90] Fukushima K, Yamazaki T, Hasegawa R, Ito Y, Sugioka N, Takada K. Pharmacokinetic and pharmacodynamic evaluation of insulin dissolving microneedles in dogs. Diabetes Technol Ther 2010; 12(6): 465-74. [http://dx.doi.org/10.1089/dia.2009.0176] [PMID: 20470231]

[91] Ito Y, Yamazaki T, Sugioka N, Takada K. Self-dissolving micropile array tips for percutaneous administration of insulin. J Mater Sci Mater Med 2010; 21(2): 835-41. [http://dx.doi.org/10.1007/s10856-009-3923-x] [PMID: 19915962]

[92] Heinemann L, Hompesch M, Kapitza C, *et al.* Intra-dermal insulin lispro application with a new microneedle delivery system led to a substantially more rapid insulin absorption than subcutaneous insulin injection. Diabet Med 2006; 23: 329.

[93] Pettis RJ, Ginsberg B, Hirsch L, *et al.* Intradermal microneedle delivery of insulin lispro achieves faster insulin absorption and insulin action than subcutaneous injection. Diabetes Technol Ther 2011; 13(4): 435-42. [http://dx.doi.org/10.1089/dia.2010.0184] [PMID: 21355718]

[94] Pettis RJ, Hirsch L, Kapitza C, *et al.* Microneedle-based intradermal *versus* subcutaneous administration of regular human insulin or insulin lispro: pharmacokinetics and postprandial glycemic excursions in patients with type 1 diabetes. Diabetes Technol Ther 2011; 13(4): 443-50. [http://dx.doi.org/10.1089/dia.2010.0183] [PMID: 21355716]

[95] Gupta J, Felner EI, Prausnitz MR. Rapid pharmacokinetics of intradermal insulin administered using microneedles in type 1 diabetes subjects. Diabetes Technol Ther 2011; 13(4): 451-6. [http://dx.doi.org/10.1089/dia.2010.0204] [PMID: 21355717]

[96] Qiu Y, Gao Y, Zhang S, Guo L, Chen J, Xu B. Immunological effects of microneedle-mediated insulin

delivery: preliminary rat studies. Int J Pharm 2013; 444(1-2): 103-5.
[http://dx.doi.org/10.1016/j.ijpharm.2013.01.020] [PMID: 23340326]

[97] Cosman F, Lane NE, Bolognese MA, *et al.* Effect of transdermal teriparatide administration on bone mineral density in postmenopausal women. J Clin Endocrinol Metab 2010; 95(1): 151-8.
[http://dx.doi.org/10.1210/jc.2009-0358] [PMID: 19858319]

[98] Peters EE, Ameri M, Wang X, Maa YF, Daddona PE. Erythropoietin-coated ZP-microneedle transdermal system: preclinical formulation, stability, and delivery. Pharm Res 2012; 29(6): 1618-26.
[http://dx.doi.org/10.1007/s11095-012-0674-z] [PMID: 22258935]

[99] Zhang Y, Brown K, Siebenaler K, Determan A, Dohmeier D, Hansen K. Development of lidocaine-coated microneedle product for rapid, safe, and prolonged local analgesic action. Pharm Res 2012; 29(1): 170-7.
[http://dx.doi.org/10.1007/s11095-011-0524-4] [PMID: 21735335]

[100] Gupta J, Denson DD, Felner EI, Prausnitz MR. Rapid local anesthesia in humans using minimally invasive microneedles. Clin J Pain 2012; 28(2): 129-35.
[http://dx.doi.org/10.1097/AJP.0b013e318225dbe9] [PMID: 21712713]

[101] Li X, Zhao R, Qin Z, *et al.* Microneedle pretreatment improves efficacy of cutaneous topical anesthesia. Am J Emerg Med 2010; 28(2): 130-4.
[http://dx.doi.org/10.1016/j.ajem.2008.10.001] [PMID: 20159380]

[102] Aust MC, Fernandes D, Kolokythas P, Kaplan HM, Vogt PM. Percutaneous collagen induction therapy: an alternative treatment for scars, wrinkles, and skin laxity. Plast Reconstr Surg 2008; 121(4): 1421-9.
[http://dx.doi.org/10.1097/01.prs.0000304612.72899.02] [PMID: 18349665]

[103] Clementoni MT, B-Roscher M, Munavalli GS. Photodynamic photorejuvenation of the face with a combination of microneedling, red light, and broadband pulsed light. Lasers Surg Med 2010; 42(2): 150-9.
[http://dx.doi.org/10.1002/lsm.20905] [PMID: 20166166]

[104] Majid I. Microneedling therapy in atrophic facial scars: an objective assessment. J Cutan Aesthet Surg 2009; 2(1): 26-30.
[http://dx.doi.org/10.4103/0974-2077.53096] [PMID: 20300368]

[105] Arora S, Bhandaree Gupta P. Automated microneedling device – a new tool in dermatologist's kit. J Pak Assoc Dermatol 2012; 22(4): 354-7.

[106] Kim JH, Park HY, Jung M, Choi EH. Automicroneedle therapy system combined with topical tretinoin shows better regenerative effects compared with each individual treatment. Clin Exp Dermatol 2013; 38(1): 57-65.
[http://dx.doi.org/10.1111/j.1365-2230.2012.04405.x] [PMID: 23252753]

[107] Reed ML, Wu C, Kneller J, *et al.* Micromechanical devices for intravascular drug delivery. J Pharm Sci 1998; 87(11): 1387-94.
[http://dx.doi.org/10.1021/js980085q] [PMID: 9811495]

[108] Smart WH, Subramanian K. The use of silicon microfabrication technology in painless blood glucose monitoring. Diabetes Technol Ther 2000; 2(4): 549-59.

[http://dx.doi.org/10.1089/15209150050501961] [PMID: 11469618]

[109] Mukerjee EV, Collins SD, Isseroff RR, Smith RL. Microneedle array for transdermal biological fluid extraction and *in situ* analysis. Sens Actuators A Phys 2004; 114: 267-75. [http://dx.doi.org/10.1016/j.sna.2003.11.008]

[110] Gittard SD, Miller PR, Boehm RD, *et al.* Multiphoton microscopy of transdermal quantum dot delivery using two photon polymerization-fabricated polymer microneedles. Faraday Discuss 2011; 149: 171-85. [http://dx.doi.org/10.1039/C005374K] [PMID: 21413181]

[111] Romani N, Thurnher M, Idoyaga J, Steinman RM, Flacher V. Targeting of antigens to skin dendritic cells: possibilities to enhance vaccine efficacy. Immunol Cell Biol 2010; 88(4): 424-30. [http://dx.doi.org/10.1038/icb.2010.39] [PMID: 20368713]

[112] Weldon WC, Zarnitsyn VG, Esser ES, *et al.* Effect of adjuvants on responses to skin immunization by microneedles coated with influenza subunit vaccine. PLoS One 2012; 7(7): e41501. [http://dx.doi.org/10.1371/journal.pone.0041501] [PMID: 22848514]

[113] Koutsonanos DG, Vassilieva EV, Stavropoulou A, *et al.* Delivery of subunit influenza vaccine to skin with microneedles improves immunogenicity and long-lived protection. Sci Rep 2012; 2: 357. [http://dx.doi.org/10.1038/srep00357] [PMID: 22500210]

[114] Choi HJ, Bondy BJ, Yoo DG, Compans RW, Kang SM, Prausnitz MR. Stability of whole inactivated influenza virus vaccine during coating onto metal microneedles. J Control Release 2013; 166(2): 159-71. [http://dx.doi.org/10.1016/j.jconrel.2012.12.002] [PMID: 23246470]

[115] Choi HJ, Yoo DG, Bondy BJ, *et al.* Stability of influenza vaccine coated onto microneedles. Biomaterials 2012; 33(14): 3756-69. [http://dx.doi.org/10.1016/j.biomaterials.2012.01.054] [PMID: 22361098]

[116] Kim YC, Quan FS, Compans RW, Kang SM, Prausnitz MR. Stability kinetics of influenza vaccine coated onto microneedles during drying and storage. Pharm Res 2011; 28(1): 135-44. [http://dx.doi.org/10.1007/s11095-010-0134-6] [PMID: 20387097]

[117] Kim YC, Yoo DG, Compans RW, Kang SM, Prausnitz MR. Cross-protection by co-immunization with influenza hemagglutinin DNA and inactivated virus vaccine using coated microneedles. J Control Release 2013; 172(2): 579-88. [http://dx.doi.org/10.1016/j.jconrel.2013.04.016] [PMID: 23643528]

[118] Kommareddy S, Baudner BC, Bonificio A, *et al.* Influenza subunit vaccine coated microneedle patches elicit comparable immune responses to intramuscular injection in guinea pigs. Vaccine 2013; 31(34): 3435-41. [http://dx.doi.org/10.1016/j.vaccine.2013.01.050] [PMID: 23398932]

[119] Kommareddy S, Baudner BC, Oh S, Kwon SY, Singh M, O'Hagan DT. Dissolvable microneedle patches for the delivery of cell-culture-derived influenza vaccine antigens. J Pharm Sci 2012; 101(3): 1021-7. [http://dx.doi.org/10.1002/jps.23019] [PMID: 22190403]

[120] Koutsonanos DG, Compans RW, Skountzou I. Targeting the skin for microneedle delivery of

influenza vaccine. Adv Exp Med Biol 2013; 785: 121-32.
[http://dx.doi.org/10.1007/978-1-4614-6217-0_13] [PMID: 23456844]

[121] Leroux RI, Weber F. Intanza (®) 9 µg intradermal seasonal influenza vaccine for adults 18 to 59 years of age. Hum Vaccin Immunother 2014; 10: 1427-30.

[122] Martin MP, Weldon WC, Zarnitsyn VG, *et al.* Local Response to Microneedle-Based Influenza Immunization in the Skin. MBio 2012; 3.

[123] Matsuo K, Hirobe S, Yokota Y, *et al.* Transcutaneous immunization using a dissolving microneedle array protects against tetanus, diphtheria, malaria, and influenza. J Control Release 2012; 160(3): 495-501.
[http://dx.doi.org/10.1016/j.jconrel.2012.04.001] [PMID: 22516091]

[124] Matsuo K. Hirobe, Yokota Y, Ayabe Y, Seto M, Quan YS. Transcutaneous immunization using a dissolving microneedle array protects against tetanus, diphtheria, malaria, and influenza. J Control Release 2014; 184: 18-9. [Erratum to document cited in CA158:456292].
[http://dx.doi.org/10.1016/j.jconrel.2014.04.001]

[125] Weldon WC, Martin MP, Zarnitsyn V, *et al.* Microneedle vaccination with stabilized recombinant influenza virus hemagglutinin induces improved protective immunity. Clin Vaccine Immunol 2011; 18(4): 647-54.
[http://dx.doi.org/10.1128/CVI.00435-10] [PMID: 21288996]

[126] Zhu Q, Zarnitsyn VG, Ye L, *et al.* Immunization by vaccine-coated microneedle arrays protects against lethal influenza virus challenge. Proc Natl Acad Sci USA 2009; 106(19): 7968-73.
[http://dx.doi.org/10.1073/pnas.0812652106] [PMID: 19416832]

[127] Moon S, Wang Y, Edens C, Gentsch JR, Prausnitz MR, Jiang B. Dose sparing and enhanced immunogenicity of inactivated rotavirus vaccine administered by skin vaccination using a microneedle patch. Vaccine 2013; 31(34): 3396-402.
[http://dx.doi.org/10.1016/j.vaccine.2012.11.027] [PMID: 23174199]

[128] Pattani A, McKay PF, Garland MJ, *et al.* Microneedle mediated intradermal delivery of adjuvanted recombinant HIV-1 CN54gp140 effectively primes mucosal boost inoculations. J Control Release 2012; 162(3): 529-37.
[http://dx.doi.org/10.1016/j.jconrel.2012.07.039] [PMID: 22960496]

[129] Prow TW, Chen X, Prow NA, *et al.* Nanopatch-targeted skin vaccination against West Nile Virus and Chikungunya virus in mice. Small 2010; 6(16): 1776-84.
[http://dx.doi.org/10.1002/smll.201000331] [PMID: 20665754]

[130] Laurent PE, Bourhy H, Fantino M, Alchas P, Mikszta JA. Safety and efficacy of novel dermal and epidermal microneedle delivery systems for rabies vaccination in healthy adults. Vaccine 2010; 28(36): 5850-6.
[http://dx.doi.org/10.1016/j.vaccine.2010.06.062] [PMID: 20600481]

[131] Quan FS, Kim YC, Compans RW, Prausnitz MR, Kang SM. Dose sparing enabled by skin immunization with influenza virus-like particle vaccine using microneedles. J Control Release 2010; 147(3): 326-32.
[http://dx.doi.org/10.1016/j.jconrel.2010.07.125] [PMID: 20692307]

[132] Pearton M, Pirri D, Kang SM, Compans RW, Birchall JC. Host responses in human skin after conventional intradermal injection or microneedle administration of virus-like-particle influenza vaccine. Adv Healthc Mater 2013; 2(10): 1401-10.
[http://dx.doi.org/10.1002/adhm.201300006] [PMID: 23564440]

[133] Song JM, Kim YC, Barlow PG, *et al.* Improved protection against avian influenza H5N1 virus by a single vaccination with virus-like particles in skin using microneedles. Antiviral Res 2010; 88(2): 244-7.
[http://dx.doi.org/10.1016/j.antiviral.2010.09.001] [PMID: 20851715]

[134] Pearton M, Kang SM, Song JM, *et al.* Influenza virus-like particles coated onto microneedles can elicit stimulatory effects on Langerhans cells in human skin. Vaccine 2010; 28(37): 6104-13.
[http://dx.doi.org/10.1016/j.vaccine.2010.05.055] [PMID: 20685601]

[135] Kim YC, Quan FS, Compans RW, Kang SM, Prausnitz MR. Formulation of microneedles coated with influenza virus-like particle vaccine. AAPS PharmSciTech 2010; 11(3): 1193-201.
[http://dx.doi.org/10.1208/s12249-010-9471-3] [PMID: 20676947]

[136] Song JM, Kim YC, Lipatov AS, *et al.* Microneedle delivery of H5N1 influenza virus-like particles to the skin induces long-lasting B- and T-cell responses in mice. Clin Vaccine Immunol 2010; 17(9): 1381-9.
[http://dx.doi.org/10.1128/CVI.00100-10] [PMID: 20631330]

[137] Quan FS, Kim YC, Vunnava A, *et al.* Intradermal vaccination with influenza virus-like particles by using microneedles induces protection superior to that with intramuscular immunization. J Virol 2010; 84(15): 7760-9.
[http://dx.doi.org/10.1128/JVI.01849-09] [PMID: 20484519]

[138] Corbett HJ, Fernando GJ, Chen X, Frazer IH, Kendall MA. Skin vaccination against cervical cancer associated human papillomavirus with a novel micro-projection array in a mouse model. PLoS One 2010; 5(10): e13460.
[http://dx.doi.org/10.1371/journal.pone.0013460] [PMID: 20976136]

[139] Matsuo K, Yokota Y, Zhai Y, *et al.* A low-invasive and effective transcutaneous immunization system using a novel dissolving microneedle array for soluble and particulate antigens. J Control Release 2012; 161(1): 10-7.
[http://dx.doi.org/10.1016/j.jconrel.2012.01.033] [PMID: 22306332]

[140] Bachy V, Hervouet C, Becker PD, *et al.* Langerin negative dendritic cells promote potent CD8+ T-cell priming by skin delivery of live adenovirus vaccine microneedle arrays. Proc Natl Acad Sci USA 2013; 110(8): 3041-6.
[http://dx.doi.org/10.1073/pnas.1214449110] [PMID: 23386724]

[141] Vrdoljak A, McGrath MG, Carey JB, *et al.* Coated microneedle arrays for transcutaneous delivery of live virus vaccines. J Control Release 2012; 159(1): 34-42.
[http://dx.doi.org/10.1016/j.jconrel.2011.12.026] [PMID: 22245683]

[142] Carey JB, Pearson FE, Vrdoljak A, *et al.* Microneedle array design determines the induction of protective memory CD8+ T cell responses induced by a recombinant live malaria vaccine in mice. PLoS One 2011; 6(7): e22442.
[http://dx.doi.org/10.1371/journal.pone.0022442] [PMID: 21799855]

[143] Edens C, Collins ML, Ayers J, Rota PA, Prausnitz MR. Measles vaccination using a microneedle patch. Vaccine 2013; 31(34): 3403-9. [http://dx.doi.org/10.1016/j.vaccine.2012.09.062] [PMID: 23044406]

[144] Hiraishi Y, Nandakumar S, Choi SO, *et al.* Bacillus Calmette-Guérin vaccination using a microneedle patch. Vaccine 2011; 29(14): 2626-36. [http://dx.doi.org/10.1016/j.vaccine.2011.01.042] [PMID: 21277407]

[145] Ding Z, Verbaan FJ, Bivas-Benita M, *et al.* Microneedle arrays for the transcutaneous immunization of diphtheria and influenza in BALB/c mice. J Control Release 2009; 136(1): 71-8. [http://dx.doi.org/10.1016/j.jconrel.2009.01.025] [PMID: 19331846]

[146] Bal SM, Ding Z, Kersten GF, Jiskoot W, Bouwstra JA. Microneedle-based transcutaneous immunisation in mice with N-trimethyl chitosan adjuvanted diphtheria toxoid formulations. Pharm Res 2010; 27(9): 1837-47. [http://dx.doi.org/10.1007/s11095-010-0182-y] [PMID: 20559701]

[147] Ding Z, Bal SM, Romeijn S, Kersten GF, Jiskoot W, Bouwstra JA. Transcutaneous immunization studies in mice using diphtheria toxoid-loaded vesicle formulations and a microneedle array. Pharm Res 2011; 28(1): 145-58. [http://dx.doi.org/10.1007/s11095-010-0093-y] [PMID: 20237826]

[148] Ding Z, Van Riet E, Romeijn S, Kersten GF, Jiskoot W, Bouwstra JA. Immune modulation by adjuvants combined with diphtheria toxoid administered topically in BALB/c mice after microneedle array pretreatment. Pharm Res 2009; 26(7): 1635-43. [http://dx.doi.org/10.1007/s11095-009-9874-6] [PMID: 19326190]

[149] Morefield GL, Tammariello RF, Purcell BK, *et al.* An alternative approach to combination vaccines: intradermal administration of isolated components for control of anthrax, botulism, plague and staphylococcal toxic shock. J Immune Based Ther Vaccines 2008; 6: 5. [http://dx.doi.org/10.1186/1476-8518-6-5] [PMID: 18768085]

[150] Huang J, D'Souza AJ, Alarcon JB, *et al.* Protective immunity in mice achieved with dry powder formulation and alternative delivery of plague F1-V vaccine. Clin Vaccine Immunol 2009; 16(5): 719-25. [http://dx.doi.org/10.1128/CVI.00447-08] [PMID: 19261773]

[151] Mikszta JA, Dekker JP III, Harvey NG, *et al.* Microneedle-based intradermal delivery of the anthrax recombinant protective antigen vaccine. Infect Immun 2006; 74(12): 6806-10. [http://dx.doi.org/10.1128/IAI.01210-06] [PMID: 17030580]

[152] Yin D, Liang W, Xing S, *et al.* Hepatitis B DNA vaccine-polycation nano-complexes enhancing immune response by percutaneous administration with microneedle. Biol Pharm Bull 2013; 36(8): 1283-91. [http://dx.doi.org/10.1248/bpb.b13-00050] [PMID: 23676787]

[153] Gill HS, Söderholm J, Prausnitz MR, Sällberg M. Cutaneous vaccination using microneedles coated with hepatitis C DNA vaccine. Gene Ther 2010; 17(6): 811-4. [http://dx.doi.org/10.1038/gt.2010.22] [PMID: 20200562]

[154] Song JM, Kim YC, O E, Compans RW, Prausnitz MR, Kang SM. DNA vaccination in the skin using

microneedles improves protection against influenza. Mol Ther 2012; 20(7): 1472-80. [http://dx.doi.org/10.1038/mt.2012.69] [PMID: 22508490]

[155] Kim YC, Song JM, Lipatov AS, *et al.* Increased immunogenicity of avian influenza DNA vaccine delivered to the skin using a microneedle patch. Eur J Pharm Biopharm 2012; 81(2): 239-47. [http://dx.doi.org/10.1016/j.ejpb.2012.03.010] [PMID: 22504442]

[156] Hooper JW, Golden JW, Ferro AM, King AD. Smallpox DNA vaccine delivered by novel skin electroporation device protects mice against intranasal poxvirus challenge. Vaccine 2007; 25(10): 1814-23. [http://dx.doi.org/10.1016/j.vaccine.2006.11.017] [PMID: 17240007]

[157] Chen X, Kask AS, Crichton ML, *et al.* Improved DNA vaccination by skin-targeted delivery using dry-coated densely-packed microprojection arrays. J Control Release 2010; 148(3): 327-33. [http://dx.doi.org/10.1016/j.jconrel.2010.09.001] [PMID: 20850487]

[158] Kask AS, Chen X, Marshak JO, *et al.* DNA vaccine delivery by densely-packed and short microprojection arrays to skin protects against vaginal HSV-2 challenge. Vaccine 2010; 28(47): 7483-91. [http://dx.doi.org/10.1016/j.vaccine.2010.09.014] [PMID: 20851091]

[159] Kim YC, Quan FS, Yoo DG, Compans RW, Kang SM, Prausnitz MR. Improved influenza vaccination in the skin using vaccine coated microneedles. Vaccine 2009; 27(49): 6932-8. [http://dx.doi.org/10.1016/j.vaccine.2009.08.108] [PMID: 19761836]

[160] Quan FS, Kim YC, Yoo DG, Compans RW, Prausnitz MR, Kang SM. Stabilization of influenza vaccine enhances protection by microneedle delivery in the mouse skin. PLoS One 2009; 4(9): e7152. [http://dx.doi.org/10.1371/journal.pone.0007152] [PMID: 19779615]

[161] Laurent PE, Bonnet S, Alchas P, *et al.* Evaluation of the clinical performance of a new intradermal vaccine administration technique and associated delivery system. Vaccine 2007; 25(52): 8833-42. [http://dx.doi.org/10.1016/j.vaccine.2007.10.020] [PMID: 18023942]

[162] Atmar RL, Patel SM, Keitel WA. Intanza(®): a new intradermal vaccine for seasonal influenza. Expert Rev Vaccines 2010; 9(12): 1399-409. [http://dx.doi.org/10.1586/erv.10.134] [PMID: 21105776]

[163] Ansaldi F, de Florentiis D, Durando P, Icardi G. Fluzone(®) Intradermal vaccine: a promising new chance to increase the acceptability of influenza vaccination in adults. Expert Rev Vaccines 2012; 11(1): 17-25. [http://dx.doi.org/10.1586/erv.11.154] [PMID: 22149703]

[164] Quan FS, Vunnava A, Compans RW, Kang SM. Virus-like particle vaccine protects against 2009 H1N1 pandemic influenza virus in mice. PLoS One 2010; 5(2): e9161. [http://dx.doi.org/10.1371/journal.pone.0009161] [PMID: 20161790]

[165] Kumar A, Wonganan P, Sandoval MA, Li X, Zhu S, Cui Z. Microneedle-mediated transcutaneous immunization with plasmid DNA coated on cationic PLGA nanoparticles. J Control Release 2012; 163(2): 230-9. [http://dx.doi.org/10.1016/j.jconrel.2012.08.011] [PMID: 22921518]

[166] DeMuth PC, Min Y, Huang B, *et al.* Polymer multilayer tattooing for enhanced DNA vaccination. Nat

Mater 2013; 12(4): 367-76.
[http://dx.doi.org/10.1038/nmat3550] [PMID: 23353628]

[167] Leroux-Roels I, Vets E, Freese R, *et al.* Seasonal influenza vaccine delivered by intradermal microinjection: A randomised controlled safety and immunogenicity trial in adults. Vaccine 2008; 26(51): 6614-9.
[http://dx.doi.org/10.1016/j.vaccine.2008.09.078] [PMID: 18930093]

[168] Levin Y, Kochba E, Kenney R. Clinical evaluation of a novel microneedle device for intradermal delivery of an influenza vaccine: are all delivery methods the same? Vaccine 2014; 32(34): 4249-52.
[http://dx.doi.org/10.1016/j.vaccine.2014.03.024] [PMID: 24930715]

[169] Kolli CS, Xiao J, Parsons DL, Babu RJ. Microneedle assisted iontophoretic transdermal delivery of prochlorperazine edisylate. Drug Dev Ind Pharm 2012; 38(5): 571-6.
[http://dx.doi.org/10.3109/03639045.2011.617753] [PMID: 21980925]

[170] Lanke SS, Kolli CS, Strom JG, Banga AK. Enhanced transdermal delivery of low molecular weight heparin by barrier perturbation. Int J Pharm 2009; 365(1-2): 26-33.
[http://dx.doi.org/10.1016/j.ijpharm.2008.08.028] [PMID: 18801420]

[171] Escobar-Chávez JJ, Bonilla-Martínez D, Villegas-González MA, Rodríguez-Cruz IM, Domínguez-Delgado CL. The use of sonophoresis in the administration of drugs throughout the skin. J Pharm Pharm Sci 2009; 12(1): 88-115.
[http://dx.doi.org/10.18433/J3C30D] [PMID: 19470295]

[172] Polat BE, Hart D, Langer R, Blankschtein D. Ultrasound-mediated transdermal drug delivery: mechanisms, scope, and emerging trends. J Control Release 2011; 152(3): 330-48.
[http://dx.doi.org/10.1016/j.jconrel.2011.01.006] [PMID: 21238514]

[173] Chen B, Wei J, Iliescu C. Sonophoretic enhanced microneedles array (SEMA) – improving the efficiency of transdermal drug delivery. Sens Actuators B Chem 2010; 145: 54-60.
[http://dx.doi.org/10.1016/j.snb.2009.11.013]

[174] Han T, Das DB. Permeability enhancement for transdermal delivery of large molecule using low-frequency sonophoresis combined with microneedles. J Pharm Sci 2013; 102(10): 3614-22.
[http://dx.doi.org/10.1002/jps.23662] [PMID: 23873449]

[175] Daugimont L, Baron N, Vandermeulen G, *et al.* Hollow microneedle arrays for intradermal drug delivery and DNA electroporation. J Membr Biol 2010; 236(1): 117-25.
[http://dx.doi.org/10.1007/s00232-010-9283-0] [PMID: 20652559]

[176] Yan K, Todo H, Sugibayashi K. Transdermal drug delivery by in-skin electroporation using a microneedle array. Int J Pharm 2010; 397(1-2): 77-83.
[http://dx.doi.org/10.1016/j.ijpharm.2010.06.052] [PMID: 20619329]

[177] Choi SO, Kim YC, Park JH, *et al.* An electrically active microneedle array for electroporation. Biomed Microdevices 2010; 12(2): 263-73.
[http://dx.doi.org/10.1007/s10544-009-9381-x] [PMID: 20012696]

[178] Choi SO, Kim YC, Lee JW, Park JH, Prausnitz MR, Allen MG. Intracellular protein delivery and gene transfection by electroporation using a microneedle electrode array. Small 2012; 8(7): 1081-91.
[http://dx.doi.org/10.1002/smll.201101747] [PMID: 22328093]

[179] Frenck RW Jr, Belshe R, Brady RC, *et al.* Comparison of the immunogenicity and safety of a split-virion, inactivated, trivalent influenza vaccine (Fluzone®) administered by intradermal and intramuscular route in healthy adults. Vaccine 2011; 29(34): 5666-74. [http://dx.doi.org/10.1016/j.vaccine.2011.06.010] [PMID: 21699951]

[180] Ameri M, Wang X, Maa YF. Effect of irradiation on parathyroid hormone PTH(1-34) coated on a novel transdermal microprojection delivery system to produce a sterile product--adhesive compatibility. J Pharm Sci 2010; 99(4): 2123-34. [http://dx.doi.org/10.1002/jps.21985] [PMID: 19894273]

CHAPTER 7

Nanocarrier Systems with the Use of Physical Enhancers

Roberto Diaz-Torres[1,*], **Isabel Marlen Rodríguez-Cruz**[2,3], **Elizabeth García-García**[4], **Clara Luisa Domínguez-Delgado**[5] and **Patricia Ramirez-Noguera**[1]

[1] *Unidad de Investigación Multidisciplinaria, Facultad de Estudios Superiores Cuautitlán, Universidad Nacional Autónoma de México, Estado de México, México*

[2] *Hospital Regional de Alta Especialidad Zumpango. Unidad de Enseñanza e Investigación. Carretera Zumpango-Jilotzingo #400. Barrio de Santiago 2da Sección. Zumpango, Estado de México. C.P. 55600, México*

[3] *Laboratorio de Investigación en Citogenética Básica del CBT Dr. Alfonso León de Garay. Calle Fresnos S/N, San Mateo, Tequixquiac, Estado de México C.P.55657, México*

[4] *Psicofarma S.A. de C.V., Calz. de Tlalpan 4369, Col. Toriello Guerra, Distrito Federal. C.P. 14050, México*

[5] *Unidad de Investigación Multidisciplinaria. Laboratorio 12: "Sistemas Transdérmicos y Nanomateriales". Facultad de Estudios Superiores Cuautitlán-Universidad Nacional Autónoma de México. Km 2.5 Carretera Cuautitlán–Teoloyucan, San Sebastián Xhala, Cuautitlán Izcalli, Estado de México, CP. 54714, México*

Abstract: At present, nanotechnology has acquired great importance. One of the fields where nanotechnology has been used with great success is medicine. This has allowed the emergence of a branch of nanotechnology called nanomedicine. Nanomedicine has been used by all known routes of administration (oral, intravenous, transdermal, *etc.*). Topical/transdermal route is one of the most used routes to administer formulated drugs in nanocarrier systems (nanoparticles, liposomes, dendrimer, transfersomes, nanoemulsion, *etc.*) in combination with the use of physical enhancers (microneedles, iontophoresis, sonophoresis, *etc.*). This route has great potential to deliver drugs, but the stratum corneum, which is the most external layer of the skin, confers properties of permeability to this organ.

* **Corresponding author Roberto Diaz-Torres:** Unidad de Investigación Multidisciplinaria, Facultad de Estudios Superiores Cuautitlán, Universidad Nacional Autónoma de México, Estado de México, México; Tel/Fax: +52 55 56231939; E-mail: diaztorres_r@hotmail.com

José Juan Escobar-Chávez (Ed.)

In order to modify the skin barrier properties and use the skin as a route to administer drugs into the body, some interesting strategies have been developed in last decades, such as the use of chemical and physical enhancers and even the combination of these enhancers with nanocarrier systems. For this reason, this chapter mainly emphasizes the applications of the 3 main physical enhancers (ultrasound, iontophoresis and microneedles) with nanocarriers for administering drugs by topical/transdermal routes, where they have been more widely used.

Keywords: Nanocarriers, Physical enhancers, Transdermal drug delivery.

1. INTRODUCTION

At the present time, nanotechnology has tremendously influenced all fields where it has been used. In the field of medicine has revolutionized many of the concepts existing up to date; for that reason, the emergence of a new hybrid concept between nanotechnology and medicine, is known as nanomedicine [1]. This new branch of medicine has changed the concept we had of treatment and diagnosis of diseases [2]. On this scale of nanometers, it is possible to treat a disease at the level of cellular organelles and adequately, control its progression. The drug path at the nanoscale is carried out by a modern version of a vehicle that protects the drug from action of the immune system, changes of pH, and it is made for the desired site of action. These so-called nanoscale vehicles are known as nanocarriers (Fig. **1**).

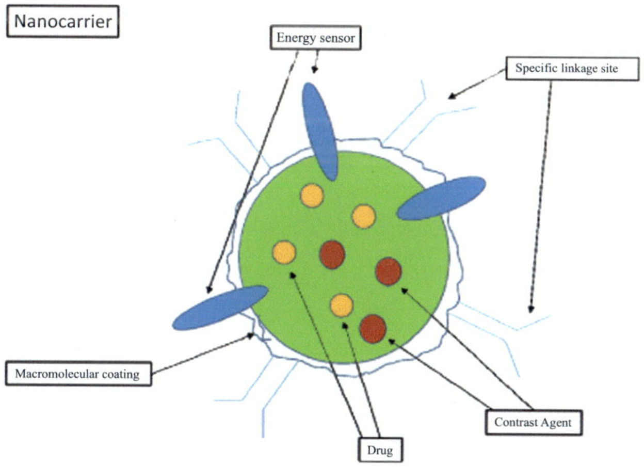

Fig. (1). Schematic representation of an ideal nanocarrier.

2. DEFINITION AND GENERALITIES OF NANOCARRIER SYSTEMS

Nanocarriers are colloidal drug delivery system in the neighborhood of 1 to 1000 nm. These systems are very tiny and they are compared to some body structures [3]. Nanocarriers are nanosized particles and they are made of different macromolecules to be able to be administered by different routes. Nanocarriers can be administered *via* different the routes. The size of nanocarriers, let them be undetectable for the immune system; for that reason, they are the perfect tool to fight again a lot of illnesses and carry the drug directly in the target organ. This fact, helps to avoid side effects and increases the effectiveness of the drug [4 - 8].

The nanocarriers have become an interesting option to deliver drugs, gene therapy [9], for increasing the bioavailability of poorly soluble drugs [10] with low permeability or for percutaneous administration. Chemicals that were unlikely to be administered, now with nanocarriers may be used in therapeutic applications [11]. There are drugs that were not feasible to use as therapeutic agents due to their low bioavailability, and by the need of high concentrations to exert a pharmacological effect with the possibility of leading to toxic levels. But now by mean of nanocarriers their application is possible.

The nanocarriers can be made with a lot of substances, for example, polysaccharides [12], natural or synthetic polymers [13], lipids [14], proteins [15], amino acids [16] and inorganic compounds (Fig. **2**). The use of different materials for nanocarriers makes these systems to have great physicochemical, pharmacological and toxicological properties. This variety of materials permits that nanocarriers can be loaded with a wide range of drugs with different physicochemical and pharmacological characteristics.

These nanostructures can be made to be very specific for the intended purpose; for example, it can be placed on the surface of these systems folic acid [17], since it is known, that many of cancers have an over expression of folate receptors. This strategy helps nanocarriers to link to the site of action and they will be joined to these receptors, making them much more targeted release of the drug directly to the tumor.

Therapeutic dose concepts used in traditional pharmacology, will change drastically using nanocarriers with specific ligands, since the maximum drug concentration will be at the target organ and if you take a sample of peripheral blood probably you will not detect a measurable concentration of the drug.

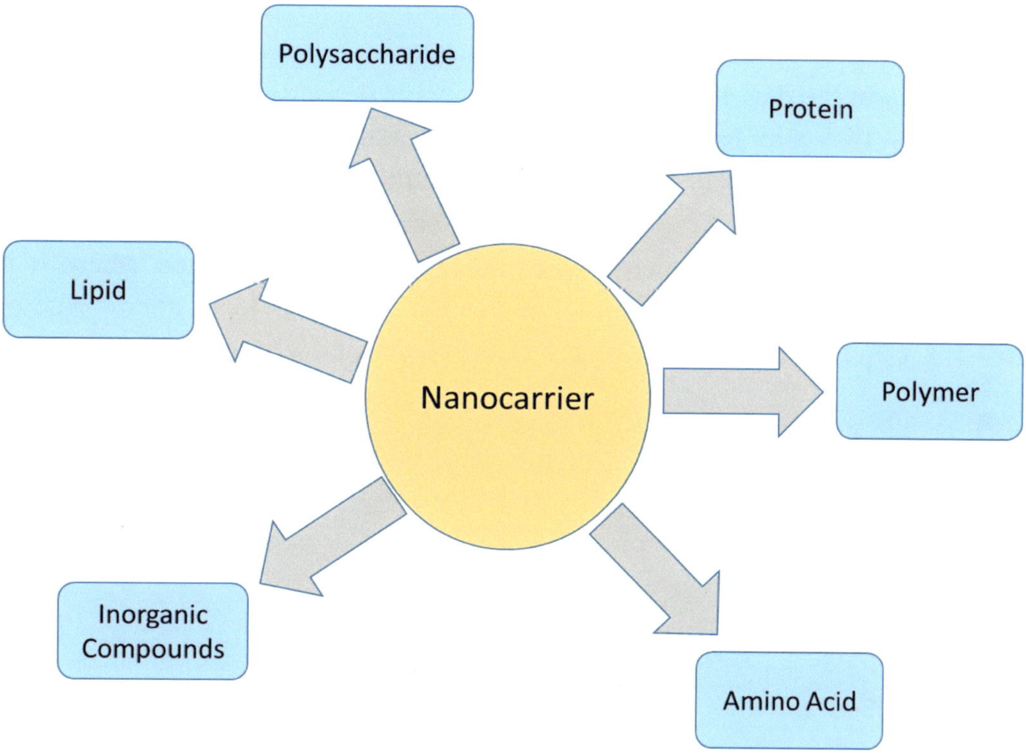

Fig. (2). Materials used to prepare nanocarriers.

The drug encapsulated into a nanocarrier system may be associated with this in different ways depending on the manufacturing process and the effect we want to give to this system. The drug may be encapsulated, entrapped, attached to the surface, conjugate or a combination of all these alternatives. The nanocarriers work like Trojans horses and are capable of carrying drugs through barriers very difficult to penetrate if the drugs were not in these vehicles [18]. Also, these nanoscale systems help some drugs pass membranes that do not have specific transporters for these drugs.

This ability to penetrate biological barriers, certain cell membranes and interacting with cell surface receptors are dependent on nanoscale architecture, which results in an accumulation in the target tissue, and regulates cellular uptake to prolong the residence time of active agents, this can increase the stability and reduce the toxicity especially compared with therapeutic agents of low molecular weight.

The next step in the development of nanocarriers is depending on the therapeutic requirements; they may have different properties and functions or a combination of them. These kind of nanocarriers are named multifunctional nanocarriers. If we think in a simple nanocarrier system, we consider some important properties [19]: a) long lasting into the bloodstream. b) Accumulation in the area where it is required. c) Sensitive to physical, biological or chemical local conditions. d) Allow for efficient intracellular delivery of drugs and also to individual cell organelles.

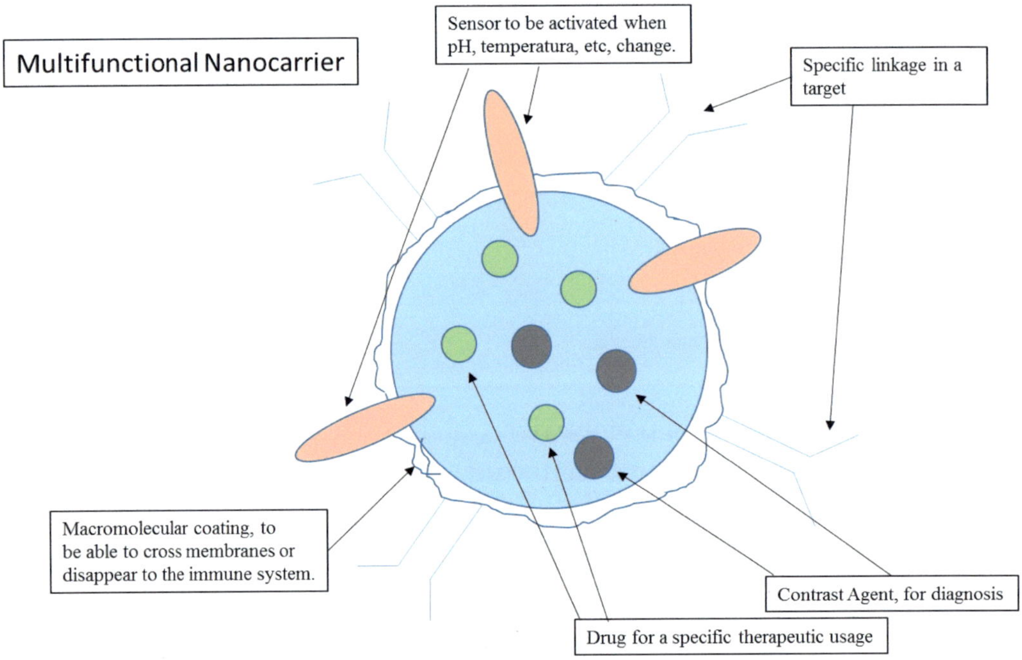

Fig. (3). Schematic representation of a pharmaceutical multifunctional nanocarrier.

Obviously, when preparing these pharmaceutical multifunctional nanocarriers, simultaneously they must be mounted on the surface and into the nanostructure to provide the required properties (Fig. **3**). There are many important reasons to make nanocarriers for long lasting into the bloodstream. For example, the maintenance of a drug into the blood between therapeutic levels for a long lasting interval [20].

The circulating nanoparticles containing drug or macromolecules remains into the bloodstream and tend to passively accumulate in pathological sites such as tumors, tissues with inflammation, *etc.* (enhanced permeability and retention, called EPR effect). After accumulation and when the nanocarrier is degraded, the drug is delivered; letting drug transporters interact more time with the target tissue [20].

Some strategies can be implemented to increase nanocarriers' longevity in bloodstream; for example, the addition of some polymers such as polyethylene glycol (PEG) to increase the hydrodynamic radius and the hydrophilicity, nanoparticles without PEG increased their accumulation in liver and spleen but these nanoparticles were excreted very fast; meanwhile, nanoparticles with PEG had increased longevity in bloodstream and decreased accumulation in organs [21]. This pegylation prevents the interaction of nanoparticles with opsonins and avoids the interaction with the reticuloendothelial system (RES); as an example, nanoparticles containing a sensitizer for photodynamic therapy of cancer were prepared with and without PEG on the surface. Those nanoparticles with PEG on the surface increased their accumulation into the tumors because those nanoparticles without PEG were captured by the RES avoiding the interaction with tumors [22].

There are nanocarriers made of block copolymers; for example, Polylactic-co-glycolic acid with Polyethylene glycol (PLGA-PEG) [23]. These nanocarriers have a solid core and they are covered with a water soluble shell.

Strategies of this type, as the use of hybrid nanocarriers coated with molecules to make them more hydrophobic or more versatile and the use of physical enhancers is a field which is being exploited significantly for drug administration.

The administration of drugs through the skin is a non-invasive path and it has certain advantages in comparison to other; this route avoids the first-pass metabolism, it has temporal delivery, *etc.* but as a disadvantage, this route is difficult for some drugs; above all, the highly hydrophilic compounds [24]. In order to increase the drug transport through membranes, one of the best approaches are the physical enhancers (ultrasound, electroporation, microneedles and iontophoresis) and those systems based on nanostructures (liposomes, niosomes, transfersomes, microemulsions, solid lipid nanoparticles, *etc.*) (Fig. **4**).

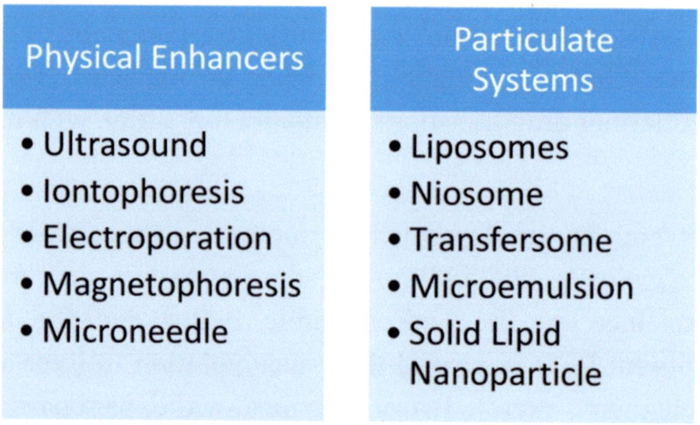

Fig. (4). Major approaches to enhance membrane delivery.

The transport of drugs through the skin is relatively low compared with transport in the membranes of the gastrointestinal tract or mucous membranes, the skin acts as a biological defense and prevents the entrance of any foreign material to the body. The low permeability of molecules through the stratum corneum is the limiting factor for the development of transdermal delivery of therapeutic agents.

Prodrugs have also been developed using the aforementioned permeation enhancers. Furthermore, the combination of physical and chemical techniques for enhancing permeation through the skin has been studied.

Using both permeability enhancers (chemical and physical), are a good strategy to increase transdermal permeability; however sometimes they may induce irritation, membrane damages and impairs the barrier function of the skin. It is recommendable to avoid using chemical permeation enhancers when we are trying to deliver a drug through a barrier, since the normal function of the barriers can be compromised. For that reason, and to avoid using chemical enhancers, nanoparticles loaded with drugs for transport through the skin have been developed.

The routes of drug administration across membranes are oral, transdermal, ocular, sublingual, *etc*. One of the most difficult membranes to penetrate is the stratum corneum. Colloids; for example, liposomes, lipid nanoparticles, nanoparticles made of polymers, micelles and inorganic nanoparticles has been used to enhance the transport of active molecules though the skin [25].

The advantages of using these types of colloidal carriers not only in percutaneous delivery but also in other different barriers are: 1. Protection of degradation of unstable therapeutic agents. 2. Controlled release of the active agent from the colloidal carrier.

The amount of combined therapies using nanocarriers and physical enhancers is gaining a very important relevance, since nanocarriers therapies sometimes are not enough to penetrate certain membranes and it is needed the usage of physical enhancers to help nanocarriers to transport drugs to the target organ or tissue.

The use of microneedles to create a path through some membranes to let nanocarriers go into the body; it is a very important therapeutic approach and also the use of an electric current to push nanocarriers through membranes, or the use of sound to help nanocarriers to deliver a pharmaceutical molecule.

All these approaches have been created to increase the nanocarriers' penetration into the body. The principle of all these systems is to create a perturbation in the membrane to let nanocarriers going deeper to increase the therapeutic effect. Sometimes, also the nanocarriers cannot transport drugs through some membranes and they need these physical enhancers to do their job.

During this work, the reader will be able to find information about the most common nanocarriers, after that, there is a brief description of physical enhancers and finally the combination of nanocarriers and physical enhancers with therapeutic applications is addressed.

3. CLASSIFICATION OF NANOCARRIERS

Every day, the number of nanocarriers increases a lot, above all in the last years. All these nanocarriers are designed with two main objectives; delivery through the time and delivery in a particular location. With all these alternatives in type of nanocarriers is difficult to decide which the better nanocarrier system is. All of them have advantages and disadvantages [26, 27].

One of the main advantages of nanoparticles is that they help drugs to be more soluble, but the behavior into the body can be very different, because the materials features may be very different too [26 - 29]. On the other hand, tailored nanoparticles can be made to reach very specific targets. This characteristic increases the effectiveness of the therapeutic system and decreases the side effects.

Physicochemical properties are very important since they are responsible of nanoparticle-biological structures interaction. The interaction of nanoparticles with biological systems depends mainly on shape, size and surface charge [26 - 29]. Nanoparticles can have solid or hollow core, when the core is solid we name them nanospheres and when the core is hollow we name them nanocapsules [14, 30]. Nanoparticles depending on the fabrication materials, they are made with a lot of processes. The process of fabrication depends on the physiochemical properties of the materials [14, 26, 27, 30]. In Table **1**, we can observe a general classification of nanocarrier systems.

Table 1. Types of nanocarriers systems.

Nanosystems	Definition	Size	Characteristics	Refs
Nanoparticles	Solid or hollow particles which have entrapped, binded or encapsulated drugs.	10-1000 nm	Nanoparticles can be composed of polymers, lipids, polysaccharides and proteins.	[31, 32]
Polymeric nanoparticles	Nanoparticles are submicron colloidal structures composed of synthetic or non-synthetic polymers.	10-1000 nm	Nanoparticles are composed by polymers.	[31, 32]

(Table 1) contd.....

Nanosystems	Definition	Size	Characteristics	Refs
Solid lipid nanoparticles	Solid lipid nanoparticles are made of lipids that are solid at room temperature.	50-100 nm	They are derived from physiologically compatible lipids such as fatty acids (*e.g.* stearic acid), fatty acid esters (*e.g.* glyceryl monostearate, glyceryl behenate), triglycerides (*e.g.* tristearin, trilaurin), steroids (*e.g.* cholesterol) and waxes (*e.g.* cetyl palmitate).	[5]
Inorganic nanoparticles	They are nanometric particles, made up of inorganic compounds such as silica, titania and alumina.	<50nm	Inorganic nanoparticles come in a wide variety of shapes and possess an array of physical properties that arise from the quantum properties of their core materials.	[33]
Quantum dots	Fluorescent semiconductor nanoparticles.	2-10nm	Made up of organic surfactants, precursors and solvents.	[34]
Lipid globules	Lipid globules.	1-100 nm	Multicomponent fluid made of water, a hydrophobic liquid, and one or several surfactants resulting in a stable system.	[5]
Microbubbles	They are gas bubbles coated with lipid, polymer, sugar or protein material.	1-10 μm	The coating reduces the surface tension, and corresponding capillary pressure which drives the gas into solution.	[35]
Lipospheres	Solid lipid core stabilized by a monolayer of phospholipids molecules embedded in their surface.	0.01-100 μm	The internal core contains the bioactive compound dissolved or dispersed in the solid fat matrix.	[36]
Aquasomes	Aquasomes are three-layered structures (*i.e.*, core, coating, and drug) that are self-assembled through no covalent bonds, ionic bonds, and van der Walls forces.	60-300 nm	The particle core is composed of non-crystalline calcium phosphate or ceramic diamond, and it is covered by a polyhydroxyl oligomeric film.	[37]
Pharmacosomes	Pure drug vesicles formed by amphiphilic drugs	<200 nm		[37]

(Table 1) contd.....

Nanosystems	Definition	Size	Characteristics	Refs
Nanoemulsions	Nanoemulsion are isotropic dispersed systems of two non-miscible liquids, normally consisting of an oily system dispersed in an aqueous system or an aqueous system dispersed in an oily system but forming droplets or other oily phases of nanometric sizes.	20-200 nm	They can be stable for long times due to the extremely small sizes and the use of adequate surfactants. Nanoemulsions can use hydrophobic and hydrophilic drugs.	[5]
Transfersomes (elastic liposomes)	Modified lipid-based soft, malleable carriers tailored for enhanced systemic delivery of drug.	100-200 nm	Noninvasive delivery of drugs into or across the deeper skin layers and/or the systemic circulation.	[5, 37]
Liposomes	Liposomes are vesicles composed of one or more concentric lipid bilayers, separated by water or aqueous buffer compartments.	25 nm- 100 μm	They are structures made of cholesterol and phospholipids.	[5, 37]
Ethosomes	Lipid-based soft, malleable vesicles containing a permeation enhancer and composed of phospholipids, ethanol, and water.	<400 nm	Ethosomes contain alcohol in the lipid bilayer to make them more flexible and be able to be deformed when pressure is applied.	[5, 37]
Niosomes	Niosomes are lamellar vesicles prepared from non-ionic surfactants.	10-3000 nm, according to lamellar vesicles.	The unique structures of niosomes make it capable of encapsulating both hydrophilic and lipophilic substances.	[38, 39]
Dendrimer	Dendrimers are highly branched symmetrical macromolecules of nanosized dimensions, have well-defined molecular mass and geometry consisting of a central core, repeating units and terminal functional groups.	Dendrimers are similar in size to a number of biological structures;~3–300 nm	The amount of branches increases exponentially and dendrimers growth is typically about 1 nm per generation. The dendrimers classification is based on the number of generations.	[40]

(Table 1) contd.....

Nanosystems	Definition	Size	Characteristics	Refs
Micelles	Micelles are nanoscopic aggregates of colloidal dimensions (*i.e.* association of colloids) formed reversibly from amphiphilic molecules. They have the ability to solubilize hydrophobic drugs and bring about site-specific delivery by passive and active targeting.	20–100 nm	Micelles are formed from surfactants or amphiphilic polymers above their critical micellar concentration (CMC) in colloidal dispersions.	[5]

The variety of nanocarriers used in the pharmaceutical sciences is very large. These systems fulfill the function of bringing the drug to its site of action in a controlled manner. The nanocarriers increase drug absorption, penetration, half-life, bioavailability, stability, *etc.*

The transport through membranes in the past was difficult because only few molecules could be administered with this objective; they will be small and lipophilic. Currently with the use of physical permeation enhancers and nanocarriers can be managed many more molecules; in this way, even large molecules and hydrophilic. Today, a wide variety of nanocarriers for transmembrane delivery are used The nanocarriers most commonly used in pharmaceutical sciences for transport across biological membranes are liposomes, nanoparticles, dendrimers and nanoemulsions. Some others nanocarriers are based on these four main nanocarriers mentioned above. For example, transformable liposomes, they are a kind of liposomes containing surface active ingredients in their membrane to let them decrease interfacial tension and enlarge/modify their structure [41]. Then, in the following paragraphs will briefly describe the different nanocarrier systems.

3.1. Liposomes

Liposomes are lipid structures formed by one or more bilayers (Fig. **5**). In the beginning of liposomes development, they only were made of phospholipids, but when times went by, they were decorated with different molecules to increase their specificity or to prolong their time in the bloodstream [36]. Due to liposomes are made of materials very similar to the biological systems, they are very useful to encapsulate drugs and protect them from the organism barriers, like immune system, pH, opsonins, *etc* [5, 9, 36]. Liposomes are pharmaceutical nanocarriers widely used for many applications. Recently many products based on liposomes have been approved for clinical use [42].

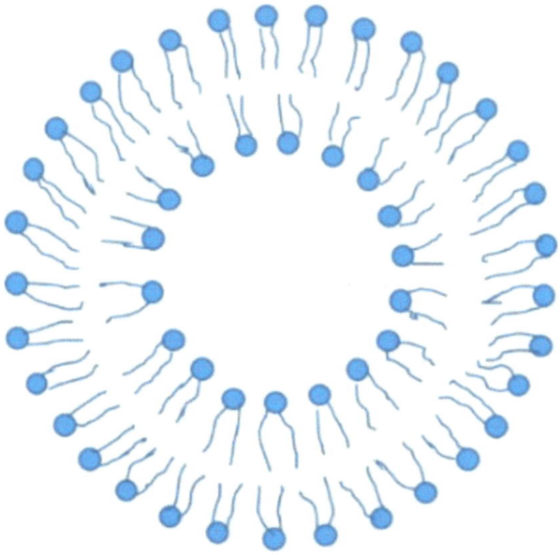

Fig. (5). Schematic representation of a liposome.

When liposomes began to be used, did not show satisfactory results *in vitro*, so they were not a good choice for new product development. Subsequently, although liposomes did not show good results *in vitro*, were shown to have very good stability and prolonged circulation time *in vivo*. The knowledge gained on the polymorphism of lipids, the physiological mechanisms of the provision of liposomes *in vivo* and lipid-drug and lipid-protein interactions changed the idea about liposomes. As a consequence of this knowledge, liposomes were obtained in a more stable manner, with a longer half-life and better biodistribution.

Liposomes have properties that make them unique, besides with the modifications that can be currently made to these systems, liposomes are one of the best drug delivery systems; for example, transporting anti-fungal drugs and in cancer treatment [43].

Liposomes can be made with negative [44], positive [45] or neutral charge [46], depending on their functional groups and the pH of the medium. This ability to modify the liposomes charge helps to have a better distribution, stability, interaction with membranes, *etc*. Neutral liposomes tend to form aggregates and due to their size they interact strongly with the cells of the reticuloendothelial system; it is recommended to add an amount of salt to reduce aggregation and stabilize the system due to proper lipid geometry packing. Negatively charged liposomes tend to have better physical stability and less aggregation due to repulsive forces. These liposomes penetrate the cells faster than neutral liposomes and they are well recognized by the receptors of certain cells including macrophages. The positively charged liposomes are used to transport DNA in gene therapy; they interact easily with serum proteins. Cationic liposomes interact with cells of the reticuloendothelial system and they are excreted through the lungs, liver and spleen. For this type of liposomes (cationic), it is used a hydrophilic polymer coating to avoid recognition by the reticuloendothelial system, and also coating decreases aggregation.

Liposomes are good carriers for drugs soluble or not soluble in water and its surface may be modified by conjugation to proteins, peptides, polymers and other molecules. Liposomes can be classified based on their size and number of layers as follows [47, 48]:

1. Small Unilamellar Vesicles (SUV) 25 to 100 nm
2. Medium-sized Unilamellar Vesicles (MUV) 100 to 500 nm
3. Large Unilamellar Vesicles (LUV) few hundred nanometers to several microns
4. Giant Unilamellar Vesicles (GUV) few hundred nanometers to several microns
5. Oligolamellar Vesicles (OLV) few hundred nanometers to several microns
6. Large Multilamellar Vesicles (LMV) few hundred nanometers to several microns
7. Multivesicular Vesicles (MVV) few hundred nanometers to several microns

Liposomes can have different performance both *in vitro* and *in vivo* depending on its size, type and position of the liposome lamellae. These differences may be important in the process of opsonization, availability, release profiles, half-life time, *etc*.

Liposomes can also be classified according to the components of the membrane:

1. Conventional: These liposomes are formed primarily from phospholipids. They are negatively or neutrally charged.
2. Stealth: These liposomes are covered with polymer to increase their blood circulation time.
3. Targeted: These liposomes have antibodies or antibody fragments on their surface.
4. Cationic: These are made of cationic surfactants to transport negatively charged DNA.

Liposomes were one of the first strategies for drug delivery through membranes. Features like size, formulation, the use of penetration enhancers and physical condition of the membrane affect the degree of penetration of the drug. Other factors that can affect are: lamellarity, lipid composition, surface charge of the liposomes, how liposomes are administered and the total lipid concentration.

Liposomes have been used for administration of analgesics through skin such as ketoprofen in combination with cyclodextrins to improve its permeability; this combination potentiated the permeation of ketoprofen through rat skin [49]. Another type of drugs have been incorporated in liposomal systems like lamivudine, which is an antiretroviral administered orally, but in this way has many side effects, including hepatotoxicity, hyperglycemia, *etc.* Therefore it sought an alternative way of administering the drug and it was found that transdermal pathway had very good results [50].

3.2. Lipospheres

These systems are in the neighborhood of 0.01 and 100 μm of diameter and they are composed of a liquid core made of lipids and surrounded by phospholipids. The active ingredient generally is located in the core. The advantages of lipospheres over other drug delivery systems are related to its better stability, their superior features like better encapsulation of lipophilic drugs, better controlled release and it is possible to obtain very good water dispersions. Additionally, they show very low toxicity [36]; and they can be administered through different routes; oral, parenteral and through the skin [5, 9, 36].

The use of lipospheres in transdermal delivery can be illustrated by the aceclofenac, which is preferably administered orally, but has some adverse effects by this route, which makes it a suitable candidate to be administered transdermally. In a work published in 2008, scientists treated a group of rats with paw edema with aceclofenac lipospheres and two topical presentations, lotion and paste; yielding, better analgesic effects with the formulation of lipospheres than with commercial presentations [51].

3.3. Dendrimers

Dendrimers are novel three dimensional systems (Fig. **6**); they are highly branched polymeric structures. They have sizes in the neighborhood of nanometers, very low polydispersity and they can be decorated with different molecules to increase their versatility as drug delivery systems [5, 52 - 54]. Dendrimers have been used in anticancer and antiviral therapies, also has spread their use as vaccines.

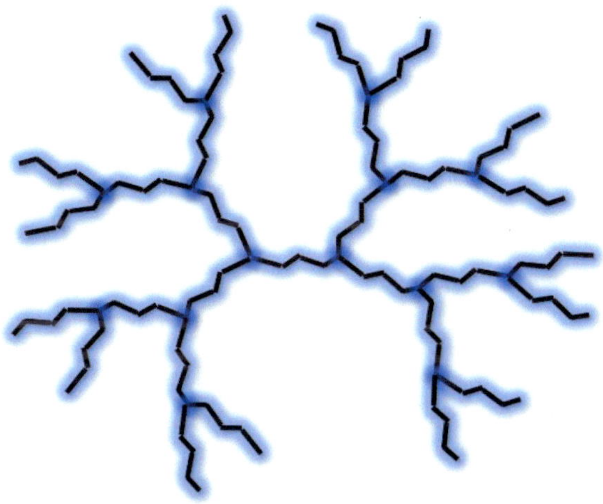

Fig. (6). Schematic representation of a dendrimer.

One of the first materials used for the manufacture of dendrimers were polyamine amides (PAMAM) [55]. Outside the pharmaceutical field, dendrimers have been used as catalysts, chemical sensors and crosslinking agents. In the context of controlled release of drugs, have been used in gene therapy and like contrast release agents.

Dendrimers classification is based on the number of generations. Once the center is created, the next chemical synthesis step to add the first monomer layer to create the first branch is called first generation; thereafter, each reaction step for adding a new monomer layer will be one more generation. Thus polymerization allows control of the homogeneity in molecular weight, size and architecture of dendrimers. However, when a critical branched state is reached dendrimers cannot grow because of lack of space. This phenomenon is called the 'starburst effect'. At this time, we can use the steric hindrance to saturate dendrimer core with various sized shell dendrimers to create a megamer resulting in precise novel nanostructure (quantized building block –generated from dendrimers-).

The fractal structure of dendrimers confers very good solubility compared with other non- polymeric structure fractals. This feature helps the dendrimers to be easily characterized and purified. Dendrimers have a low intrinsic viscosity compared to linear polymers. Also, due to their branched structure have the peculiarity of having loci tailored for a specific molecular recognition and encapsulation of molecules. As previously mentioned, the characteristic structure of dendrimers increases the solubility of the molecules encapsulated within them; moreover, the toxicity of the encapsulated molecules tends to decrease.

The trapping of molecules in a carrier, is a concept from many years ago. The dendritic structures have gaps within their structure compared to linear polymers, which confers very useful and important features. Dendrimers can join molecules in their internal and external structure. Functional groups present in the dendrimers, are easily ionized, which helps to bind by electrostatic forces many drugs regardless of stoichiometry. This dendrimer-drug association gives better drug solubility, improves transport across biological membranes and sometimes increases stability.

The amount of drug molecules that can be attached to the dendrimers, depend on the amount of functional groups on the dendrimers; therefore the greater the generation of the dendrimer, the greater number of linked drug molecules.

Dendrimers can have negative or positive charges, which makes them versatile to be able to join a variety of drugs. They can be used for transport across biological membranes and have proven be effective for transporting drugs such as tamsulosin [56], indomethacin [57], ketoprofeno [58], diflunisal and 5-fluorouracil [59]. The problem with such systems is the low biodegradability and an inherent cytotoxicity. By contrast, the dendrimer-peptide systems have the advantage of a low toxicity, which is achieved by attaching the amine groups of the branches of dendrimers with amino acids, resulting in peptide-amine linkages [60]. When a peptide amine system is biotransformed, the result is aminoacid derivatives.

Permeability studies of peptide dendrimer systems are rare [61] because the analytical methods for the quantification of these in biological membranes have not been developed for different types of dendrimers.

The main advantage of dendrimers is their multivalence and because of this, it is possible to control the amount of drug that binds to the functional groups. Due to their shape and size, dendrimers can transport drugs and contrast agents. These systems may interact with the lipids in the membrane and they have shown a very good penetration in cell culture and the intestinal membrane. The mechanisms by which the dendrimers can move and interact with the skin are not well known yet.

A chemotherapeutic drug widely used to treat skin cancer is 5-fluorouracil (5FU), whose permeation was evaluated using iontophoresis, sonophoresis and laser ablation. Also, dendrimers have been used to increase the permeability through the skin of 5FU [62].

3.4. Nanoparticles

The fundamental objective of pharmaceutical scientist is to deliver drug to its site of action. Using nanotechnology, this objective is closer every day. Nanotecsthnology has helped to combat pathogens or syndromes difficult to treat; in fact, there are many diseases that in the past without the use of nanotechnology could not be treated. The nanoscale carriers used for the treatment of diseases, are called nanoparticles, ranging from 1 to 1000 nm (Fig. **7**).

Materials that can be loaded into the nanoparticles are varied, but for therapeutic applications we can mention drugs [63], proteins, peptides, DNA, *etc*. Many therapeutic agents by conventional therapeutic systems exhibit low bioavailability and/or high toxicity; in these cases, the nanoparticles offer great advantages because they considerably increase the bioavailability and decrease the toxicity.

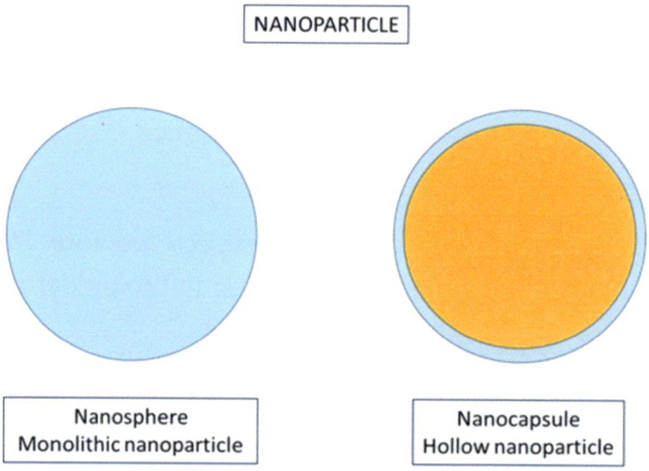

Fig. (7). Representation of nanoparticles (nanosphere and nanocapsule).

The nanoparticles are made with materials that resist pH, temperature, enzyme attack and other problems, which protects the drug from these factors, since the degradation of some molecules may results in toxic degradation products.

Nanoparticles have the ability to penetrate biological barriers and can survive in the bloodstream. These systems release the drug at the site of action and at a desired time; because of these characteristics, adverse effects diminish or disappear and the therapeutic effect increases. The size of nanoparticles makes them virtually undetectable to the immune system and this feature is very well spent when strategies against cells infected with the human immunodeficiency virus (HIV) are developed [64].

Nanoparticles made from a single material and having only the function to carry a drug through the bloodstream are called first generation nanoparticles. Those nanoparticles that are conferred; for example, the ability to remain for longer in the bloodstream by coating with a material to prevent the immune system attack (stealth), they are known as a second generation nanoparticles. Finally, in addition to the nanoparticles having a coating to avoid the immune system attack; the third generation nanoparticles are decorated with a material to bind to a specific target tissue. This division for generations is a result of the advancement of science in this field, since nanoparticles were initially made of non- biodegradable polymers; subsequently manufacturing of nanoparticles was performed by using biodegradable polymers, beginning to add new materials trying to prevent further interaction of nanoparticles with plasma proteins. Researchers began to better understand diseases and for example, it was discovered that there are cancers overexpressing receptors for vitamins [65] and amino acids. These substances were used to decorate the nanoparticles with molecules of this type or with specific antibodies for any component of the tumor membrane.

Nanoparticles can be used as adjuvants in vaccine development [66], since they have advantages over traditional adjuvants. Nanoparticles are chemically stable and reproducible. Besides the above mentioned, the nanoparticles are very versatile and could be used as adjuvants while could be given another function. It can also develop sensitive systems to physical, chemical or biological variables, generated as a result of illness [67].

Nanoparticles can be classified depending on the materials they were made; for example, if they are made of lipids or polymers, the name is lipid or polymeric nanoparticles. Nanoparticles can be made using polymers, lipids, polysaccharides, proteins, *etc.* [68 - 70].

There are two main types of nanoparticles for transmembrane drug delivery; the solid lipid nanoparticles (SLNs) [71] and nanostructured lipid carriers (NLCs) [72]. Aside from lipid nanoparticles, polymeric nanoparticles are very good options for transport through biological membranes because they can be tailor-made in different sizes and it is possible to modify surface polarity in order to improve and increase membrane penetration. From the outside region of a membrane, nanoparticles can reach the inner regions because they exhibit mechanical flexion. Nanoparticles can even travel from the skin to lymph nodes, representing a promising tool for immunomodulation. Some of the most important types of nanoparticles are listed below.

3.4.1. Solid Lipid Nanoparticles (SLN)

These nanoparticles were created due to the need of having a nanostructure with lipophilic characteristics like liposomes but with the stability of polymeric nanoparticles. They are a very good alternative to other colloidal systems and have the advantage of carrying lipophilic drugs [6]. SLN have very high drug encapsulation yields and they are made of triglycerides, fatty acids and waxes. Their fabrication can be done by different techniques; for that reason they are very versatile [6]. The drugs that can be administered transdermally can be local application and systemic application. An example might be, flurbiprofen, which is an analgesic that was administered in solid lipid nanoparticles to exert a local action [73]. Another type of drugs that have been administered through solid lipid nanoparticles is lornoxicam which is effective for pain and inflammation [74].

3.4.2. Magnetic Nanoparticles (MNPs)

These nanostructures can be use in both diagnostic and therapeutic fields. Their use has been widely reported because they have demonstrated being very good to reach cell targets. One of the main uses of these systems is the magnetic hyperthermia directly in the cancer tumor. These kinds of particles in combination with an external magnetic field or magnetic implants have very good performance in drug delivery. Magnetic nanoparticles are charged with organic molecules or metallic oxides [75, 76]. In 2008, some scientists developed an emulsified system containing a magnetic fluid of maguemita citrate derivative with biodegradable surfactants. These magnetic nanoparticles were loaded with a photosensitizer drug used in photodynamic therapy [77].

3.4.3. Gold Nanoparticles (GNPs)

The Gold nanoparticles (GNPs) are one of the most antique nanoparticles with more than one hundred years of usage. The nanoparticles made of gold are used in its metallic form [78]. These nanoparticles have very good performance in delivering drugs, gene therapy, diagnosis and cancer therapy. May be the main disadvantage of these nanoparticles is their accumulation. Some nanoparticles have been used for gene delivery through the skin. SiRNA has been administered using gold nanoparticles through keratinocytes *in vitro* [79].

3.5. Nanoemulsions

The nanoemulsions are heterogeneous isotropic systems considered thermodynamically unstable; they are made by two immiscible liquid usually in the form of oil droplets dispersed in an aqueous system (o/w). The inherent instability of nanoemulsions is due to the fact that during its manufacture requires a lot of energy. When nanoemulsions lose their structure, they are very susceptible to form creams, floccules, *etc*. These stability problems can be attacked by using efficient surfactant systems and decrease globule size at nanoscale.

The nanoemulsions can be used for both formulations of hydrophilic and lipophilic drugs, since we can develop o/w nanoemulsions; and w/o nanoemulsions. Nanoemulsions are considered non-toxic and non-irritating systems, which can be used to transport drugs through biological membranes and for parenteral and non-parenteral administration.

Nanoemulsions have a particle size between 20 and 200 nm and they are widely used in the fields of cosmetics and pharmaceutical products. The performance of these systems is dependent on manufacturing materials as well as the electric charge. Nanoemulsions are associated with polymers and other macromolecules and are also used as nanoreactors for making other nanostructures [80].

In the field of transmembrane drug delivery, nanoemulsions are a promising alternative for their physicochemical properties and they are suitable for transporting drugs through biological membranes both locally and systemically [81]. Currently, the nanoemulsions are not used as much as nanoparticles and liposomes and the main reason is because of their inherent stability problems. By using nanoemulsions, drug availability is much faster because the drug has no barriers to cross, in comparison with drugs contained in a polymeric nanoparticle or a dendrimer. This advantage has been used for the delivery of analgesics, corticosteroids, anticancer agents, *etc* [82].

3.6. Micelles

The main advantages of micelles are: a) high capacity of load drugs, b) increment in drug solubility, c) very low cytotoxicity and genotoxicity, d) small particle size

(20 to 100nm) [83]. To create polymeric micelles we take advantage of the capacity of polymers to self-assemble. For that reason, amphiphilic polymers are used to create micelles [83]. Polymeric micelles are widely used for anticancer therapies taking advantage of an increase of the efficacy in pharmacokinetic performance [84]. However, polymeric micelles have some disadvantages; for example, they deliver the drug very fast, the amount of drug inside micelles in low and it is difficult to decorate micelles to make them more site specific [83, 85].

3.7. Niosomes

Niosomes are bilayer structures made with cholesterol or derivatives of it and a non-ionic surfactant. Niosomes can carry either hydrophilic or lipophilic molecules [39, 86]. They can have lipophilic drugs inside the lipid bilayer and hydrophilic drugs in the core. The production of Niosomes is very similar to liposomes and they were used firstly in the cosmetic industry but day to day the use of Niosomes in pharmaceutical industry increases a lot [38, 39, 87 - 90]. Niosomes have many advantages such as: they can be loaded with different types of molecules; in comparison to liposomes, they are very stable and can be storage for longer time; they can be decorated with different molecules to increase site specificity and they have a bilayer much more flexible than liposomes [38, 39, 87, 89, 90]. The main disadvantages are that in aqueous media they can be hydrolyzed and degraded. Also they have instabilities like emulsions; for example, aggregation or flocculation [89].

3.8. Transfersomes (TF)

Transfersomes are (elastic or ultra-flexible liposomes) ultra-flexible deformable lipid supramolecular aggregates consisting of phospholipids and surfactants. This surfactant gives the flexibility to transfersomes. They have a bilayer like and a liquid core like liposomes [91]. Transfersomes have very good skin permeation due to their flexibility; they are innocuous and safety to skin. Transfersomes can pass through the intercellular spaces due to their ultra-flexible layer [90 - 92].

3.9. Quantum Dots (QDs)

Quantum dots (QDs) are fluorescent semiconductor nanoparticles (nanocrystals).

Their size is in the neighborhood of 2 to 10 nm and they are used to transport some drugs. Their main characteristics are their size and the optical properties, since they are capable to transport drugs and emit a fluorescent signal to be follow into de body. The QDs are frequently used within another particle system due to their toxicity. QDs also can be loaded with gold or magnetic materials to be used for clinical in photo thermal therapy and magneto-transfection [34].

QDs have fluoresced size-dependent and this is very convenient for image analysis in diagnosis [93 - 96]. They can be decorated to give them more versatility and sometimes to increase stability under different conditions of pH, electrolyte concentration, *etc.* [33]. Actually, the use of QDs in the treatment of cancer has taken an important role and QDs in combination with other nanoparticles confers to those systems multifunctional characteristics [33, 34].

3.10. Aquasomes

Aquasomes are systems formed by three layers (core, layer and drug, for example). Due to their size in the range of nanometers, the surface properties give to Aquasomes the possibility of self-assembling. They were created to transport peptides and proteins, including enzymes or antigens. The core of Aquasomes is made of ceramic materials, the layer is a carbohydrate and finally a peptide or protein is attached on the surface [37, 97]. Due to their particular structure Aquasomes are more stable than liposomes and the proteins and peptides attached do not suffer denaturalization [97].

3.11. Nanotoxicology

Due to the nature of this kind of structures, they can reach sites where drugs alone cannot reach. For that reason, nanostructures can change functions in a cellular system. They can affect organelles, gene material and also the immune system. Due to this, it is common when some group develop a new nanosystem, the study of cytotoxicity, genotoxicity and immunotoxicity.

4. PHYSICAL ENHANCERS

4.1. Ultrasound

When a tissue is subjected to ultrasound, the tissue can be heated and this can be used for therapeutic purposes. There are other benefits that occur when interacting with ultrasound no attributed to warming of tissues, and this can be used to exert therapeutic effects. Ultrasound therapies are divided into high and low power. Regarding to high power ultrasound we can mention therapies as targeted lithotripsy and those of low power as: Sonophoresis, sonoporation, bone healing and gene therapy.

One of the main mechanisms of action of ultrasound is cavitation, which is the formation of bubbles of gas in the medium after ultrasound exposure due to a pressure change [98]. Ultrasound is able to form micro strong currents that increase the bioavailability of drugs [99, 100].

An important ultrasound application is transfection. Initial attempts *in vitro* transfection dates back to 1987 when Fechheimer *et al.* [101] reported a low level of transfected murine fibroblasts using 3 half-second pulses with an intensity of 20 kHz with a sonicator used to homogenize tissues. Techniques were improved and today transfections are performed in a variety of eukaryotic cells.

The use of ultrasound in gene therapy has recently been a very useful tool and has become an alternative to viral gene therapy and other non-viral therapies. The ultrasound increases the permeability of the cell membrane and hence can be administered plasmids and other genetic material. This technique is usually performed by injection of plasmids of DNA and subsequently applying ultrasonic waves to assist the migration and penetration of the material into cells to be treated.

The effectiveness of the sonoporation may depend on the cellular cycle phase wherein cell is sonoporated, since these have different viscoelastic properties of the membrane depending upon the stage in the cycle they are [102, 103].

The approximations of non-viral gene therapy in biological membranes results in a transient gene expression varying levels due to rapid replacement and renewal of epithelial cells [104]. In addition, they are up to 1000 times less efficient than viral therapies, as well as cause cellular acute toxicity and cell death in many cases.

The sonothrombolysis method is based on the use of very low frequency ultrasound to destroy clots obstructing brain arteries. This treatment is only experimental and used with patients who cannot be treated by the administration of conventional thrombolytic agents, but it can be used with any patient within the time window for the treatment of stroke, which is the first six hours after the event. This methodology is considered non-invasive and safe for the patient and has almost no contraindications.

One of the approved therapies for acute ischemic attack is intravenous tissue plasmogen activator (tPA) whose successful thrombolysis highly dependent on the release of tPA around the obstruction. The wave pulse of transcranial Doppler (TCD) can expose obstruction to an ultrasonic pressure. Using these methodologies was carried out a clinical trial called CLOTBUST (Combined Lysis of Thrombus with Transcranial Ultrasound 2 MHz and systemic tPA) obtaining very encouraging results [105, 106].

One of the first applications of ultrasound in medicine was called ultrasonic massage that was used for the first time in Berlin in 1938. Pohlman Raimar demonstrated therapeutic effects of ultrasound waves in human tissues and began to perform physical therapy ultrasound as a routine procedure in medical practice [107]. The use of ultrasound for the treatment of sports injuries [108] and tennis elbow [109] is very common nowadays.

The use of ultrasound in physical therapy focuses primarily on the treatment of soft tissue injuries [110], for the acceleration of wound healing [111], reduction of edema and makes the scar tissue stronger and more elastic. It is also used in bone injuries and circulatory disorders. In 2002 Robertson conducted a randomized trial of physiotherapy with ultrasound but was unable to find a dose-effect relationship [112].

Sonophoresis has been used in sports medicine from the sixties. Studies have shown that this technique has no adverse effects or very small within the range considered therapeutic (1-3 MHz frequency, intensity of 1-2 W/cm2, lasting 5-10 minutes, continuous or pulsed mode).

Recent research has shown the therapeutic benefits of ultrasound on damaged bone [113]. Studies using ultrasound in fresh fractures show that healing is reduced from 30% to 38% of the time. When applied to unbound bone fractures, it is noted that ultrasonic therapy stimulates recovery in 86% of cases. These benefits were obtained with low-intensity ultrasound (<0.1 W/cm2) using pulses (LIPUS) [114].

The use of ultrasound as a therapy for the calcification of the shoulder tendinitis is another application that occurs in sports medicine. Studies have reported promising data using shock waves. The intensity of ultrasound used as therapy for painful conditions of the musculoskeletal system varies from 0.5 to 2.0 W per square centimeter.

Ultrasound has also been used for the treatment of chronic tendinopathy of the Achilles tendon, although the results are heterogeneous in different clinical studies [115], it has been seen that ultrasound may be a promising therapy for this condition.

4.2. Iontophoresis

Applying an electric current (0.5 mA/cm^2 or less) in order to facilitate the transport of drugs through membranes, it is known as iontophoresis (Fig. **8**). Which is applied with a low current density, low voltage, through an electric circuit consisting of two drug reservoirs placed on the membrane. When electric current is applied, the drug is pushed on by the electrode to pass through the membrane. The three mechanisms by which a drug may pass through membranes by iontophoresis are: electromigration, electroosmosis and passive diffusion.

Biological membranes by its constitution of lipids, proteins and polysaccharides are very complex and control the passage of molecules. For example, above the isoelectric point of the skin (4-4.5) the carboxylic acid groups are ionized. Thus at higher pH than the isoelectric point, the skin becomes very selective to permeation and attracts cations repelled by the anode, favoring the transport of molecules by electrophoresis. Movement of sodium through the skin generates a flow of solvent that can drag small uncharged molecules (electroosmosis). Mobility decreases when molecular weight increases. Therefore, the electroosmosis plays a fundamental role in the permeability of larger molecules. The pathways that drugs use to penetrate the skin are sebaceous glands, hair follicles and imperfections.

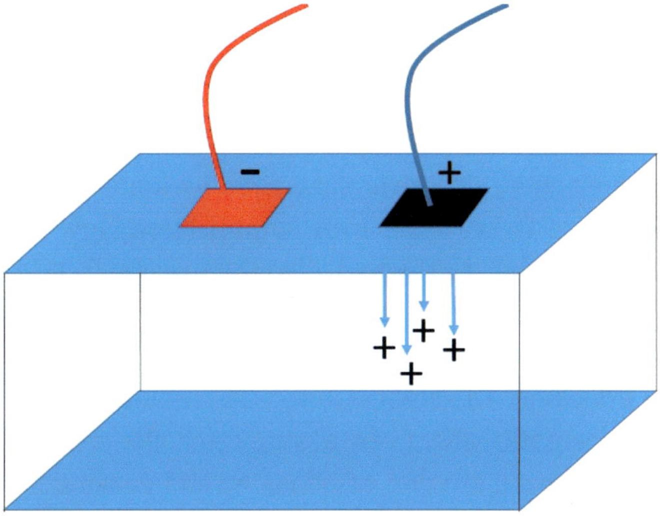

Fig. (8). Iontophoresis device.

There has been great progress in the transdermal administration by iontophoresis using peptides, antioxidants, hormones, oligonucleotides, *etc.* The use of other permeability enhancers in combination with iontophoresis has increased the range of molecules that can be administered through the skin. The increase in permeability which is achieved with iontophoresis compared to the diffusion is huge; permeability data of insulin using iontophoresis in comparison to passive diffusion are in the order of 713 fold and was also observed a significant decrease in blood glucose levels, which opens the possibility of administering this molecule for the treatment of diabetes mellitus by dermal route [116].

Molecules migration through iontophoresis is based on the charge/mass ratio, since if charge/mass ratio of a molecule is large; iontophoresis is a promoter that significantly will increase the permeability of that molecule. It has also been seen that neutral molecules can increase their permeability through iontophoresis, such as glucose, which can be extracted by means of iontophoresis for quantification in diabetic patients [117].

The use of iontophoresis may be combined with the use of a microprocessor to release drug at time intervals in desired amounts, generating release profiles which would otherwise be impossible [118].

The use of corticosteroids for physical therapy is one of the most used drugs with iontophoresis [119]. Corticosteroids are anti-inflammatory negatively charged, which migrate with the help of a negative field. In these cases, must take care to evaluate formulations administered by iontophoresis, since some of the formulation components may also be administered by iontophoresis without being this the main objective. It has also been administered, low molecular weight molecules such as lidocaine [120] and dexamethasone [121]. In the case of lidocaine, it was administered by iontophoresis as a local anesthetic, obtaining very promising results. Dexamethasone is often administered *via* iontophoresis in combination with lidocaine. Dexamethasone was administered from the positive electrode by electroosmotic effect. In a study for the treatment of shoulder tendinitis, it was found that a mixture of lidocaine and dexamethasone applied by iontophoresis, had the same effect as the same mixture administered by intramuscular injection [118].

As we mentioned, lidocaine has also been administered by iontophoresis. It is a hydrochloride salt form and dissociates into a positive ion which is administered from the anode. By using iontophoresis, the effect is localized and the amounts given are very small, this avoids a systemic effect of this drug and the adverse effects that this entails.

In the diagnosis of cystic fibrosis, iontophoresis is used to administer pilocarpine and cause sweating, which is analyzed to give a diagnostic [118].

4.3. Microneedles

In the oral route some drugs have low absorption and suffer enzymatic degradation in the gastrointestinal tract and liver, as a first alternative arises parenteral administration using injections, but in some cases this route is very painful, which is not liked by most people. From this need arose primarily the patches, but drugs that cannot penetrate the stratum corneum, found in microneedles an excellent alternative of administration. The microneedles generate holes sufficiently large to allow penetrating small molecules and some macromolecules, in a controlled manner without infringing damage of clinical importance to the skin. The microneedles are arrays of small needles used for transdermal administration and they can be classified in four types:

1. Solid microneedles.
2. Solid microneedles having a powdered drug adhered.
3. Polymeric microneedles.
4. Hollow microneedles releasing a drug infusion.

It has been shown that the microneedles (Fig. **9**) can generate perforations large enough to penetrate the stratum corneum with small molecules, large molecules and nanoparticles. Some experiments conducted in animals have shown that this methodology can be used to deliver oligonucleotides [122], insulin [123], human growth hormone [124], *etc.* Protein vaccines can be administered using microneedles [125].

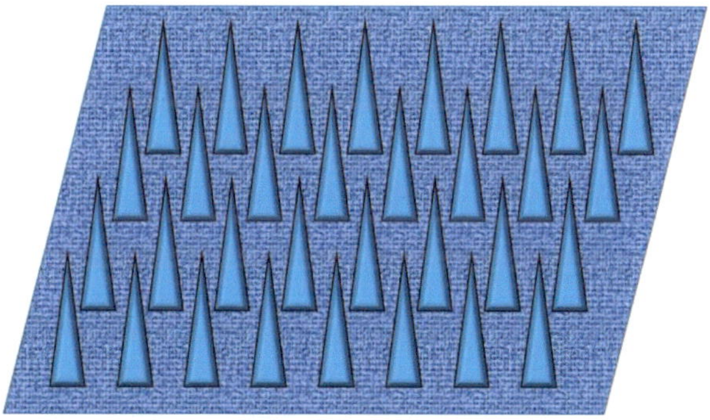

Fig. (9). Schematic representation of microneedles.

The microneedles are made of silicon, metals, polymers and other materials and they can be of different sizes ranging from submicronic size up to several microns.

Among the modalities of administration by means of solid microneedles are the following:

1. Poke with patch [126]: In this case, the holes are made and after that, the drug is administered in the form of solution, gel or patch. Examples of drug administered with this type of procedure are the oligonucleotides and insulin. This technique can be combined with iontophoresis to enhance drug penetration into the skin.
2. Coat and poke [127]: With this procedure solid microneedles are coated with the drug to form a powder or film and then the holes are made, leaving the substances adhered to the microneedles in the skin, thus the dissolved drug exerts a therapeutic effect; the example most representative of this type of methodology is protein-based vaccines.
3. Dip and scrape [128]: This methodology is adapted to deliver vaccines and DNA, it is carried out by immersing the array of microneedles in a solution of DNA to subsequently make multiple passes to create skin abrasion.

There are also hollow microneedles; in this kind of microneedles, the drug is released by simple diffusion [129]. This type of needles have been used to deliver insulin and actually there are few publications of this type of needles and their application in skin.

5. PHYSICAL ENHANCERS IN COMBINATION WITH THE USE OF NANOCARRIERS

5.1. Microneedles and Nanocarriers

One of the drugs that have been tested using this dual approach of skin permeation is ketoprofen, which has a log P = 2.94, which is more appropriate than other NSAIDs. Despite this log P, ketoprofen have not the ability to reach deeper layers of the skin and also it is deactivated at the site of action where inflammation occurs, which makes this molecule an ideal candidate to be administered encapsulated into nanoparticles. In a study reported, it was used Polylactic acid (PLA) as nanocarrier for ketoprofen, because this polymer is lipophilic, biodegradable, biocompatible and it is approved by the FDA for clinical use [130].

The use of microneedles with polylactic acid nanoparticles to enhance the permeability of ketoprofen, allowed to generate pores for passage of nanoparticles with ketoprofen and avoided the passage through the stratum corneum, which is a very selective barrier.

This combination, has also been used with anticancer agents such as docetaxel, which is a molecule of high molecular weight and very slightly soluble in water. Liposome permeability of the drug through rat and pig skin was evaluated; it was found to be better the administration of ultra-flexible liposomes than the combination of liposomes and microneedles. However, the combination of methodologies using microneedles and ultra- flexible liposomes increased the permeability in comparison to ultra-flexible liposomes alone [131].

An important strategy for drug delivery in skin is to incorporate nanoparticulated drug carriers. Antigens have been incorporated into such polymeric carriers to allow controlled release to the skin dendritic cells.

Lipid nanocarriers as solid lipid nanoparticles (SLN) and nanostructured lipid carriers (NLC) have been incorporated within water soluble polymeric matrices for lipid drug formulation and due to this lipophilic character, there is not immune rejection. By incorporating lipid nanocarriers into polymer matrices, allows to incorporate lipophilic drugs into polymeric microneedles (Fig. **10**) made of polylactic acid and hyaluronic acid. These strategies have been developed to maintain an adequate concentration of drug into the skin in order to combat diseases such as vitiligo, pigmentation, psoriasis and some tropical infections [132].

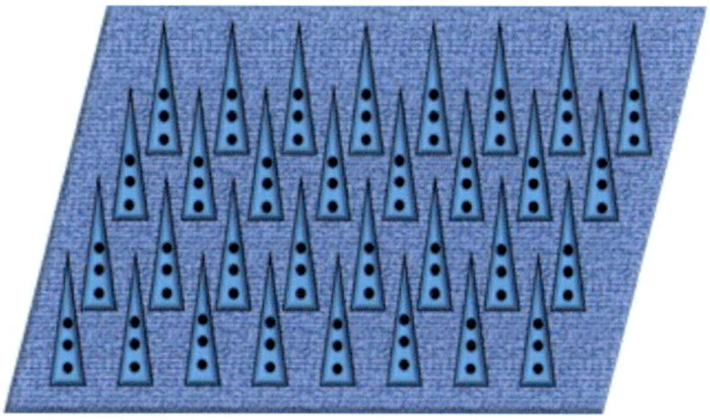

Fig. (10). Microneedles and nanoparticles.

The fact to create micro channels in the stratum corneum to deliver nanocarriers for local or systemic effect is a fact still not well understood. The interaction of nanocarriers with the ducts has multiple components; for example, the charge ratio of nanocarriers and the diameter of the channels; the composition of the nanocarriers per se, the size and the ability to penetrate the skin cells, *etc*. The complexity of this new alternative to improve the permeability of nanoparticles through the skin is amazing but offers many advantages and opens the way for the administration of drugs that had previously been impossible to be administered through the skin [133].

One of the most promising applications for the combination of nanocarriers and microneedles is the delivery of vaccines. There is substantial improvement by combining the manufacture of poly electrolyte multilayer (PEM) with the vaccine, which is administered forming a film of PEM in the microneedles, thus the system is placed to let the skin components disintegrate the PEM film and go releasing the vaccine [134].

It has also been found that the dermal administration of naked DNA plasmids supported on cationic nanocarriers using solid microneedles gives better results than intramuscular administration of the same DNA plasmid. Why the therapy using microneedles works better than an intramuscular administration with a syringe and needle; it is still not known, but such strategies are being implemented more each day. In a research study, nanoparticles were used for immunization with DNA plasmids and nanoparticles were manufactured using polylactic-co-glycolic acid (PLGA) and 1, 2 dioleoyl-3-trimethylammonium propane (DOTAP), which are biocompatible and generate a positive charge nanocarrier which interacts with the negatively charged DNA [135].

To deliver drugs through the stratum corneum without the use of nanocarriers or microneedles; drugs must have molecular weights below 500 Da and they need to be lipophilic. Using nanocarriers without microneedles we need to manufacture nanoparticles below 100 nm, and many of the drugs of large molecular weight do not allow to produce such small nanoparticles and some are trapped in the stratum corneum, and finally with the use of nanoparticles and microneedles, we can administer nanocarriers of larger particle sizes (although it is not known what size) directly into the epidermis.

As can be seen, the combination of nanocarriers with microneedles results in very efficient drug delivery systems, with great future, since the skin for its size allows a large area of administration and for different purposes. It has also been shown that the distance of penetration of microneedles, generates no pain or damage of clinical importance, which is a big advantage over the intramuscular administration.

5.2. Iontophoresis and Nanocarriers

The use of an electric current for administration of nanoparticles is a widely used methodology. Recently, *in vivo* studies have been made through the abdominal skin of rats, the administration of indomethacin for polylactic-co-glycolic acid (PLGA) nanoparticles having an average size of 100nm. Using iontophoresis (3 V/cm) resulted in a substantial improvement compared to the administration of the indomethacin molecule by passive diffusion.

There are studies using PLGA nanoparticles loaded with estradiol (average size of 150nm). The administration was also made in rat skin *in vitro* and *in vivo*, using a constant voltage of 3 V/cm.

The use of nanocarriers for transport drugs across the skin is very extensive. Liposomes, transfersomes, lipid nanoparticles, polymeric nanoparticles (PLGA, PLA, *etc.*) and other types of nanocarriers as dendrimers have been used. Dendrimers permeability is dependent on their size and their generation. The smaller size (generation) the greater penetration. The relevance of using dendrimers loaded in combination with iontophoresis for transdermal drug delivery has been studied. The studies were done using pig skin and dendrimers loaded with fluoroisothiocyanate (FITC), the transport was characterized using confocal laser scanning microscopy. In this case, the cationic dendrimers also had greater penetration than anionic and neutral dendrimers [136].

The use of iontophoresis combined with nanocarriers, is a very convenient strategy (Fig. **11**). Neutral drugs can be encapsulated in charged nanocarriers to be used with iontophoresis. In a work reported, colchicine was encapsulated in liposomes with neutral charge and its permeation was enhanced using iontophoresis [137]. In another study, it is suggested that to prevent the proteolytic breakdown of peptides, a good strategy is encapsulate them [138].

The use of nanocarriers is a very fruitful strategy for transport drugs through the skin, some of nanocarriers most used were the liposomes and microemulsions; however, these systems have an inherent instability problem. For this reason, this type of nanocarriers has been replaced by Solid Lipid Nanoparticles (SLN), which has better stability and helps improving the stability of some inherently unstable drugs. Another advantage is the drug control release since some of the drugs are very irritating and need to be dosed in small quantities over prolonged periods. The use of hydrogels with this type of nanocarriers is a good strategy to improve the use of Solid Lipid Nanoparticles in clinical studies and improving rheological properties and tissue compatibility. In addition, hydrogels are an appropriate means for applying iontophoresis [139].

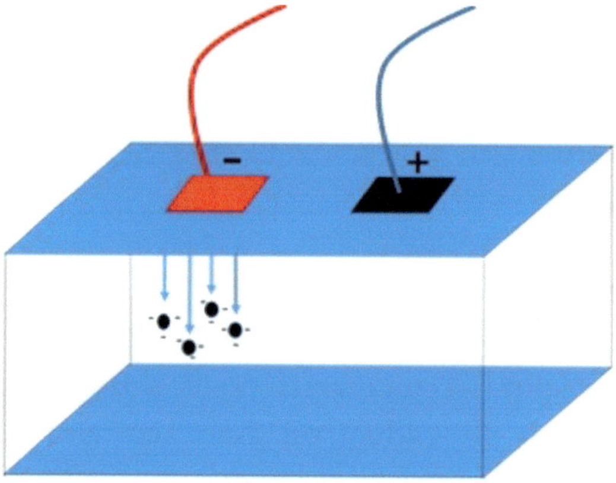

Fig. (11). Iontophoresis and nanoparticles.

The use of iontophoresis in combination with microneedles for transporting high molecular weight molecules like insulin (6 kDa) is a strategy that has proved successful results. Furthermore, nanovesicles have been incorporated to improve the permeation of drugs with high molecular weight. Nanovesicles, has proven being very useful in the encapsulation of cyclosporin A and ascorbyl palmitate and increase the permeability through skin of these compounds using iontophoresis [140].

In order to increase the loads of polymeric nanoparticles of polylactic-co-glycolic acid (PLGA) with indomethacin, two types of nanoparticles were produced; first made by the traditional method of emulsification and solvent evaporation and another produced by anti- solvent diffusion. Nanoparticles produced by the second method are not stabilized with any surfactant, but the first one is stabilized with poly vinyl alcohol (PVA). Manufactured nanoparticles by anti-solvent diffusion have higher load, which improves iontophoretic flux at 68 fold compared to the stabilized with PVA [141].

Another application of the combination of nanocarriers and iontophoresis is in transdermal delivery of superoxide dismutase (SOD); which is a powerful antioxidant that is used to protect the skin against damage caused by UV rays. SOD is a high molecular weight molecule so transdermal administration of this molecule without the aid of physical promoters as iontophoresis and liposomes, would be unthinkable. The permeation study of SOD was performed in rats to prevent skin damage caused by UV radiation. Superoxide dismutase was encapsulated in cationic liposomes and thereafter iontophoresis applied. Liposomes were observed that adequately permeate into the viable skin layer around hair follicles. As a negative control, was used no iontophoresis treatment, which does not adequately permeate. With the combination of liposomes and iontophoresis a marked decrease in oxidation products such as malondialdehyde, haxanoyl lysine and 8-hydroxi-2- deoxyguanosine, was observed after skin irradiation with UV light. It was possible to develop an intradermal SOD system that could be used for other macromolecules [142].

5.3. Ultrasound and Nanocarriers

Currently, cancer therapies have intrinsic systemic toxicity. Therefore, nanomedicine has opened new alternatives to administer these therapies decre-asing adverse and toxic effects. The problem with the application of nanotechnology in anti-cancer therapies is the low permeability of nanoparticles into the tissues and blood vessels. On the contrary, between the endothelial cells of tumors are spaces that allow extravasation into surrounding tissues, which is very important to chemotherapy, as well allows the passage of drugs into the tumor by passive transport. Nanostructures such as liposomes, micelles, polymeric nanoparticles, *etc.* can penetrate tumors through these spaces between the cells of the endothelial tissue and accumulate in the tumors. This effect is known as Enhanced Permeability and Retention (EPR). As we mentioned in this paper, physical penetration enhancers have been incorporated to improve permeability of nanometric systems through membranes, particularly in this case, we will talk about the sound effect. The development of ultrasonic devices is very important to enhance the permeability of nanocarriers and they have certain advantages over other physical promoters. For example, ultrasound can reach deeper tumors and many factors can be modified to optimize treatment. In the case of cancer, combination of nanoparticles and ultrasound is widely used; here, passive targeting of nanoparticles helps them to accumulate in tumor and as a second part of the therapy, it is used a stimulation by ultrasound for a controlled drug release [143].

Within nanoparticles we can find two types: the rigid nanoparticles and soft nanoparticles. In particular, speaking of rigid nanoparticles can be found information in the literature about their design as transmembrane nanocarriers. Actually, some authors are studying the mechanism of penetration and biocompatibility.

Although rigid nanoparticles can be used as transmembrane nanocarriers; The stratum corneum is one of the most difficult barrier to penetrate and permeability of nanoparticles through the skin is a topic of debate, because the objective of increase the penetration of nanoparticles through the skin has been achieved but in very small quantities. The success of therapy based on nanoparticles through the skin depends on how deep and amount they can penetrate. Different physical penetration enhancers on skin have been tested. In a work reported, chemical enhancer (sodium lauryl sulfate) and application of low frequency ultrasound were used simultaneously. For the mentioned study, as a rigid nanoparticle model was used quantum dots with different charges (cationic, anionic and neutral), since it has been found that the penetration of nanocarriers in skin, depends on the charge. The results show that there was an increase in the penetration of quantum dots using low frequency ultrasound and sodium lauryl sulfate; surprisingly, the best penetration was not for the most cationic quantum dots. It is suggested that the charge has to be optimized [144].

The combination of low frequency ultrasound and chemical enhancers such as sodium lauryl sulfate, allow:

1. Reduce treatment times.
2. Decrease input power requirements.
3. Increase skin permeability.
4. Increase connectivity of lacular region in the stratum corneum.
5. Less physical disturbance of the skin compared with only low frequency ultrasound.

Low frequency ultrasound can increase the penetration and dispersion of the chemical enhancers and hence a marked synergism [145].

There are mainly two types of sonophoresis:

1. Simultaneous sonophoresis: On the membrane the drug is administered, and ultrasound is applied simultaneously. In this case, the patient uses the device during treatment.
2. Pretreatment with sonophoresis: In this method the ultrasound is applied previously to the drug administration. In this case the skin is treated to increase its permeability and so remains for a long time and the drug can then permeate.

In the method number two, is required knowing the skin permeability, for that reason, conductance measurements are used because it has much correlation with the permeability of the skin.

In a study, diclofenac was encapsulated in liposomes to be used with a sonophoretic release system. Topically administered in rats its systemic availability was evaluated. Diclofenac liposomes were applied and they were located at the site of application with a very slow systemic availability. Subsequently, ultrasonic pulses were applied and systemic availability was increased noticeably.

Ultrasound has also been used to increase the efficiency of gene therapy using liposomes. These liposomes are cationic and acoustic and they allow reflex ultrasound.

Another use of ultrasound therapy combined with carriers, it is shown using encapsulated testosterone in lipid solid microparticles. Testosterone alone causes irritation but using testosterone lipid solid microparticles, skin irritation decreases a lot. It has been found that low frequency ultrasound produces greater penetration of testosterone encapsulated than high frequency ultrasound, but the low frequency ultrasound requires a more careful selection of parameters to perform safe administration of testosterone [146].

6. PHYSICAL ENHANCERS AND NANOPARTICLES DEVICES

The strategy for administering drugs into nanocarriers and helping to penetrate different membranes by physical enhancers has had great success. In the bibliographic research to write this work, we found many devices used to improve the penetration of drugs through different membranes.

In this work; as the reader will have noticed, we focused on the three main physical enhancers used to administered drugs in nanoparticles; microneedles, iontophoresis and ultrasound. We found different devices using these three physical enhancers, which can be used to enhance the permeability of certain drugs or nanocarriers. Here are some of the systems found and mainly those for which there is already a patent.

6.1. Microneedles Devices

The microneedles devices to administer nanocarriers have been extensively studied. There are different types of systems depending on the manufacture material and the microneedles form, as we previously mentioned. In 2008, was patented a system for administration of nanoparticles at a certain depth of the skin without touching pain receptors. The patent has the name of microarray device [147]. In the same year, came another device whose patent was named; microdevice and method for transdermal delivery and sampling of active substances, which was developed to prevent, treat or ameliorate any specific medical condition [148], using drugs alone or in a nanocarrier. The development of drug delivery systems using microneedles has been extended to administration of COX inhibitors through the skin [149].

Not only in the skin can delivered drugs or nanocarriers, also through the ocular route using only a single microneedle [150].

A device made of biocompatible, dissolving microneedles, containing nanoparticles with drug and biomolecules for delivery through the skin and other epithelia was patented in 2014 [151].

As shown, the use of physical enhancers' devices in combination with nanocarriers is a topic that is under development and features of both systems are taken to create a synergetic system and dramatically improve drug penetration through the epithelia.

6.2. Iontophoretic Devices

For the usage of iontophoretic devices in combination with nanocarriers, the most important characteristic is the presence of a charge on the nanocarriers. In the literature we can find very interesting systems using the combination of both penetration enhancers.

A system developed and patented in 1998, refers to the use of hydrogels or lipogels for drug delivery by iontophoresis. Drugs may be administered alone or within a liposome, nanoparticle, *etc* [152].

In 2003 a system using both iontophoresis and nanocarriers (liposomes and niosomes), for administration botulinum toxin was also patented [153]. In 2007, other device that released drug by an iontophoretic system associated with nanoparticles was developed [154]. In that same year, another system using ionic nanoparticles to transport drugs across a membrane by the action of an iontophoretic system was patented [155].

Across the ocular route, the use of iontophoretic devices in combination with nanoparticles, liposomes and nanocrystals has also been developed very successfully [156].

The use of more than one physical enhancer in combination with nanocarriers is also a strategy that has been used to release molecules through the skin. In an invention of 2009, the use of iontophoresis and ultrasound for the administration of melanin within liposomes and polymeric nanoparticles was developed [157]. In the same year, a system that also used the combination of iontophoresis, ultrasound and nanocarriers loaded with melanin for laser hair removal was patented [158].

The use of ionized nanoparticles for drug release in combination with iontophoretic systems is a very successful strategy for transport through the tissue of the oral cavity. Drugs that have been used to support the patent of this invention are; gentamicin, ketoconazole, ibuprofen, dexamethasone, mitomycin C, *etc* [159].

6.3. Ultrasound Devices

Using the combination of ultrasound with nanocarriers is mainly used in drug delivery by destroying nanocarriers' structure by ultrasonic effect and then we obtain drug release.

In 2007, was patented a system based on ultrasound and it may or may not contain nanocarriers. This device was used for hair removal, skin rejuvenation, reduction of scars, varicose veins, *etc*. The patent claimed was not limited to treatment of skin but also subcutaneous fat, connective tissue, muscle tissue, blood vessels, *etc* [160]. Also this combination has been used in ultrasound and nanocarriers to deliver drugs *via* the ocular route (transcleral). The device is designed to manage free drug and dendrimers, liposomes, nanoparticles, *etc* [161]. The drug release for the treatment of thrombosis can also be developed with a device containing nanocarriers and ultrasound. In an invention patented in 2008, it is proposed to use this device for the treatment of thrombosis and other applications [162].

The use of ultrasound to activate the drug delivery is evidenced by an invention patented in 2012, where nanocarriers that can be tracked by MRI are administered. Once the nanocarriers reach their site of action, drug release is triggered by ultrasound [163]. This is one of the most common applications of combination of nanocarriers and ultrasound and is designed for this purpose. The devices are designed with adequate ultrasonic penetration to trigger drug release.

Another use of ultrasound is the ablation of stratum corneum to facilitate penetration of nanocarriers. In a patent of 2013, a device was developed to facilitate ablation of the stratum corneum and allow entry of drugs encapsulated in nanoparticles of hyaluronic acid [164].

CONCLUSION

The usage of nanocarriers in combination with physical permeation enhancers is a field that has great potential. Many of nanoparticles currently developed for systemic drug delivery, have the disadvantage of not being able to pass through stratum corneum and this limits some therapeutic applications. The improvement in permeability of nanocarriers provided by physical enhancers is very important because they are the driven force necessary to carry these drug delivery systems beyond the stratum corneum.

Combination of physical enhancers and nanocarriers opens the possibility to treat diseases that previously would not be possible to deal. Many of the drugs applied in the skin can generate immunological reactions or be degraded; however, if the drug is transported into a nanocarrier, the effects of the immune system are avoided and increase its stability and half-life.

The use in combination of physical enhancers and nanocarriers has been increased over the years and according to the number of publications found, there is a very promising future for this type of therapy.

CONFLICT OF INTEREST

The authors confirm that they have no conflict of interest to declare for this publication.

ACKNOWLEDGEMENTS

Authors acknowledge to the projects UNAM-DGAPA, PAPIIT IN219715 and UNAM-FESC, PIAPIC-18.

REFERENCES

[1] Moghimi SM, Hunter AC, Murray JC. Nanomedicine: current status and future prospects. FASEB J 2005; 19(3): 311-30.
[http://dx.doi.org/10.1096/fj.04-2747rev] [PMID: 15746175]

[2] Freitas RA Jr. What is nanomedicine? Nanomedicine 2005; 1(1): 2-9.
[PMID: 17292052]

[3] Jain S, Hirst DG, O'Sullivan JM. Gold nanoparticles as novel agents for cancer therapy. Br J Radiol 2012; 85(1010): 101-13.
[http://dx.doi.org/10.1259/bjr/59448833] [PMID: 22010024]

[4] Rodríguez-Cruz IM, Domínguez-Delgado CL, Escobar-Chávez JJ, Leyva-Gómez G, Ganem-Quintanar A, Quintanar-Guerrero D. Nanoparticle infiltration to prepare solvent-free controlled drug delivery systems. Int J Pharm 2009; 371(1-2): 177-81.
[http://dx.doi.org/10.1016/j.ijpharm.2008.12.024] [PMID: 19150491]

[5] Tonga GY, Moyano DF, Kim CS, Rotello VM. Inorganic nanoparticles for therapeutic delivery: Trials, tribulations and promise. Curr Opin Colloid Interface Sci 2014; 19(2): 49-55.
[http://dx.doi.org/10.1016/j.cocis.2014.03.004] [PMID: 24955019]

[6] Manchun S, Dass CR, Sriamornsak P. Targeted therapy for cancer using pH-responsive nanocarrier systems. Life Sci 2012; 90(11-12): 381-7.
[http://dx.doi.org/10.1016/j.lfs.2012.01.008] [PMID: 22326503]

[7] Kataoka K, Harada A, Nagasaki Y. Block copolymer micelles for drug delivery: design, characterization and biological significance. Adv Drug Deliv Rev 2001; 47(1): 113-31.
[http://dx.doi.org/10.1016/S0169-409X(00)00124-1] [PMID: 11251249]

[8] Oberdörster G, Oberdörster E, Oberdörster J. Nanotoxicology: an emerging discipline evolving from studies of ultrafine particles. Environ Health Perspect 2005; 113(7): 823-39.
[http://dx.doi.org/10.1289/ehp.7339] [PMID: 16002369]

[9] Ganta S, Devalapally H, Shahiwala A, Amiji M. A review of stimuli-responsive nanocarriers for drug and gene delivery. J Control Release 2008; 126(3): 187-204.
[http://dx.doi.org/10.1016/j.jconrel.2007.12.017] [PMID: 18261822]

[10] Kumari A, Yadav SK, Yadav SC. Biodegradable polymeric nanoparticles based drug delivery systems. Colloids Surf B Biointerfaces 2010; 75(1): 1-18.
[http://dx.doi.org/10.1016/j.colsurfb.2009.09.001] [PMID: 19782542]

[11] Merisko-Liversidge EM, Liversidge GG. Drug nanoparticles: formulating poorly water-soluble compounds. Toxicol Pathol 2008; 36(1): 43-8.
[http://dx.doi.org/10.1177/0192623307310946] [PMID: 18337220]

[12] Liu Z, Jiao Y, Wang Y, Zhou C, Zhang Z. Polysaccharides-based nanoparticles as drug delivery systems. Adv Drug Deliv Rev 2008; 60(15): 1650-62.
[http://dx.doi.org/10.1016/j.addr.2008.09.001] [PMID: 18848591]

[13] Owens DE III, Peppas NA. Opsonization, biodistribution, and pharmacokinetics of polymeric nanoparticles. Int J Pharm 2006; 307(1): 93-102.
[http://dx.doi.org/10.1016/j.ijpharm.2005.10.010] [PMID: 16303268]

[14] Pardeike J, Hommoss A, Müller RH. Lipid nanoparticles (SLN, NLC) in cosmetic and pharmaceutical dermal products. Int J Pharm 2009; 366(1-2): 170-84.
[http://dx.doi.org/10.1016/j.ijpharm.2008.10.003] [PMID: 18992314]

[15] Hawkins MJ, Soon-Shiong P, Desai N. Protein nanoparticles as drug carriers in clinical medicine. Adv Drug Deliv Rev 2008; 60(8): 876-85.
[http://dx.doi.org/10.1016/j.addr.2007.08.044] [PMID: 18423779]

[16] Osada K, Christie RJ, Kataoka K. Polymeric micelles from poly(ethylene glycol)-poly(amino acid) block copolymer for drug and gene delivery. J R Soc Interface 2009; 6 (Suppl. 3): S325-39.
[http://dx.doi.org/10.1098/rsif.2008.0547.focus] [PMID: 19364722]

[17] Liu Y, Li K, Pan J, Liu B, Feng SS. Folic acid conjugated nanoparticles of mixed lipid monolayer shell and biodegradable polymer core for targeted delivery of Docetaxel. Biomaterials 2010; 31(2): 330-8.
[http://dx.doi.org/10.1016/j.biomaterials.2009.09.036] [PMID: 19783040]

[18] Roney C, Kulkarni P, Arora V, *et al.* Targeted nanoparticles for drug delivery through the blood-brain barrier for Alzheimer's disease. J Control Release 2005; 108(2-3): 193-214.
[http://dx.doi.org/10.1016/j.jconrel.2005.07.024] [PMID: 16246446]

[19] Fleige E, Quadir MA, Haag R. Stimuli-responsive polymeric nanocarriers for the controlled transport of active compounds: concepts and applications. Adv Drug Deliv Rev 2012; 64(9): 866-84.
[http://dx.doi.org/10.1016/j.addr.2012.01.020] [PMID: 22349241]

[20] Torchilin VP. Multifunctional nanocarriers. Adv Drug Deliv Rev 2012; 64: 302-15.
[http://dx.doi.org/10.1016/j.addr.2012.09.031] [PMID: 17092599]

[21] Lee CM, Choi Y, Huh EJ, *et al.* Polyethylene glycol (PEG) modified 99mTc-HMPAO-liposome for improving blood circulation and biodistribution: the effect of the extent of PEGylation. Cancer Biother Radiopharm 2005; 20(6): 620-8.
[http://dx.doi.org/10.1089/cbr.2005.20.620] [PMID: 16398614]

[22] Allémann E, Brasseur N, Benrezzak O, *et al.* PEG-coated poly(lactic acid) nanoparticles for the delivery of hexadecafluoro zinc phthalocyanine to EMT-6 mouse mammary tumours. J Pharm Pharmacol 1995; 47(5): 382-7.
[http://dx.doi.org/10.1111/j.2042-7158.1995.tb05815.x] [PMID: 7494187]

[23] Cheng J, Teply BA, Sherifi I, *et al.* Formulation of functionalized PLGA-PEG nanoparticles for *in vivo* targeted drug delivery. Biomaterials 2007; 28(5): 869-76.
[http://dx.doi.org/10.1016/j.biomaterials.2006.09.047] [PMID: 17055572]

[24] Prausnitz MR, Langer R. Transdermal drug delivery. Nat Biotechnol 2008; 26(11): 1261-8.
[http://dx.doi.org/10.1038/nbt.1504] [PMID: 18997767]

[25] Tomoda K, Terashima H, Suzuki K, Inagi T, Terada H, Makino K. Enhanced transdermal delivery of indomethacin-loaded PLGA nanoparticles by iontophoresis. Colloids Surf B Biointerfaces 2011; 88(2): 706-10.
[http://dx.doi.org/10.1016/j.colsurfb.2011.08.004] [PMID: 21885261]

[26] Escobar-Chávez JJ, Rodríguez-Cruz IM, Domínguez-Delgado CL. Chemical and physical enhancers for transdermal drug delivery. Rijeka, Croatia: INTECH Open Access Publisher 2012.

[27] Domínguez-Delgado CL, Rodríguez-Cruz IM, López-Cervantes M. The Skin as a Valuable Route for Administration of Drugs. Escobar-Chávez JJ Current technologies to increase the transdermal delivery of drugs. Bentham Science 2010.

[28] Bernkop-Schnürch A. Nanocarrier systems for oral drug delivery: do we really need them? Eur J Pharm Sci 2013; 49(2): 272-7.
[http://dx.doi.org/10.1016/j.ejps.2013.03.008] [PMID: 23537503]

[29] Vega-Villa KR, Takemoto JK, Yáñez JA, Remsberg CM, Forrest ML, Davies NM. Clinical toxicities of nanocarrier systems. Adv Drug Deliv Rev 2008; 60(8): 929-38.
[http://dx.doi.org/10.1016/j.addr.2007.11.007] [PMID: 18313790]

[30] Domínguez-Delgado CL, Rodríguez-Cruz IM, Fuentes-Prado E, *et al.* Drug carrier systems using chitosan for non-parenteral routes. Lee, Pharmacology. Europe, InTech 2014; p. 54.
[http://dx.doi.org/10.5772/57235]

[31] Rodríguez-Cruz IM, Merino V, Merino M, *et al.* Polymeric nanospheres as strategy to increase the amount of triclosan retained in the skin: passive diffusion *vs.* iontophoresis. J Microencapsul 2013; 30(1): 72-80.
[http://dx.doi.org/10.3109/02652048.2012.700956] [PMID: 22746545]

[32] Rodríguez-Cruz IM, Domínguez-Delgado CL, Escobar-Chávez JJ, Leyva-Gómez G, Ganem-Quintanar A, Quintanar-Guerrero D. Nanoparticle infiltration to prepare solvent-free controlled drug delivery systems. Int J Pharm 2009; 371(1-2): 177-81.
[http://dx.doi.org/10.1016/j.ijpharm.2008.12.024] [PMID: 19150491]

[33] Tonga GY, Moyano DF, Kim CS, Rotello VM. Inorganic nanoparticles for therapeutic delivery: Trials, tribulations and promise. Curr Opin Colloid Interface Sci 2014; 19(2): 49-55.
[http://dx.doi.org/10.1016/j.cocis.2014.03.004] [PMID: 24955019]

[34] Probst CE, Zrazhevskiy P, Bagalkot V, Gao X. Quantum dots as a platform for nanoparticle drug delivery vehicle design. Adv Drug Deliv Rev 2013; 65(5): 703-18.
[http://dx.doi.org/10.1016/j.addr.2012.09.036] [PMID: 23000745]

[35] Kooiman K, Vos HJ, Versluis M, de Jong N. Acoustic behavior of microbubbles and implications for drug delivery. Adv Drug Deliv Rev 2014; 72: 28-48.
[http://dx.doi.org/10.1016/j.addr.2014.03.003] [PMID: 24667643]

[36] Elgart A, Cherniakov I, Aldouby Y, Domb AJ, Hoffman A. Lipospheres and pro-nano lipospheres for delivery of poorly water soluble compounds. Chem Phys Lipids 2012; 165(4): 438-53.
[http://dx.doi.org/10.1016/j.chemphyslip.2012.01.007] [PMID: 22342324]

[37] Umashankar MS, Sachdeva RK, Gulati M. Aquasomes: a promising carrier for peptides and protein delivery. Nanomedicine (Lond) 2010; 6(3): 419-26.
[PMID: 19931422]

[38] Escudero I, Geanta RM, Ruiz MO, Benito JM. Formulation and characterization of Tween 80/cholestherol niosomesmodified with tri-n-octylmethylammonium chloride (TOMAC) for carboxylic acids entrapment. Colloids Surf A Physicochem Eng Asp 2014; 461: 167-77.
[http://dx.doi.org/10.1016/j.colsurfa.2014.07.042]

[39] Moghassemi S, Hadjizadeh A. Nano-niosomes as nanoscale drug delivery systems: an illustrated review. J Control Release 2014; 185: 22-36.
[http://dx.doi.org/10.1016/j.jconrel.2014.04.015] [PMID: 24747765]

[40] Manchun S, Dass CR, Sriamornsak P. Targeted therapy for cancer using pH-responsive nanocarrier

systems. Life Sci 2012; 90(11-12): 381-7.
[http://dx.doi.org/10.1016/j.lfs.2012.01.008] [PMID: 22326503]

[41] Benson HA. Transfersomes for transdermal drug delivery. Expert Opin Drug Deliv 2006; 3(6): 727-37.
[http://dx.doi.org/10.1517/17425247.3.6.727] [PMID: 17076595]

[42] Immordino ML, Dosio F, Cattel L. Stealth liposomes: review of the basic science, rationale, and clinical applications, existing and potential. Int J Nanomedicine 2006; 1(3): 297-315.
[PMID: 17717971]

[43] Gaitanis A, Staal S. Liposomal doxorubicin and nab-paclitaxel: nanoparticle cancer chemotherapy In current clinical use Cancer Nanotechnology. Springer 2010; pp. 385-92.

[44] Zhong Z, Shi S, Han J, Zhang Z, Sun X. Anionic liposomes increase the efficiency of adenovirus-mediated gene transfer to coxsackie-adenovirus receptor deficient cells. Mol Pharm 2010; 7(1): 105-15.
[http://dx.doi.org/10.1021/mp900151k] [PMID: 19968324]

[45] Karmali PP, Chaudhuri A. Cationic liposomes as non-viral carriers of gene medicines: resolved issues, open questions, and future promises. Med Res Rev 2007; 27(5): 696-722.
[http://dx.doi.org/10.1002/med.20090] [PMID: 17022036]

[46] Halder J, Kamat AA, Landen CN Jr, *et al.* Focal adhesion kinase targeting using *in vivo* short interfering RNA delivery in neutral liposomes for ovarian carcinoma therapy. Clin Cancer Res 2006; 12(16): 4916-24.
[http://dx.doi.org/10.1158/1078-0432.CCR-06-0021] [PMID: 16914580]

[47] Akbarzadeh A, Rezaei-Sadabady R, Davaran S, *et al.* Liposome: classification, preparation, and applications. Nanoscale Res Lett 2013; 8(1): 102.
[http://dx.doi.org/10.1186/1556-276X-8-102] [PMID: 23432972]

[48] Mura P, Bragagni M, Mennini N, Cirri M, Maestrelli F. Development of liposomal and microemulsion formulations for transdermal delivery of clonazepam: effect of randomly methylated β-cyclodextrin. Int J Pharm 2014; 475(1-2): 306-14.
[http://dx.doi.org/10.1016/j.ijpharm.2014.08.066] [PMID: 25194352]

[49] Maestrelli F. GonzálezRodríguez ML, Rabasco AM, Mura P. Preparation and characterization of liposomes encapsulating ketoprofen–cyclodextrin complexes for transdermal drug delivery. Int J Pharm 2005; 298(1): 5567.
[http://dx.doi.org/10.1016/j.ijpharm.2005.03.033] [PMID: 15941634]

[50] Pai R, Devi K. Lamivudine liposomes for transdermal deliveryformulation, characterization, stability and *in vitro* evaluation. Int J Pharm Sci Nanotechnol 2009; 1: 31726.

[51] Nasr M, Mansour S, Mortada ND, El Shamy AA. Lipospheres as carriers for topical delivery of aceclofenac: preparation, characterization and *in vivo* evaluation. AAPS PharmSciTech 2008; 9(1): 154-62.
[http://dx.doi.org/10.1208/s12249-007-9028-2] [PMID: 18446476]

[52] Kesharwani P, Jain K, Kumar Jain N. Dendrimer as nanocarrier for drug delivery. Prog Polym Sci 2014; 39: 268-307.

[http://dx.doi.org/10.1016/j.progpolymsci.2013.07.005]

[53] Yang Y, Sunoqrot S, Stowell C, *et al.* Effect of size, surface charge, and hydrophobicity of poly(amidoamine) dendrimers on their skin penetration. Biomacromolecules 2012; 13(7): 2154-62. [http://dx.doi.org/10.1021/bm300545b] [PMID: 22621160]

[54] Filipowicz A, Wołowiec S. Solubility and *in vitro* transdermal diffusion of riboflavin assisted by PAMAM dendrimers. Int J Pharm 2011; 408(1-2): 152-6. [http://dx.doi.org/10.1016/j.ijpharm.2011.01.033] [PMID: 21272625]

[55] Tomalia DA, Reyna LA, Svenson S. Dendrimers as multi-purpose nanodevices for oncology drug delivery and diagnostic imaging. Biochem Soc Trans 2007; 35(Pt 1): 61-7. [http://dx.doi.org/10.1042/BST0350061] [PMID: 17233602]

[56] Gupta U, Agashe HB, Asthana A, Jain NK. A review of *in vitro–in vivo* investigations on dendrimers: the novel nanoscopic drug carriers. Nanomedicine: Nanotechnology. Biol Med 2006; 2(2): 66-73.

[57] Gupta U, Agashe HB, Asthana A, Jain NK. Dendrimers: novel polymeric nanoarchitectures for solubility enhancement. Biomacromolecules 2006; 7(3): 649-58. [http://dx.doi.org/10.1021/bm050802s] [PMID: 16529394]

[58] Díaz-Torres R. Transdermal nanocarriers. In: José JE, Merino V, Eds. Current Technologies to deliver drugs through the skin. Bentham Science Publishers 2010.

[59] Venuganti VV, Perumal OP. Effect of poly(amidoamine) (PAMAM) dendrimer on skin permeation of 5-fluorouracil. Int J Pharm 2008; 361(1-2): 230-8. [http://dx.doi.org/10.1016/j.ijpharm.2008.05.034] [PMID: 18582550]

[60] Klementieva O, Benseny-Cases N, Gella A, Appelhans D, Voit B, Cladera J. Dense shell glycodendrimers as potential nontoxic anti-amyloidogenic agents in Alzheimer's disease. Amyloid-dendrimer aggregates morphology and cell toxicity. Biomacromolecules 2011; 12(11): 3903-9. [http://dx.doi.org/10.1021/bm2008636] [PMID: 21936579]

[61] Venuganti VV, Perumal OP. Poly(amidoamine) dendrimers as skin penetration enhancers: Influence of charge, generation, and concentration. J Pharm Sci 2009; 98(7): 2345-56. [http://dx.doi.org/10.1002/jps.21603] [PMID: 18937369]

[62] Mutalik S, Nayak UY, Kalra R, Kumar A, Kulkarni RV, Parekh HS. Sonophoresis-mediated permeation and retention of peptide dendrimers across human epidermis. Skin Res Technol 2012; 18(1): 101-7. [http://dx.doi.org/10.1111/j.1600-0846.2011.00539.x] [PMID: 21507071]

[63] Petros RA, DeSimone JM. Strategies in the design of nanoparticles for therapeutic applications. Nat Rev Drug Discov 2010; 9(8): 615-27. [http://dx.doi.org/10.1038/nrd2591] [PMID: 20616808]

[64] das Neves J, Araújo F, Andrade F, *et al. In vitro* and *ex vivo* evaluation of polymeric nanoparticles for vaginal and rectal delivery of the anti-HIV drug dapivirine. Mol Pharm 2013; 10(7): 2793-807. [http://dx.doi.org/10.1021/mp4002365] [PMID: 23738946]

[65] Zhang Z, Huey Lee S, Feng SS. Folate-decorated poly(lactide-co-glycolide)-vitamin E TPGS nanoparticles for targeted drug delivery. Biomaterials 2007; 28(10): 1889-99. [http://dx.doi.org/10.1016/j.biomaterials.2006.12.018] [PMID: 17197019]

[66] des Rieux A, Fievez V, Garinot M, Schneider YJ, Préat V. Nanoparticles as potential oral delivery systems of proteins and vaccines: a mechanistic approach. J Control Release 2006; 116(1): 1-27. [http://dx.doi.org/10.1016/j.jconrel.2006.08.013] [PMID: 17050027]

[67] Lin YH, Sonaje K, Lin KM, *et al.* Multi-ion-crosslinked nanoparticles with pH-responsive characteristics for oral delivery of protein drugs. J Control Release 2008; 132(2): 141-9. [http://dx.doi.org/10.1016/j.jconrel.2008.08.020] [PMID: 18817821]

[68] Poree DE, Giles MD, Lawson LB, He J, Grayson SM. Synthesis of amphiphilic star block copolymers and their evaluation as transdermal carriers. Biomacromolecules 2011; 12(4): 898-906. [http://dx.doi.org/10.1021/bm101185t] [PMID: 21341702]

[69] Shah PP, Desai PR, Singh M. Effect of oleic acid modified polymeric bilayered nanoparticles on percutaneous delivery of spantide II and ketoprofen. J Control Release 2012; 158(2): 336-45. [http://dx.doi.org/10.1016/j.jconrel.2011.11.016] [PMID: 22134117]

[70] Yang Y, Bugno J, Hong S. Nanoscale polymeric penetration enhancers in topical drug delivery. Polym Chem 2013; 4: 2651-7. [http://dx.doi.org/10.1039/c3py00049d]

[71] Shah KA, Date AA, Joshi MD, Patravale VB. Solid lipid nanoparticles (SLN) of tretinoin: potential in topical delivery. Int J Pharm 2007; 345(1-2): 163-71. [http://dx.doi.org/10.1016/j.ijpharm.2007.05.061] [PMID: 17644288]

[72] Schäfer-Korting M, Mehnert W, Korting HC. Lipid nanoparticles for improved topical application of drugs for skin diseases. Adv Drug Deliv Rev 2007; 59(6): 427-43. [http://dx.doi.org/10.1016/j.addr.2007.04.006] [PMID: 17544165]

[73] Jain SK, Chourasia MK, Masuriha R, *et al.* Solid lipid nanoparticles bearing flurbiprofen for transdermal delivery. Drug Deliv 2005; 12(4): 207-15. [http://dx.doi.org/10.1080/10717540590952591] [PMID: 16036715]

[74] Gönüllü Ü, Üner M, Yener G, Karaman EF, Aydoğmuş Z. Formulation and characterization of solid lipid nanoparticles, nanostructured lipid carriers and nanoemulsion of lornoxicam for transdermal delivery. Acta Pharm 2015; 65(1): 1-13. [http://dx.doi.org/10.1515/acph-2015-0009] [PMID: 25781700]

[75] Domínguez-Delgado CL, Rodríguez-Cruz IM, Escobar-Chávez JJ, Calderón-Lojero IO, Quintanar-Guerrero D, Ganem A. Preparation and characterization of triclosan nanoparticles intended to be used for the treatment of acne. Eur J Pharm Biopharm 2011; 79(1): 102-7. [http://dx.doi.org/10.1016/j.ejpb.2011.01.017] [PMID: 21295142]

[76] Baroli B, Ennas MG, Loffredo F, Isola M, Pinna R, López-Quintela MA. Penetration of metallic nanoparticles in human full-thickness skin. J Invest Dermatol 2007; 127(7): 1701-12. [http://dx.doi.org/10.1038/sj.jid.5700733] [PMID: 17380118]

[77] Primo FL, Rodrigues MM, Simioni AR, Bentley MV, Morais PC, Tedesco AC. *In vitro* studies of cutaneous retention of magnetic nanoemulsion loaded with zinc phthalocyanine for synergic use in skin cancer treatment. J Magn Magn Mater 2008; 320(14): e2114. [http://dx.doi.org/10.1016/j.jmmm.2008.02.050]

[78] Jain S, Hirst DG, O'Sullivan JM. Gold nanoparticles as novel agents for cancer therapy. Br J Radiol

2012; 85(1010): 101-13.
[http://dx.doi.org/10.1259/bjr/59448833] [PMID: 22010024]

[79] Zheng D, Giljohann DA, Chen DL, *et al.* Topical delivery of siRNA-based spherical nucleic acid nanoparticle conjugates for gene regulation. Proc Natl Acad Sci USA 2012; 109(30): 11975-80.
[http://dx.doi.org/10.1073/pnas.1118425109] [PMID: 22773805]

[80] Solans C, Izquierdo P, Nolla J, Azemar N, Garcia-Celma M. Nano-emulsions. Curr Opin Colloid Interface Sci 2005; 10(3): 102-10.
[http://dx.doi.org/10.1016/j.cocis.2005.06.004]

[81] Shakeel F, Baboota S, Ahuja A, Ali J, Aqil M, Shafiq S. Nanoemulsions as vehicles for transdermal delivery of aceclofenac. AAPS PharmSciTech 2007; 8(4): E104.
[http://dx.doi.org/10.1208/pt0804104] [PMID: 18181525]

[82] Shakeel F, Shafiq S, Haq N, Alanazi FK, Alsarra IA. Nanoemulsions as potential vehicles for transdermal and dermal delivery of hydrophobic compounds: an overview. Expert Opin Drug Deliv 2012; 9(8): 953-74.
[http://dx.doi.org/10.1517/17425247.2012.696605] [PMID: 22703228]

[83] Kataoka K, Harada A, Nagasaki Y. Block copolymer micelles for drug delivery: design, characterization and biological significance. Adv Drug Deliv Rev 2001; 47(1): 113-31.
[http://dx.doi.org/10.1016/S0169-409X(00)00124-1] [PMID: 11251249]

[84] Yang Y, Pearson RM, Lee O, *et al.* Dendron-based micelles for topical delivery of endoxifen: a potential chemo-preventive medicine for breast cancer. Adv Funct Mater 2014; 24: 2442-9.
[http://dx.doi.org/10.1002/adfm.201303253]

[85] Manchun S, Dass CR, Sriamornsak P. Targeted therapy for cancer using pH-responsive nanocarrier systems. Life Sci 2012; 90(11-12): 381-7.
[http://dx.doi.org/10.1016/j.lfs.2012.01.008] [PMID: 22326503]

[86] Voigt J, Wendelken M, Driver V, Alvarez OM. Low-frequency ultrasound (20-40 kHz) as an adjunctive therapy for chronic wound healing: a systematic review of the literature and meta-analysis of eight randomized controlled trials. Int J Low Extrem Wounds 2011; 10(4): 190-9.
[http://dx.doi.org/10.1177/1534734611424648] [PMID: 22184750]

[87] Gupta PN, Mishra V, Rawat A, *et al.* Non-invasive vaccine delivery in transfersomes, niosomes and liposomes: a comparative study. Int J Pharm 2005; 293(1-2): 73-82.
[http://dx.doi.org/10.1016/j.ijpharm.2004.12.022] [PMID: 15778046]

[88] Oberdörster G, Sharp Z, Atudorei V, *et al.* Extrapulmonary translocation of ultrafine carbon particles following whole-body inhalation exposure of rats. J Toxicol Environ Health A 2002; 65(20): 1531-43.
[http://dx.doi.org/10.1080/00984100290071658] [PMID: 12396867]

[89] Yeom S, Shin BS, Han S. An electron spin resonance study of non-ionic surfactant vesicles (niosomes). Chem Phys Lipids 2014; 181: 83-9.
[http://dx.doi.org/10.1016/j.chemphyslip.2014.03.004] [PMID: 24721595]

[90] Leo AL, Shearwood C, Ng KC. Transdermal microneedles for drug delivery applications. Mater Sci Eng 2006; 132: 151-4.
[http://dx.doi.org/10.1016/j.mseb.2006.02.008]

[91] Chaudhary H, Kohli K, Kumar V. Nano-transfersomes as a novel carrier for transdermal delivery. Int J Pharm 2013; 454(1): 367-80.
[http://dx.doi.org/10.1016/j.ijpharm.2013.07.031] [PMID: 23871739]

[92] Lei W, Yu C, Lin H, Zhou X. Development of tacrolimus-loaded transfersomes for deeper skin penetration enhancement and therapeutic effect improvement *in vivo*. Asian J Pharm Sci 2013; 8: 336-45.
[http://dx.doi.org/10.1016/j.ajps.2013.09.005]

[93] Grieve K, Mulvaney P, Grieser F. Synthesis and electronic properties of semiconductor nanoparticles/quantum dots. Curr Opin Colloid Interface Sci 2000; 5: 168-72.
[http://dx.doi.org/10.1016/S1359-0294(00)00050-9]

[94] Zhan N, Palui G, Grise H, Tang H, Alabugin I, Mattoussi H. Combining ligand design with photoligation to provide compact, colloidally stable, and easy to conjugate quantum dots. ACS Appl Mater Interfaces 2013; 5(8): 2861-9.
[http://dx.doi.org/10.1021/am302788q] [PMID: 23421991]

[95] Zhong X, Han M, Dong Z, White TJ, Knoll W. Composition-tunable Zn(x)Cd(1-x)Se nanocrystals with high luminescence and stability. J Am Chem Soc 2003; 125(28): 8589-94.
[http://dx.doi.org/10.1021/ja035096m] [PMID: 12848567]

[96] Xu BB, Zhang YL, Zhang R, *et al.* Programmable assembly of CdTe quantum dots into microstructures by femtosecond laser direct writing. J Mater Chem C Mater Opt Electron Devices 2013; 1: 4699-704.
[http://dx.doi.org/10.1039/c3tc30666f]

[97] Rojas-Oviedo I, Salazar-López RA, Reyes-Gasga J, Quirino-Barreda CT. Elaboration and structural analysis of aquasomes loaded with indomethacin. Eur J Pharm Sci 2007; 32(3): 223-30.
[http://dx.doi.org/10.1016/j.ejps.2007.07.008] [PMID: 17905573]

[98] Clark DJ, Lessio S, O'Donoghue M, Schainfeld R, Rosenfield K. Safety and utility of intravascular ultrasound-guided carotid artery stenting. Catheter Cardiovasc Interv 2004; 63(3): 355-62.
[http://dx.doi.org/10.1002/ccd.20188] [PMID: 15505835]

[99] Tachibana K, Tachibana S. [Application of ultrasound energy as a new drug delivery system]. Nippon Yakurigaku Zasshi 1999; 114(5S) (Suppl. 1): 138P-41P.
[http://dx.doi.org/10.1254/fpj.114.supplement_138] [PMID: 10629870]

[100] Tang OS, Ng EH, So WW, Ho PC. Ultrasound-guided embryo transfer: a prospective randomized controlled trial. Hum Reprod 2001; 16(11): 2310-5.
[http://dx.doi.org/10.1093/humrep/16.11.2310] [PMID: 11679510]

[101] Fechheimer M, Boylan JF, Parker S, Sisken JE, Patel GL, Zimmer SG. Transfection of mammalian cells with plasmid DNA by scrape loading and sonication loading. Proc Natl Acad Sci USA 1987; 84(23): 8463-7.
[http://dx.doi.org/10.1073/pnas.84.23.8463] [PMID: 2446324]

[102] Zhong W, Sit WH, Wan JM, Yu AC. Sonoporation induces apoptosis and cell cycle arrest in human promyelocytic leukemia cells. Ultrasound Med Biol 2011; 37(12): 2149-59.
[http://dx.doi.org/10.1016/j.ultrasmedbio.2011.09.012] [PMID: 22033133]

[103] Hernot S, Klibanov AL. Microbubbles in ultrasound-triggered drug and gene delivery. Adv Drug Deliv Rev 2008; 60(10): 1153-66.
[http://dx.doi.org/10.1016/j.addr.2008.03.005] [PMID: 18486268]

[104] Wells DJ. Electroporation and ultrasound enhanced non-viral gene delivery *in vitro* and *in vivo*. Cell Biol Toxicol 2010; 26(1): 21-8.
[http://dx.doi.org/10.1007/s10565-009-9144-8] [PMID: 19949971]

[105] Alonso A, Dempfle CE, Della Martina A, *et al. In vivo* clot lysis of human thrombus with intravenous abciximab immunobubbles and ultrasound. Thromb Res 2009; 124(1): 70-4.
[http://dx.doi.org/10.1016/j.thromres.2008.11.019] [PMID: 19349068]

[106] Martin RC II, Reuter NP, Woodall C. Intra-operative contrast-enhanced ultrasound improves image enhancement in the evaluation of liver tumors. J Surg Oncol 2010; 101(5): 370-5.
[PMID: 20191613]

[107] Jagannathan J, Sanghvi NT, Crum LA, *et al.* High-intensity focused ultrasound surgery of the brain: part 1--A historical perspective with modern applications. Neurosurgery 2009; 64(2): 201-10.
[http://dx.doi.org/10.1227/01.NEU.0000336766.18197.8E] [PMID: 19190451]

[108] Allen GM, Wilson DJ. Ultrasound in sports medicine--a critical evaluation. Eur J Radiol 2007; 62(1): 79-85.
[http://dx.doi.org/10.1016/j.ejrad.2007.01.029] [PMID: 17329055]

[109] D'Vaz AP, Ostor AJ, Speed CA, *et al.* Pulsed low-intensity ultrasound therapy for chronic lateral epicondylitis: a randomized controlled trial. Rheumatology (Oxford) 2006; 45(5): 566-70.
[http://dx.doi.org/10.1093/rheumatology/kei210] [PMID: 16303817]

[110] Khanna A, Nelmes RT, Gougoulias N, Maffulli N, Gray J. The effects of LIPUS on soft-tissue healing: a review of literature. Br Med Bull 2009; 89: 169-82.
[http://dx.doi.org/10.1093/bmb/ldn040] [PMID: 19011263]

[111] Kavros SJ, Liedl DA, Boon AJ, Miller JL, Hobbs JA, Andrews KL. Expedited wound healing with noncontact, low-frequency ultrasound therapy in chronic wounds: a retrospective analysis. Adv Skin Wound Care 2008; 21(9): 416-23.
[http://dx.doi.org/10.1097/01.ASW.0000323546.04734.31] [PMID: 18769168]

[112] Robertson VJ. Dosage and treatment response in randomized clinical trials of therapeutic ultrasound. Phys Ther Sport 2002; 3(3): 124-33.
[http://dx.doi.org/10.1016/S1466-853X(02)90107-0]

[113] Malizos KN, Hantes ME, Protopappas V, Papachristos A. Low-intensity pulsed ultrasound for bone healing: an overview. Injury 2006; 37(1) (Suppl. 1): S56-62.
[http://dx.doi.org/10.1016/j.injury.2006.02.037] [PMID: 16581076]

[114] Walsh WR, Stephens P, Vizesi F, Bruce W, Huckle J, Yu Y. Effects of low-intensity pulsed ultrasound on tendon-bone healing in an intra-articular sheep knee model. Arthroscopy 2007; 23(2): 197-204.
[http://dx.doi.org/10.1016/j.arthro.2006.09.003] [PMID: 17276228]

[115] Yeung CK, Guo X, Ng YF. Pulsed ultrasound treatment accelerates the repair of Achilles tendon rupture in rats. J Orthop Res 2006; 24(2): 193-201.
[http://dx.doi.org/10.1002/jor.20020] [PMID: 16435348]

[116] Shaji J, Varkey D. Recent Advances in Physical Approaches for Transdermal Penetration Enhancement. Curr Drug Ther 2012; 7(3): 184-97.
[http://dx.doi.org/10.2174/157488550703160121191905]

[117] Mitragotri S. Devices for overcoming biological barriers: the use of physical forces to disrupt the barriers. Adv Drug Deliv Rev 2013; 65(1): 100-3.
[http://dx.doi.org/10.1016/j.addr.2012.07.016] [PMID: 22960787]

[118] Lakshmanan S, Gupta GK, Avci P, *et al.* Physical energy for drug delivery; poration, concentration and activation. Adv Drug Deliv Rev 2014; 71: 98-114.
[http://dx.doi.org/10.1016/j.addr.2013.05.010] [PMID: 23751778]

[119] Gökoğlu F, Fındıkoğlu G, Yorgancoğlu ZR, Okumuş M, Ceceli E, Kocaoğlu S. Evaluation of iontophoresis and local corticosteroid injection in the treatment of carpal tunnel syndrome. Am J Phys Med Rehabil 2005; 84(2): 92-6.
[http://dx.doi.org/10.1097/01.PHM.0000151942.49031.DD] [PMID: 15668556]

[120] Sintov AC, Brandys-Sitton R. Facilitated skin penetration of lidocaine: combination of a short-term iontophoresis and microemulsion formulation. Int J Pharm 2006; 316(1-2): 58-67.
[http://dx.doi.org/10.1016/j.ijpharm.2006.02.034] [PMID: 16564144]

[121] Sylvestre JP, Díaz-Marín C, Delgado-Charro MB, Guy RH. Iontophoresis of dexamethasone phosphate: competition with chloride ions. J Control Release 2008; 131(1): 41-6.
[http://dx.doi.org/10.1016/j.jconrel.2008.07.002] [PMID: 18662729]

[122] Kim YC, Park JH, Prausnitz MR. Microneedles for drug and vaccine delivery. Adv Drug Deliv Rev 2012; 64(14): 1547-68.
[http://dx.doi.org/10.1016/j.addr.2012.04.005] [PMID: 22575858]

[123] Ito Y, Hagiwara E, Saeki A, Sugioka N, Takada K. Feasibility of microneedles for percutaneous absorption of insulin. Eur J Pharm Sci 2006; 29(1): 82-8.
[http://dx.doi.org/10.1016/j.ejps.2006.05.011] [PMID: 16828268]

[124] Lee JW, Choi SO, Felner EI, Prausnitz MR. Dissolving microneedle patch for transdermal delivery of human growth hormone. Small 2011; 7(4): 531-9.
[http://dx.doi.org/10.1002/smll.201001091] [PMID: 21360810]

[125] Prausnitz MR, Mikszta JA, Cormier M, Andrianov AK. Microneedle-based vaccines Vaccines for Pandemic Influenza. Springer 2009; pp. 369-93.
[http://dx.doi.org/10.1007/978-3-540-92165-3_18]

[126] Prausnitz MR. Microneedles for transdermal drug delivery. Adv Drug Deliv Rev 2004; 56(5): 581-7.
[http://dx.doi.org/10.1016/j.addr.2003.10.023] [PMID: 15019747]

[127] van der Maaden K, Jiskoot W, Bouwstra J. Microneedle technologies for (trans)dermal drug and vaccine delivery. J Control Release 2012; 161(2): 645-55.
[http://dx.doi.org/10.1016/j.jconrel.2012.01.042] [PMID: 22342643]

[128] Bora P, Kumar L, Bansal AK. Microneedle technology for advanced drug delivery: Evolving vistas. Curr Res Inf Pharm Sci 2009; 9(1): 7-10.

[129] Davis SP, Martanto W, Allen MG, Prausnitz MR. Hollow metal microneedles for insulin delivery to diabetic rats. Biomed Engineering. IEEE Transactions on 2005; 52(5): 909-15.

[130] Vučen SR, Vuleta G, Crean AM, Moore AC, Ignjatović N, Uskoković D. Improved percutaneous delivery of ketoprofen using combined application of nanocarriers and silicon microneedles. J Pharm Pharmacol 2013; 65(10): 1451-62.
[http://dx.doi.org/10.1111/jphp.12118] [PMID: 24028612]

[131] Marchetti JM, de Souza MC, Marotta-Oliveira SS. Nanocarriers and cancer therapy: approaches to topical and transdermal delivery Nanocosmetics and Nanomedicines. Springer 2011; pp. 269-86.

[132] Lee SG, Jeong JH, Lee KM, *et al.* Nanostructured lipid carrier-loaded hyaluronic acid microneedles for controlled dermal delivery of a lipophilic molecule. Int J Nanomedicine 2014; 9: 289-99.
[PMID: 24403833]

[133] Coulman SA, Anstey A, Gateley C, *et al.* Microneedle mediated delivery of nanoparticles into human skin. Int J Pharm 2009; 366(1-2): 190-200.
[http://dx.doi.org/10.1016/j.ijpharm.2008.08.040] [PMID: 18812218]

[134] DeMuth PC, Su X, Samuel RE, Hammond PT, Irvine DJ. Nano-layered microneedles for transcutaneous delivery of polymer nanoparticles and plasmid DNA. Adv Mater 2010; 22(43): 4851-6.
[http://dx.doi.org/10.1002/adma.201001525] [PMID: 20859938]

[135] Kumar A, Wonganan P, Sandoval MA, Li X, Zhu S, Cui Z. Microneedle-mediated transcutaneous immunization with plasmid DNA coated on cationic PLGA nanoparticles. J Control Release 2012; 163(2): 230-9.
[http://dx.doi.org/10.1016/j.jconrel.2012.08.011] [PMID: 22921518]

[136] Venuganti VV, Sahdev P, Hildreth M, Guan X, Perumal O. Structure-skin permeability relationship of dendrimers. Pharm Res 2011; 28(9): 2246-60.
[http://dx.doi.org/10.1007/s11095-011-0455-0] [PMID: 21633876]

[137] Kulkarni SB, Banga AK, Betageri GV. Transdermal lontophoretic delivery of colchicine encapsulated in liposomes. Drug Deliv 1996; 3(4): 245-50.
[http://dx.doi.org/10.3109/10717549609029456]

[138] Vutla NB, Betageri GV, Banga AK. Transdermal iontophoretic delivery of enkephalin formulated in liposomes. J Pharm Sci 1996; 85(1): 5-8.
[http://dx.doi.org/10.1021/js950349y] [PMID: 8926583]

[139] Lee S, Lee J, Choi YW. Skin permeation enhancement of ascorbyl palmitate by liposomal hydrogel (lipogel) formulation and electrical assistance. Biol Pharm Bull 2007; 30(2): 393-6.
[http://dx.doi.org/10.1248/bpb.30.393] [PMID: 17268089]

[140] Chen H, Zhu H, Zheng J, *et al.* Iontophoresis-driven penetration of nanovesicles through microneedle-induced skin microchannels for enhancing transdermal delivery of insulin. J Control Release 2009; 139(1): 63-72.
[http://dx.doi.org/10.1016/j.jconrel.2009.05.031] [PMID: 19481577]

[141] Tomoda K, Yabuki N, Terada H, Makino K. Application of polymeric nanoparticles prepared by an antisolvent diffusion with preferential solvation for iontophoretic transdermal drug delivery. Colloid Polym Sci 2014; 292(12): 3195-203.
[http://dx.doi.org/10.1007/s00396-014-3342-5]

[142] Kigasawa K, Miyashita M, Kajimoto K, Kanamura K, Harashima H, Kogure K. Efficient intradermal

delivery of superoxide dismutase using a combination of liposomes and iontophoresis for protection against UV-induced skin damage. Biol Pharm Bull 2012; 35(5): 781-5. [http://dx.doi.org/10.1248/bpb.35.781] [PMID: 22687417]

[143] Rapoport NY, Nam KH, Gao Z, Kennedy A. Application of ultrasound for targeted nanotherapy of malignant tumors. Acoust Phys 2009; 55(4-5): 594-601.

[144] Lopez RF, Seto JE, Blankschtein D, Langer R. Enhancing the transdermal delivery of rigid nanoparticles using the simultaneous application of ultrasound and sodium lauryl sulfate. Biomaterials 2011; 32(3): 933-41. [http://dx.doi.org/10.1016/j.biomaterials.2010.09.060] [PMID: 20971504]

[145] Polat BE, Deen WM, Langer R, Blankschtein D. A physical mechanism to explain the delivery of chemical penetration enhancers into skin during transdermal sonophoresis - Insight into the observed synergism. J Control Release 2012; 158(2): 250-60.

[146] Rao R, Nanda S. Sonophoresis: recent advancements and future trends. J Pharm Pharmacol 2009; 61(6): 689-705. [http://dx.doi.org/10.1211/jpp.61.06.0001] [PMID: 19505359]

[147] Binks PN, Critchley MM, Irving RA, Pouton CW, White PJ. Microarray device. US Patent 2008/0312610 A1, 2008.

[148] Xu B. Microdevice and method for transdermal delivery and sampling of active substances. US Patent 2008/0214987 A1, 2008.

[149] Banks SL, Stinchcomb AL. Methods and compositions for enhancing the viability of microneedle pores. US Patent 2009/0143762 A1, 2009.

[150] Edelhauser HF, Jiang N, Prausnitz MR. Method for drug delivery to ocular tissue using microneedle. US Patent 7918814 B2, 2011.

[151] Yan L, Chen X. Mechanically robust fast-dissolving microneedles for transdermal drug and vaccine delivery. US Patent 2014/0142541 A1, 2014.

[152] Edwards DA. Hydrogels or lipogels with enhanced mass transfer for transdermal drug delivery. US Patent 5833647, 1998.

[153] Coleman W. Topically applied clostridium botulinum toxin compositions and treatment methods. US Patent 2003/0113349 A1, 2003.

[154] Smith G. Iontophoretic delivery of active agents conjugated to nanoparticles. US Patent 2007/0078375 A1, 2007.

[155] Akiyama H, Matsumura T, Matsumura A, Nakayama M. Electrode assembly for iontophoresis for administering active agent enclosed in nanoparticle and iontophoresis device using the same. US Patent 2007/0135754 A1, 2007.

[156] Peyman GA. Delivery of an ocular agent using iontophoresis. US Patent 2007/0299386 A1, 2007.

[157] Jones DR. Use of iontophoresis or electrotherapy and ultrasound to deliver melanin for skin rejuvenation. US Patent 2009/0192438 A1, 2009.

[158] Jones DR, Parker ED. Use of iontophoresis and ultrasound to deliver melanin or other chromophores for laser hair removal. US Patent 2009/0149796 A1, 2009.

[159] Domb AJ. Device, methods and sponges for iontophoretic drug delivery. US Patent 8290579 B2, 2012.

[160] Esenaliev R. Ultrasound-based treatment methods for therapeutic treatment of skin and subcutaneous tissues. US Patent 2007/0078290 A1, 2007.

[161] Lindgren D, Mitra AK. Ultrasound-mediated transscleral drug delivery. US Patent 2008/0177220 A1, 2008.

[162] Entis AC, Goldman M, Zusman L. Ultrasonic drug-delivery system. US Patent 2008/0097281 A1, 2008.

[163] Liu T. Ultrasonically-triggered drug vehicle with magnetic resonance imaging function. US Patent 2012/0045397 A1, 2012.

[164] Mohapatra SS, Kumar A, Sahoo B. Method of transdermal drug delivery. US Patent 8467868 B1, 2013.

Glossary

Cavitation = formation of vapour cavities in a medium upon ultrasound exposure.

Dendrimers = monodisperse populations those are structurally and chemically uniform. They allow conjugation with numerous functional groups due to the nature of their branches.

Electroporation = phenomenon in which cell membrane permeability to ions and macromolecules is increased by exposing the cell to short high electric field pulses.

Gene delivery = is a therapeutic technique, in which a functional gene is inserted into a patient's cells to correct a genetic defect or to provide the cells a new function.

Iontophoresis = consists of the application of a low density current and low voltage (typically 0.5 A/cm^2) *via* an electrical circuit constituted by two drug reservoirs (anode and cathode) deposited on skin surface.

Liposomes = are hollow lipid bilayer structures that can transport hydrophilic drugs inside the core and hydrophobic drugs between the bilayer.

Microneedles = is a drug delivery device for use in the percutaneous administration of a drug for local therapy or systemic therapy.

Nanoemulsions = are isotropic dispersed systems of two non-miscible liquids, normally consisting of an oily system dispersed in an aqueous system (o/w nanoemulsion), or an aqueous system dispersed in an oily system but forming droplets or other oily phases of nanometric sizes (100 nm).

Nanoparticles = is a small object that behaves as a whole unit in terms of its transport and properties.

Physical penetration enhancers = Enhancement technologies that increase the passage of drugs throughout the skin.

Radiofrequency = is a versatile technology commonly used to generate therapeutic levels of heat by using various forms of alternating current.

Reverse iontophoresis = convenient non-invasive method for extracting substances through skin, allowing this way sampling body fluids to monitor them efficiently.

Sonolysis = therapy that involves administration of microbubbles with ultrasound, but without the administration of a thrombolytic drug.

Sonophoresis = absorption of ultrasonic energy that has been used with therapeutic intent in many conditions.

Transcorneal iontophoresis = delivery of a high concentration of drug to the anterior segment of the eye: cornea, ciliary body, aqueous humors and lens.

Ultrasound = a form of mechanical energy that is propagated from one point to another by the interaction between neighboring oscillating particles.

SUBJECT INDEX

A

B

C

José Juan Escobar-Chávez (Ed.)

D

E

F

G

H

I

J

K

L

M

N

O

P

Q

R

S

V

W

Made in the USA
Las Vegas, NV
03 November 2026

57422775R00205